Certification
and Core Review *for*
High Acuity, Progressive, *and* Critical Care Nursing

SEVENTH EDITION

Edited by

Lisa M. Stone, BSN, RN, CCRN-CMC
Staff Nurse
Coronary Care Unit
Einstein Healthcare Network
Philadelphia, Pennsylvania

ELSEVIER

ELSEVIER

3251 Riverport Lane
St. Louis, Missouri 63043

CERTIFICATION AND CORE REVIEW FOR HIGH ACUITY,
PROGRESSIVE, AND CRITICAL CARE NURSING, SEVENTH EDITION   ISBN-13: 978-0-323-44640-2

Library of Congress Cataloging-in-Publication Data

Names: Stone, Lisa M., editor. | American Association of Critical-Care
    Nurses, issuing body.
Title: Certification & core review for high acuity, progressive, and critical
    care nursing / edited by Lisa M. Stone.
Other titles: Core review for critical care nursing. | Certification and core
    review for high acuity, progressive, and critical care nursing | Guide to
    (expression): Core curriculum for high acuity, progressive, and critical
    care nursing. Seventh edition.
Description: 7th edition. | St. Louis, Missouri : Elsevier, Inc., [2018] |
    Preceded by AACN certification and core review for high acuity and
    critical care nursing / edited by JoAnn Grif Alspach. 6th ed. c2008. |
    Guide to Core curriculum for high acuity, progressive, and critical care
    nursing / American Association of Critical-Care Nurses; edited by Tonja
    M. Hartjes. Seventh edition. 2018. | Includes bibliographical references.
Identifiers: LCCN 2017028504 | ISBN 9780323446402
Subjects: | MESH: Critical Care Nursing | Examination Questions
Classification: LCC RT120.I5 | NLM WY 18.2 | DDC 616.02/8--dc23 LC record
    available at https://lccn.loc.gov/2017028504

Executive Content Strategist: Lee Henderson
Senior Content Development Manager: Laurie Gower
Senior Content Development Specialist: Heather Bays
Publishing Services Manager: Deepthi Unni
Senior Book Project Manager: Kamatchi Madhavan
Designer: Bridget Hoette

Printed in the United States of America

Last digit is the print number: 9 8 7 6 5 4 3 2 1

Reviewers

Marcia Bixby, RN, MS, CCRN, APRN-BC
Critical Care Clinical Nurse Specialist
Consultant for Critical Care Education
Randolph, Massachusetts

Tina Deatherage, DNP, NEA-BC, CCRN, CNRN, CCNS
Director of Nursing
Novant Health Presbyterian Medical Center
Tega Cay, South Carolina

Diane Glowacki, MSN, RN, CNRN-ABNN, CMC-AACN
Clinical Nurse Specialist
Catholic Health Mercy Hospital of Buffalo
Buffalo, New York

Mary Ann House-Fancher, ACNP, MSN, CCRN, CMC-CSC, PCCN
Acute Care Nurse Practitioner
Division of Critical Care Medicine
University of Florida;
President
CCAMI
Education for Medical Professionals
Gainesville, Florida

Ankur Jain, MD, FACP
Assistant Professor and Medical Director
Division of Hospital Medicine
Department of Internal Medicine
University of Florida
Gainesville, Florida

Sara M. Knippa, MS, RN, ACCNS-AG, CCRN, PCCN
Clinical Nurse Specialist/Educator
ICU Educator Supervisor
University of Colorado Hospital
Aurora, Colorado

Preface

Quality care of the critically ill patient requires that the nurse be competent in critical care nursing practice. The American Association of Critical-Care Nurses (AACN) denotes competency in critical care nursing by means of its CCRN® certification program. Certification in critical care nursing demands both a clinical practice requirement as well as the successful completion of the CCRN examination, which is a written test on the cognitive elements that underlie critical care nursing practice. AACN's *Core Curriculum for Critical Care Nursing* defines the knowledge base for critical care nursing, and the *Certification and Core Review for High Acuity, Progressive, and Critical Care Nursing* provides a means to verify acquisition of that knowledge base.

In addition to its usefulness as a study guide for critical care nursing practice, the *Certification and Core Review* is also designed to assist nurses who are preparing to take the Adult CCRN certification examination administered by the AACN Certification Corporation. Each CCRN certification examination is based on a job analysis study that defines the dimensions of acute and critical care nursing practice. Using the AACN Synergy Model for Patient Care as an organizing framework, those dimensions of care are then reviewed in order to define the knowledge, skills, and abilities required for critical care nursing practice. CCRN certification examinations are based on these skills and abilities and the knowledge necessary to perform them. The *Certification and Core Review* provides three complete practice CCRN examinations based on the latest edition of the *AACN Core Curriculum*. The test items in this book evaluate the knowledge, skills, and abilities identified as crucial for nursing care of patients with acute and life-threatening health problems. Achievement of these dual purposes necessitates retention of many aspects of the prior edition of this work as well as inauguration of some new features.

Similarities with the sixth edition include comprehensive coverage of topics contained in the most recent version of the *Core Curriculum*. This edition of the *Certification and Core Review* is based on the seventh edition of the *Core Curriculum*.

As with prior versions of the *Certification and Core Review*, test items cover revised, continued, expanded, additional, and updated content from the most recent *Core Curriculum* and integrate psychosocial aspects of care. The test items still consist of four-option, multiple-choice questions with explanations for both correct and incorrect answers, and the test items are again divided into three separate practice CCRN examinations. Content areas and their distributions precisely match those detailed in the adult portion of the CCRN examination blueprint (available at www.aacn.org/~/media/aacn-website/certification/get-certified/handbooks/ccrnexamhandbook.pdf). Feedback on answers is again located at the end of each examination so that test completion and timing are not disrupted and item responses may more closely resemble completion of the actual CCRN examination. References for each correct and incorrect answer are again provided to assist readers in identifying relevant references for each content area in the CCRN examination blueprint.

Most of the new features of this edition of the *Certification and Core Review* were introduced to ensure that each practice examination matches the content areas, content distribution, item numbers, cognitive levels, and format used in the actual CCRN examination. Content new to this edition features expanded coverage of pain and palliative and end-of-life care, nutritional support for the critically ill patient, and transplantation. Content distributions precisely match those designated in the latest blueprint for the adult CCRN examination, including 80% of items pertaining to the nurse competency of Clinical Judgment and 20% of items now related to the other seven nurse competencies (Advocacy–Moral Agency, Caring Practices, Collaboration, Systems Thinking, Response to Diversity, Clinical Inquiry, and Facilitation of Learning) grouped under the umbrella of Professional Caring and Ethical Practice. Because the CCRN examination now tests critical thinking using higher cognitive levels, the majority of items contained in the *Certification and Core Review* now test at the application or analysis cognitive level. Consistency with the actual CCRN examination is also the rationale for including 150 rather than 200 items per test and for no longer incorporating use of clinical scenarios that apply to more than one test item. The accompanying Evolve site includes 100 extra examination questions and provides the ability to review body systems and to take the examinations electronically.

Although these review tests are intended to simulate the CCRN examination, none of the test questions were or will be actual CCRN examination items. Because changes in the CCRN examination occur from time to time, candidates preparing for this examination are strongly encouraged to contact the AACN Certification Corporation and check its website (www.certcorp.org) to obtain the current CCRN certification examination handbook and blueprint that will be in effect for the date on which they plan to take the examination.

The author of this book has made every attempt to provide a study guide that is helpful in validating a nurse's ability to apply the content of the *Core Curriculum* to critical care nursing practice and in assisting nurses to prepare for the CCRN certification examination. Your comments regarding how well these objectives have been achieved are welcome.

Lisa M. Stone, BSN, RN, CCRN-CMC

Instructions

Each of the three tests in this book consists of 150 four-option, multiple choice questions. To simulate taking a CCRN examination, mark your answer to each question on the reproducible answer sheet and allow a maximum of 3 hours to complete each test. After you have completed each test, compare your answers to those that appear in the answer key that follows that test.

Core Review Test
Answer Sheet

1. ❏ A ❏ B ❏ C ❏ D   26. ❏ A ❏ B ❏ C ❏ D   51. ❏ A ❏ B ❏ C ❏ D

2. ❏ A ❏ B ❏ C ❏ D   27. ❏ A ❏ B ❏ C ❏ D   52. ❏ A ❏ B ❏ C ❏ D

3. ❏ A ❏ B ❏ C ❏ D   28. ❏ A ❏ B ❏ C ❏ D   53. ❏ A ❏ B ❏ C ❏ D

4. ❏ A ❏ B ❏ C ❏ D   29. ❏ A ❏ B ❏ C ❏ D   54. ❏ A ❏ B ❏ C ❏ D

5. ❏ A ❏ B ❏ C ❏ D   30. ❏ A ❏ B ❏ C ❏ D   55. ❏ A ❏ B ❏ C ❏ D

6. ❏ A ❏ B ❏ C ❏ D   31. ❏ A ❏ B ❏ C ❏ D   56. ❏ A ❏ B ❏ C ❏ D

7. ❏ A ❏ B ❏ C ❏ D   32. ❏ A ❏ B ❏ C ❏ D   57. ❏ A ❏ B ❏ C ❏ D

8. ❏ A ❏ B ❏ C ❏ D   33. ❏ A ❏ B ❏ C ❏ D   58. ❏ A ❏ B ❏ C ❏ D

9. ❏ A ❏ B ❏ C ❏ D   34. ❏ A ❏ B ❏ C ❏ D   59. ❏ A ❏ B ❏ C ❏ D

10. ❏ A ❏ B ❏ C ❏ D   35. ❏ A ❏ B ❏ C ❏ D   60. ❏ A ❏ B ❏ C ❏ D

11. ❏ A ❏ B ❏ C ❏ D   36. ❏ A ❏ B ❏ C ❏ D   61. ❏ A ❏ B ❏ C ❏ D

12. ❏ A ❏ B ❏ C ❏ D   37. ❏ A ❏ B ❏ C ❏ D   62. ❏ A ❏ B ❏ C ❏ D

13. ❏ A ❏ B ❏ C ❏ D   38. ❏ A ❏ B ❏ C ❏ D   63. ❏ A ❏ B ❏ C ❏ D

14. ❏ A ❏ B ❏ C ❏ D   39. ❏ A ❏ B ❏ C ❏ D   64. ❏ A ❏ B ❏ C ❏ D

15. ❏ A ❏ B ❏ C ❏ D   40. ❏ A ❏ B ❏ C ❏ D   65. ❏ A ❏ B ❏ C ❏ D

16. ❏ A ❏ B ❏ C ❏ D   41. ❏ A ❏ B ❏ C ❏ D   66. ❏ A ❏ B ❏ C ❏ D

17. ❏ A ❏ B ❏ C ❏ D   42. ❏ A ❏ B ❏ C ❏ D   67. ❏ A ❏ B ❏ C ❏ D

18. ❏ A ❏ B ❏ C ❏ D   43. ❏ A ❏ B ❏ C ❏ D   68. ❏ A ❏ B ❏ C ❏ D

19. ❏ A ❏ B ❏ C ❏ D   44. ❏ A ❏ B ❏ C ❏ D   69. ❏ A ❏ B ❏ C ❏ D

20. ❏ A ❏ B ❏ C ❏ D   45. ❏ A ❏ B ❏ C ❏ D   70. ❏ A ❏ B ❏ C ❏ D

21. ❏ A ❏ B ❏ C ❏ D   46. ❏ A ❏ B ❏ C ❏ D   71. ❏ A ❏ B ❏ C ❏ D

22. ❏ A ❏ B ❏ C ❏ D   47. ❏ A ❏ B ❏ C ❏ D   72. ❏ A ❏ B ❏ C ❏ D

23. ❏ A ❏ B ❏ C ❏ D   48. ❏ A ❏ B ❏ C ❏ D   73. ❏ A ❏ B ❏ C ❏ D

24. ❏ A ❏ B ❏ C ❏ D   49. ❏ A ❏ B ❏ C ❏ D   74. ❏ A ❏ B ❏ C ❏ D

25. ❏ A ❏ B ❏ C ❏ D   50. ❏ A ❏ B ❏ C ❏ D   75. ❏ A ❏ B ❏ C ❏ D

Core Review Test
Answer Sheet *(Continued)*

76.	❏A	❏B	❏C	❏D	101.	❏A	❏B	❏C	❏D	126.	❏A	❏B	❏C	❏D
77.	❏A	❏B	❏C	❏D	102.	❏A	❏B	❏C	❏D	127.	❏A	❏B	❏C	❏D
78.	❏A	❏B	❏C	❏D	103.	❏A	❏B	❏C	❏D	128.	❏A	❏B	❏C	❏D
79.	❏A	❏B	❏C	❏D	104.	❏A	❏B	❏C	❏D	129.	❏A	❏B	❏C	❏D
80.	❏A	❏B	❏C	❏D	105.	❏A	❏B	❏C	❏D	130.	❏A	❏B	❏C	❏D
81.	❏A	❏B	❏C	❏D	106.	❏A	❏B	❏C	❏D	131.	❏A	❏B	❏C	❏D
82.	❏A	❏B	❏C	❏D	107.	❏A	❏B	❏C	❏D	132.	❏A	❏B	❏C	❏D
83.	❏A	❏B	❏C	❏D	108.	❏A	❏B	❏C	❏D	133.	❏A	❏B	❏C	❏D
84.	❏A	❏B	❏C	❏D	109.	❏A	❏B	❏C	❏D	134.	❏A	❏B	❏C	❏D
85.	❏A	❏B	❏C	❏D	110.	❏A	❏B	❏C	❏D	135.	❏A	❏B	❏C	❏D
86.	❏A	❏B	❏C	❏D	111.	❏A	❏B	❏C	❏D	136.	❏A	❏B	❏C	❏D
87.	❏A	❏B	❏C	❏D	112.	❏A	❏B	❏C	❏D	137.	❏A	❏B	❏C	❏D
88.	❏A	❏B	❏C	❏D	113.	❏A	❏B	❏C	❏D	138.	❏A	❏B	❏C	❏D
89.	❏A	❏B	❏C	❏D	114.	❏A	❏B	❏C	❏D	139.	❏A	❏B	❏C	❏D
90.	❏A	❏B	❏C	❏D	115.	❏A	❏B	❏C	❏D	140.	❏A	❏B	❏C	❏D
91.	❏A	❏B	❏C	❏D	116.	❏A	❏B	❏C	❏D	141.	❏A	❏B	❏C	❏D
92.	❏A	❏B	❏C	❏D	117.	❏A	❏B	❏C	❏D	142.	❏A	❏B	❏C	❏D
93.	❏A	❏B	❏C	❏D	118.	❏A	❏B	❏C	❏D	143.	❏A	❏B	❏C	❏D
94.	❏A	❏B	❏C	❏D	119.	❏A	❏B	❏C	❏D	144.	❏A	❏B	❏C	❏D
95.	❏A	❏B	❏C	❏D	120.	❏A	❏B	❏C	❏D	145.	❏A	❏B	❏C	❏D
96.	❏A	❏B	❏C	❏D	121.	❏A	❏B	❏C	❏D	146.	❏A	❏B	❏C	❏D
97.	❏A	❏B	❏C	❏D	122.	❏A	❏B	❏C	❏D	147.	❏A	❏B	❏C	❏D
98.	❏A	❏B	❏C	❏D	123.	❏A	❏B	❏C	❏D	148.	❏A	❏B	❏C	❏D
99.	❏A	❏B	❏C	❏D	124.	❏A	❏B	❏C	❏D	149.	❏A	❏B	❏C	❏D
100.	❏A	❏B	❏C	❏D	125.	❏A	❏B	❏C	❏D	150.	❏A	❏B	❏C	❏D

Contents

1 Core Review Test 1

1-1. A 76-year-old male has been admitted to the emergency room for shortness of breath. His vital signs are as follows: temperature 37.1°C HR 120/min (sinus tachycardia), BP 130/76 mm Hg, RR 35/min with SpO_2 89%. Upon auscultation, you hear crackles all lung fields. The chest x-ray report states that there are Kerley B lines, enlargement of the peribronchial hilar spaces, and enlarged cardiac silhouette. You anticipate that the patient will be diagnosed with which of these conditions?
  A. Pericardial tamponade
  B. Pulmonary edema
  C. Pneumonia
  D. Acute inferior wall MI with right ventricular failure

1-2. You have been informed that a research study is taking place on your unit. The study is to test a new medication for congestive heart failure. You are outside another patient's room, and you overhear a conversation between one of the research coordinators and a patient. The research coordinator asks the subject if he would like to enroll in the study because it is a quick way to make $100. The patient asks whether any risk is involved, and the staff member says, "Not really. All you have to do is sign this form." How should you respond?
  A. Report what was overheard to the ethics committee
  B. Contact the primary investigator on the study

  C. Enter the room and review the protocol with the patient
  D. Recognize that the staff member is a volunteer interested in gathering data for this important study

1-3. A patient has been admitted to the ICU after a motor vehicle accident. Radiographic imaging reveals that he sustained fractures to the pelvis, bilateral femurs, multiple ribs, and left arm. Two hours after the initial patient assessment, the nurse notes these findings: increased anxiety and confusion, BP unchanged at 148/84 mm Hg, HR increased from 120 to 146/min, respiratory rate increased from 18 to 44/min. Pulmonary artery pressure is 55/28 mm Hg, and cardiac output is decreased from 4 to 2.3 L/min. Which would be the first intervention?
  A. Obtain a stat chest x-ray
  B. Initiate sequential compression device
  C. Administer oxygen and prepare for intubation
  D. Administer thrombolytic medication

1-4. A patient undergoes emergency CABG (coronary artery bypass graft) surgery after failed thrombolysis and a percutaneous coronary intervention (PCI) during which coronary artery dissection occurred. Before surgery, the patient was alert and able to give verbal consent. Mediastinal and pleural chest tubes are present with moderate drainage. Moderate oozing is also present at the sternotomy and saphenous vein graft incisions and at the right groin sheath site. The patient has a PA catheter, an NG tube, and a urinary catheter in place. Frequent assessments by the nurse for this patient should include which of these actions?

A. Minimum of hourly pupil checks to determine whether intracranial bleeding has occurred

B. Inspecting the patient's back hourly for signs of retroperitoneal bleeding

C. Hourly groin palpation and neurovascular checks of the leg used for PCI

D. Hourly auscultation of bowel sounds to determine whether gastric bleeding is present

1-5. A trauma alert has been called in the ER. As soon as the patient arrives in the trauma room, what would be the primary assessment?

A. Breathing, circulation, and vital signs

B. Airway, breathing, and circulation

C. Disability, head-to-toe examination, and exposure

D. Vital signs, circulation, and inspection

1-6. A patient with a past medical history of hypertension, multiple MI's with stents, unstable angina, diabetes, and a 50 pack/year history of smoking is admitted to the ICU with acute coronary syndrome. Which of these leads would you choose to display on the ECG monitor?

A. II

B. V_6

C. I

D. V_3

1-7. A patient with septic shock is hypotensive and tachycardic. Which of these vasopressors would be indicated for this patient?

A. Norepinephrine (Levophed)

B. Phenylephrine (Neo-Synephrine)

C. Dopamine

D. Epinephrine

1-8. A patient with urosepsis was admitted to the ICU 12 hours ago, has received 6 L of fluid thus far, and is receiving Levophed to maintain her systolic BP higher than 90 mm Hg. She is on assist-control ventilation with a rate of 12, tidal volumes of 8 mL/kg, PEEP of +5, and FiO_2 of 50%. Over the past 2 hours, her oxygen saturation has been slowly decreasing from 99% to 90% despite increasing her FiO_2 to 80%. Her most recent ABG shows a pH of 7.30, $PaCO_2$ of 55 mm Hg, and PaO_2 of 60 mm Hg. Her pulmonary pressures are increasing, and her static pressure is now 40. What ventilator changes does the nurse anticipate?

A. Increase the PEEP to +10 and reevaluate O_2 saturation and ABG

B. Switch to a pressure support mode for greater patient comfort

C. Increase the set respiratory rate to normalize the pH

D. Decrease tidal volumes to 6 mL/kg and maintain minute ventilation

1-9. A 38-year-old male has been admitted to the hospital after he sustained significant blunt abdominal trauma during an assault. His vital signs remain stable. The nurse is monitoring the patient's bowel sounds, abdominal tenderness, and abdominal girth frequently. Which of these laboratory parameters is especially important for the nurse to closely monitor for bleeding in this patient?

A. Platelet count

B. Protime

C. Hematocrit

D. Mean corpuscular volume

1-10. A patient is admitted for elective craniotomy and clipping of a posterior communicating artery aneurysm. On the initial ICU assessment, the nurse notes that the patient's Glasgow Coma Scale (GCS) score is 15 with no focal weakness. The patient has a large, nonreactive pupil as well as ptosis in the left eye. The nurse's best course of action at this point would be to

A. Call the neurosurgeon immediately because the aneurysm may have ruptured

B. Prepare the patient for an anticipated STAT head CT scan to evaluate for expansion of the aneurysm

C. Review the medical record to identify the patient's presenting symptoms and examination before admission

D. Call anesthesia STAT for emergent intubation in response to the altered neuro assessment

1-11. Approximately 3 minutes after the first CRRT treatment is initiated, a patient complains of severe back pain and itching. The patient's vital signs are BP 84/50 mm Hg, HR 115 beats/min, and RR 26/min. The nurse's initial intervention for this patient would be to
   A. Administer 100 mL of normal saline fluid bolus
   B. Check for bleeding at the access site
   C. Administer diphenhydramine (Benadryl) 12.5 mg IV
   D. Disconnect the patient from the machine

1-12. A patient is admitted to the ICU from the medical floor complaining of palpitations. He denies chest pain or shortness of breath. Initial vital signs are temp 36.9°C respirations 22/min; BP 140/84 mm Hg; SpO$_2$ 97%. A 12-lead ECG is obtained and posted below. What would be the most appropriate immediate intervention?
   A. Have the patient perform a vagal maneuver
   B. Administer adenosine 6 mg IV rapidly
   C. Administer diltiazem 0.25 mg/kg IV over 2 minutes
   D. Perform immediate synchronized cardioversion

1-13. A 48-year-old male complaining of severe chest and back pain has arrived in the emergency room. His vital signs on arrival are unstable with a current blood pressure of 80/50 mm Hg. Bedside transesophageal echocardiography reveals a dissecting aortic aneurysm with pericardial effusion. Emergency surgery is scheduled. Before transferring the patient to the operating room, which of the following does the nurse need to prepare for?
   A. Immediate pericardiocentesis to relieve tamponade
   B. Administration of labetalol to decrease afterload and contractility
   C. Administration of norepinephrine at 4 mcg/min to raise BP
   D. Insertion of two large-bore IVs to obtain laboratory samples and administer fluids

1-14. One of the most common psychological effects experienced by patients who have received an implantable cardioverter defibrillator (ICD) is
   A. Fear of being shocked by the device
   B. Anxiety over being awakened from sleep by the device
   C. Worry that electronic interference will trigger the device
   D. Depression over dependence on the device

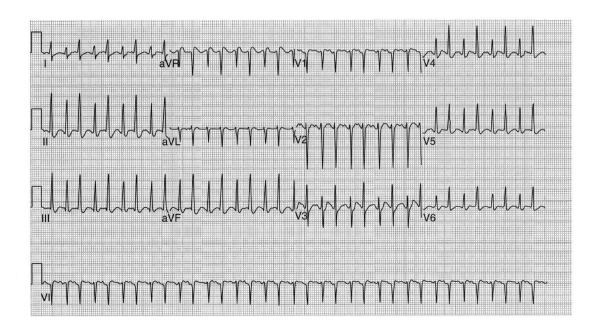

1-15. A patient admitted for acute alcohol ingestion was intubated by paramedics at the scene because of a decreased level of consciousness. The paramedics reported that the patient vomited a large amount of emesis during the intubation. On admission to the ICU, the patient's vital signs are as follows: temperature 38.5°C HR 120/min; BP 90/60 mm Hg; RR 28/min; S_aO_2 94% on FiO_2 100%. A chest x-ray shows infiltrates in the patient's right lower lobe. Which of these interventions should the critical care nurse anticipate?
A. Aggressive broad-spectrum antibiotics
B. Bronchoalveolar lavage to clear the distal airways
C. Steroid therapy to mitigate the inflammatory cascade
D. Aggressive pulmonary hygiene and culturing

1-16. The responsible critical care nurse delegates to unlicensed assistive personnel when appropriate. The five "rights" of delegation are: right task, right circumstances, right person, right supervision, and _____.
A. Right time
B. Right direction/communication
C. Right patient
D. Right location

1-17. A patient has been admitted to the ICU for nausea, vomiting, and electrolyte abnormalities. During her course of care, she develops respiratory distress and hypoxia, requiring intubation because of aspiration pneumonia. Despite aggressive support, she remained hypoxic. Her ICU course is now complicated by the development of acute tubular necrosis and hepatic failure. To establish appropriate priorities of care for this patient, the nurse needs to plan care for a patient with which of these conditions?
A. Systemic inflammatory response syndrome (SIRS)
B. Septic shock
C. Bacteremia
D. Multiple organ dysfunction syndrome (MODS)

1-18. A patient admitted 2 weeks ago for bilateral flail chest injuries associated with a motor vehicle collision had chest tubes inserted and has been intubated and mechanically ventilated throughout that period. His left chest tube demonstrates persistent bubbling during inspiration and expiration, although his breath sounds are clear bilaterally and the drainage system is working properly. Which of these interventions should the critical care nurse consider next?
A. Monitor tidal volumes
B. Obtain a STAT chest x-ray
C. Assess the patient for tracheal deviation
D. Place the left chest tube to water seal

1-19. A patient with end-stage renal disease (ESRD) is receiving peritoneal dialysis. He complains of severe shoulder pain after the inflow period. What is the appropriate immediate intervention?
A. Drain the effluent with the patient in the knee-chest position
B. Change the patient's position to right side-lying
C. Ensure that all future infusions are warmed to body temperature
D. Increase the dwell time

1-20. A motor vehicle trauma patient is assigned to your care. Over the past 2 hours, his urine output has increased from 125 to 900 mL/hr. Which of these assessments would be most appropriate at this time?
A. Abdominal girth measurement
B. Urine specific gravity
C. Capillary blood glucose level
D. Potassium level

1-21. A patient with no history of cardiac disease or edema is transported to the ER for acute respiratory distress. He is intubated upon arrival and transferred to your care in the ICU. Upon admission, diagnostic testing reveals:
12-lead ECG demonstrating sinus tachycardia at 120 beats/min with atrial premature contractions and 1-mm ST segment depression in leads V_3, V_4, V_5, V_6
CPK-MB 5%
Troponin 0.1 ng/mL
BNP 598 pg/mL
These findings are most consistent with
A. Acute MI with cardiogenic shock
B. Pericarditis
C. Acute heart failure
D. Tricuspid valve insufficiency

1-22. You are caring for a patient on IV heparin therapy for deep vein thrombosis (DVT). He complains of chest pain, difficulty breathing, anxiety, palpitations, and lower extremity pain. Which of these laboratory tests would be most important for determining whether this patient is experiencing heparin-induced thrombocytopenia (HIT)?

A. Enzyme-linked immunosorbent assay and platelet count

B. International normalized ratio and prothrombin time

C. Complete blood count with manual differential

D. Arterial blood gas and mixed venous blood gas

1-23. A 56-year-old man is admitted to the ICU with severe abdominal pain, elevated lipase levels, nausea, and vomiting. He denies any alcohol or smoking history. He is diagnosed with acute pancreatitis. The patient states that he never wants to suffer this way again. How can the nurse best assist this patient in better understanding his diagnosis to meet his goal?

A. Discuss the etiology of this disorder

B. Provide information on how to regain weight

C. Assess the patient's food preferences

D. Ask if a living will is on file

1-24. A 76-year-old female is transferred to the progressive care unit for treatment of acute pulmonary edema. Pulmonary edema is most likely to develop when

A. Right atrial pressure exceeds 18 mm Hg

B. Cardiac output is 4 L/min or less

C. PAOP exceeds 20 mm Hg

D. Systemic blood pressure exceeds 180/110 mm Hg

1-25. A patient who has been hospitalized for 3 days with a severe pelvic fracture is admitted to the ICU with hypotension, hypoxia, chest pain, and shortness of breath. His BP is now 88/54 mm Hg, decreased from 128/77 mm Hg in the previous unit. His pulse is 74 beats/min, and his respiratory rate is 36 breaths/min. The patient does not exhibit edema, pulses are 2+, and extremities are warm. The most likely cause of this patient's hypotension is

A. Increased afterload

B. Peripheral vasodilatation

C. Cardiomyopathy

D. Reduced preload

1-26. A patient admitted to the ICU after endovascular repair of an abdominal aortic aneurysm (AAA) has these assessment findings: BP 120/74 mm Hg; HR 90/min; RR 20/min;

temperature 36°C. Distal pulses are 2+, capillary refill is 2 seconds, and the groin site demonstrates no evidence of hematoma. Urine output is 20 mL/hr for 2 hours. The most likely cause of decreased urine output is

A. Renal toxic effects of contrast agents

B. Occlusion of the renal artery by the endograft

C. Hypovolemia because of operative blood loss

D. Hypovolemia because of retroperitoneal bleeding

1-27. A patient in the progressive care unit is recovering from a gastric resection for stomach cancer. The patient complains of a poor appetite, and his family has brought his favorite foods from home. Within minutes of eating, the patient develops diaphoresis, weakness, cramping, and palpitations. His BP is 102/70 mm Hg, pulse is 96 beats/min, and respirations are 22 breaths/min. Which of these conditions best explains these clinical findings?

A. Myocardial infarction

B. Pulmonary embolism

C. Severe rebound hyperglycemia

D. Dumping syndrome

1-28. An 88-year-old woman who lives with her grandson is admitted to the ICU with electrolyte imbalance, malnutrition, and chest pain. Upon receiving the patient from the emergency department, the ICU nurse notices the residue from a tape mark across the patient's mouth, which was documented in the patient's ED assessment. After the two nurses discuss this finding, what should be considered as the next best course of action?

A. Make a report to adult protective services

B. Carefully document assessment and patient response to tape marks

C. Call the physician to report these findings

D. Discuss these findings with the family in order to gain more information

1-29. You have received report on a patient being transferred to the ICU. She is 32 weeks' pregnant and was admitted to the maternity unit for preeclampsia and generalized edema. Her vital signs are temperature 37.1°C pulse 120 beats/min; RR 31 breaths/min; BP 210/128 mm Hg; and pulse oxygen 98% on room air. A stat chest x-ray shows evidence of pulmonary edema. IV furosemide

40 mg was given before transfer to the ICU. Which of these medications do you anticipate administering to reduce blood pressure and prevent fetal harm?

A. Sodium nitroprusside (Nipride) titrated to achieve a systolic BP of 150 mm Hg
B. Hydralazine 5 to 10 mg IV
C. Captopril (Capoten) 100 mg PO
D. Phentolamine (Regitine) 5 mg IV

1-30. A patient in the ICU is intubated and mechanically ventilated on these settings: tidal volume 600 mL; rate 12/min; FiO_2 70%; PEEP 15 cm H_2O. The peak inspiratory pressure is 50 cm H_2O, and the patient's respiratory rate is 12/min. Arterial blood gas values include pH 7.25, PaO_2 60 mm Hg, and $PaCO_2$ 48 mm Hg. Which of these findings would best indicate clinical improvement in this patient?

A. Peak inspiratory pressure 43 cm H_2O
B. $PaCO_2$ 45 mm Hg
C. PaO_2 62 mm Hg
D. Respiratory rate 14/min

1-31. The AACN expected practice for care of the ventilated patient includes evidence-based protocols for the prevention of ventilator-associated events (VAE). Which of the following will prevent VAE and possible bacteremia and sepsis?

A. Elevating the HOB 30 to 45 degrees
B. Providing oral care every 4 to 6 hours
C. Changing ventilator circuit every 24 hours
D. Keeping oral mucosa dry

1-32. Upon arrival to the critical care unit after coronary artery bypass graft surgery, the patient has a BP of 180/110 mm Hg, a heart rate of 70 beats/min 100% paced, a RAP of 6 mm Hg, a PAD of 10 mm Hg, a temperature of 36°C and cardiac output of 3.5 LPM. Urine output for the first hour is 60 mL. Which of these interventions should the nurse perform first?

A. Bolus the patient with 250 mL to increase the RAP and PAD
B. Increase the nitroglycerin infusion by 6.6 mcg/min to decrease BP
C. Increase the pacing rate to 75 to improve cardiac output
D. Administer propranolol 1 mg IV to decrease blood pressure

1-33. A 42-year-old male with a history of severe asthma and of 1 pack per day smoking has been admitted to the ICU for asthma exacerbation. His work of breathing has increased, and a stat ABG was sent. ABG results on 50% Venturi mask are pH 7.25; CO_2 65 mm Hg; PaO_2 60 mm Hg; and HCO_3 25 mEq/L. Which of these interventions would the critical care nurse anticipate?

A. Addition of steroids to the bronchodilator regime
B. Changing from beta agonists to leukotriene inhibitors
C. Initiation of inhaled nitric oxide
D. Immediate intubation

1-34. Hospital-acquired pneumonia and ventilator-acquired pneumonia result in increased morbidity and mortality for the inpatient population. You have created a committee to focus on decreasing the incidence of pneumonia. Which of these interventions would have the most impact on this health problem?

A. Adherence to handwashing and sterile technique
B. Prophylactic antibiotics for ventilator patients
C. Pneumococcal vaccines for patients older than 65 years
D. DVT prophylaxis

1-35. A patient in the ICU has been admitted with pneumonia and exacerbation of COPD. He is currently on an insulin drip and receiving IV steroids and antibiotic therapy. The patient has become irritable and agitated over the past 30 minutes. Which of the following should the nurse complete first?

A. Obtain a stat ECG
B. Administer an anxiolytic medication
C. Measure capillary glucose
D. Provide milk and crackers

1-36. A cancer patient is scheduled to have a bone marrow transplant. He remains in strict isolation, and he is tearful and anxious. He explains that he feels lonely and isolated. What would be an appropriate nursing intervention?

A. Playing music the patient enjoys and allowing photographs at the bedside
B. Allowing the patient's cat to visit for a pet therapy session

C. Encouraging the patient's school-aged grandchildren to visit

D. Asking family members to bring in fresh produce as comfort food

1-37. The ICU monitor alarms, and you find your patient displays a wide complex tachycardia at a rate of 180 beats/min. He complains of chest pain and shortness of breath. His MAP is 58 mm Hg, and he is diaphoretic. Which intervention should be performed immediately?

A. Administer amiodarone 150 mg IV over 10 minutes

B. Administer adenosine 6 mg rapid IV push

C. Perform synchronized cardioversion

D. Defibrillate with 300 joules

1-38. During a staff meeting, the unit-based performance improvement nurse provides data on stress-related mucosal disease (SRMD) in the ICU. Data for the previous 3 months suggest that, on average, 20 of the monthly census of 100 patients are developing SRMD. The nurse asks her colleagues for suggestions to decrease the incidence of SRMD. One good suggestion would be to

A. Develop a prevention protocol for high-risk patients in the ICU

B. Add a proton pump inhibitor to the standing orders for all patients

C. Deliver the data to physicians on the medical ICU committee for their consideration

D. Continue data collection to ensure sufficient evidence exists before a response is made

1-39. After cardiac catheterization with percutaneous coronary intervention, a patient develops a pulsus paradoxus. The most likely cause for this finding is

A. Pericardial tamponade

B. Coronary artery spasm

C. Dysrhythmia

D. Vasovagal reaction

1-40. A postoperative abdominal surgery patient weighing 700 lb (318 kg) develops acute onset of dyspnea and chest pain. Arterial blood gas values are pH 7.35; PaO_2 is 74 mm Hg; $PaCO_2$ is 30 mm Hg; and O_2 is saturation 90%. Chest x-ray demonstrates an enlarged cardiac silhouette, a prominent pulmonary artery, and mild right pleural effusion. The 12-lead ECG demonstrates T-wave inversions in the anterior leads. These findings suggest that this patient has most likely developed which of the following?

A. Aspiration pneumonia

B. Pulmonary embolism

C. Acute myocardial infarction

D. Pneumothorax

1-41. The critical care nurse is receiving a patient with chronic renal failure. He presents to the triage nurse complaining of abdominal cramping, nausea, diarrhea, and severe itching. Laboratory testing reveals a calcium level of 6.2 mg/dL. Which of these treatments does the nurse anticipate?

A. IV potassium supplement

B. Oral phosphate supplement

C. Oral sevelamer

D. IV sodium bicarbonate

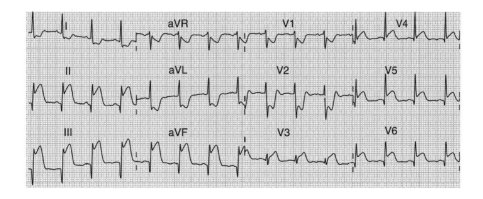

1-42. A patient has been admitted to the emergency room complaining of chest pain. A 12-lead ECG is obtained (shown on previous page). The patient is administered a tablet of 1/150 grains sublingual nitroglycerin, and his blood pressure drops from 138/84 mm Hg to 82/56 mm Hg. Which of the following is most likely identified as the cause of the decrease in blood pressure?
- A. Hypersensitivity to nitroglycerin
- B. Right ventricular MI
- C. Papillary muscle rupture
- D. Rupture of the ventricular free wall

1-43. A patient had an upper esophagogastroduodenoscopy (EGD) 30 minutes ago and is drowsy. As the patient is slowly waking up, he asks, "Can I have a drink of water?" The nurse's best response would be to say,
- A. "If you can swallow, you can have something to drink."
- B. "You cannot have anything until your gag reflex returns."
- C. "Try to rest for now; you need to recover from the procedure."
- D. "Now that you're thirsty, we can order your lunch tray for delivery in 30 minutes."

1-44. Your patient has been admitted to the ICU for the seventh time in 2 months. He has end-stage cardiomyopathy, and has refused an LVAD (implanted left ventricular assist device). He has discussed comfort care with his family and has decided that he wants comfort care interventions only. Which of these medical interventions should continue?
- A. Blood draws for laboratory values
- B. IV Lasix administration
- C. Daily chest x-ray
- D. Blood glucose monitoring AC and HS

1-45. When a patient with an implanted cardioverter defibrillator develops rapid atrial fibrillation that results in inappropriate delivery of defibrillation shocks. The nurse's first intervention should be to
- A. Perform overdrive pacing with a transcutaneous pacemaker
- B. Place a pacemaker magnet over the pacemaker generator
- C. Administer diltiazem 20 mg IV over 2 minutes
- D. Administer amiodarone 150 mg IV over 10 minutes

1-46. Your 35-year-old patient is admitted to the progressive care unit for treatment of acute exacerbation of asthma with IV steroids. During morning assessment, you find him to be obtunded. A stat blood glucose level is 624 mg/dL. Which of these conditions should you plan to manage?
- A. Diabetes insipidus
- B. Type 1 diabetes mellitus
- C. Hyperglycemic, hyperosmolar, nonketotic coma
- D. Polycythemia vera

1-47. You are caring for a heart failure patient who is a retired primary care physician. His echocardiogram was completed, and he was told by the cardiologist that he has classic diastolic dysfunction. He calls you into the room and tells you he was too embarrassed to ask the cardiologist to explain diastolic dysfunction. Which of these explanations would you provide?
- A. Ejection fraction 55% and decreased early diastolic filling time
- B. Ejection fraction 50% and increased late diastolic filling time
- C. Ejection fraction 60% and prolonged left ventricular ejection time
- D. Ejection fraction 35% and shortened left ventricular ejection time

1-48. A nurse in a 16-bed ICU that is managed with a shared governance model is currently the chair of a multidisciplinary committee that evaluates the use of medical devices for attributes such as unit costs, type, infection rate, and malfunction rate. The committee is notified that a new cardiologist coming in a few months will be implanting cardioverter-defibrillator devices, so the hospital requested that the committee develop a tool to be used to evaluate outcomes related to this device, similar to a registry (log of positive and negative outcomes). As the leader of this multidisciplinary group, how should the nurse proceed to investigate this device?
- A. Contact the sales representative from a company selling ICDs
- B. Research the current registries to identify variables measured
- C. Modify the current evaluation tool for use with the ICD
- D. Consider obtaining a consultant to help the committee with this task

1-49. An ICU nurse caring for a patient admitted with severe abdominal discomfort and fatigue notes that the patient tested positive for *Helicobacter pylori* and has a history of cigarette smoking. The patient develops nausea and abdominal tenderness. His vital signs are BP 123/80 mm Hg; pulse 89 beats/min; respirations 15 breaths/min. Within 15 minutes, the patient vomits, and his emesis contains coffee grounds. His vital signs are BP 100/68 mm Hg; pulse 120 beats/min; respirations 24 breaths/min. Which of these medical orders for this patient merits the nurse's immediate attention?
   A. Secure initial coagulation study findings and monitor each shift
   B. Insert large-bore IV
   C. Upright KUB x-ray
   D. Monitor fluid balance closely

1-50. A patient with community-acquired pneumonia has an advanced directive stating no intubation. The patient's spouse, who is also the Durable Power of Attorney (DPA) for the patient, wishes to have the patient intubated. The patient is in obvious respiratory distress, on BiPAP, but he remains alert and oriented. The nurse caring for the patient should
   A. Inform the spouse that the DPA is not in effect until the patient is no longer able to make decisions
   B. Encourage the patient to consider intubation as his spouse desires
   C. Inform the patient of the spouse's concerns and ask if the patient wishes to be intubated for a trial period
   D. Encourage the patient to discuss intubation with his spouse

1-51. A patient arrives to the unit post coronary stent via the right femoral approach. The catheterization laboratory nurse reported that the cardiology fellow performed a high femoral stick. The patient is most likely at risk for which of these vascular access site complications?
   A. Pseudoaneurysm
   B. Arteriovenous fistula
   C. Retroperitoneal hemorrhage
   D. Hematoma

1-52. Your patient is in the ICU for treatment of a ruptured cerebral aneurysm. He was stable yesterday but has progressed overnight to critical condition after developing hydrocephalus. The patient's wife is an obstetric nurse. She is tearful at the bedside and asks you to explain why her husband has developed hydrocephalus. Which of these explanations should be provided?
   A. Blood in the subarachnoid space blocks reabsorption of cerebrospinal fluid (CSF) in the arachnoid villi
   B. A thrombus may form and obstruct flow of CSF out of the ventricles
   C. Cerebral edema may lead to a mass effect that blocks CSF flow
   D. Vasospasm may limit the flow of CSF

1-53. A patient with warfarin overdose is in the ICU for treatment of a lower GI bleed. He is currently experiencing bright red blood per rectum. Which of the following is the earliest sign of impending hypovolemic shock?
   A. Systolic BP less than 90 mm Hg
   B. Capillary refill time greater than 4 seconds
   C. Decreased urine output
   D. Tachycardia greater than 120 beats/min

1-54. A 75-year-old patient presents to the ED after a head-on motor vehicle collision in which he was a belted driver. He is alert and oriented with stable vital signs and complains of mild pain to his right chest. During his trauma workup, he suddenly develops shortness of breath, his oxygen saturation drops to 85%, and his heart rate and blood pressure elevate slightly from baseline. He has decreased breath sounds in his right lung fields, and his trachea is midline. What is the most appropriate nursing action at this time?
   A. Secure a chest tube insertion kit and notify the physician that the patient may have a pneumothorax
   B. Administer oxygen via a nasal cannula and notify the physician about these assessment findings
   C. Obtain an order for and administer STAT a narcotic analgesic
   D. Document the assessment findings and prepare the patient for prompt admission to ICU

1-55. Patients' complaints of frequent venipunctures in the ICU are an ongoing issue. Patients on IV heparin therapy can have three to four venipunctures per day to monitor PTT levels. You would like to change the hospital policy to permit PTT samples to be drawn from a peripheral IV site. What should be your next course of action to promote this change in policy?
   A. Identify key stakeholders in this proposed change of practice
   B. Specify the intended change in bedside practice
   C. Modify the nursing flowsheet to accommodate the change
   D. Evaluate the success of the change in procedure

1-56. Two hours after coronary artery bypass graft surgery, a patient has these assessment findings:
   Heart rate 80/min, 100% paced
   BP 80/62 mm Hg, MAP 68 mm Hg, RAP 15 mm Hg
   PAD 14 mm Hg, CO 3.0 L/min
   Chest tube output has been 50 mL/hr for 2 hours. These findings are consistent with which of the following?
   A. Normal postoperative course after open heart surgery
   B. Myocardial stunning
   C. Cardiac tamponade
   D. Perioperative myocardial infarction

1-57. In caring for a patient admitted from the ER with a diagnosis of ingestion of N-methyl-D-aspartate (Ecstasy), the critical care nurse observes that the patient has cola-colored urine with a specific gravity of 1.028. These findings are consistent with the development of rhabdomyolysis. One of the most important interventions to prevent renal failure in patients with rhabdomyolysis includes
   A. Maintaining a urine pH lower than 5.0
   B. Inserting an indwelling urinary catheter
   C. Maintaining urine output greater than 150 mL/hr
   D. Monitoring hemodynamics closely

1-58. You are caring for a patient with complaints of intermittent chest pain. He has a past medical history of severe peripheral vascular disease, smoking, diabetes, and hypertension. His troponin levels are normal, and his ECG shows a left bundle branch block. The cardiologist has ordered an ischemia workup. Which of these testing methods would be most helpful to diagnose myocardial ischemia for this patient?
   A. Exercise treadmill stress test
   B. SPECT perfusion imaging with technetium-99m sestamibi
   C. Regadenoson (Lexiscan) stress test
   D. Magnetic resonance imaging (MRI)

1-59. A 29-year-old man is admitted to the telemetry unit with a diagnosis of unstable angina. The patient has had numerous admissions over the past year with a history of cocaine abuse and demanding demeanor. All of his cardiac workups have been negative. As soon as he is admitted, he asks for pain medication and for lunch. He states that his pain is midsternal and that the level is a 7 on a scale of 1 to 10. The patient has NTG SL and morphine 2 mg IV ordered for pain. The charge nurse tells the nurse assigned to this patient, "Just give him the morphine; you know that is what he wants." What should the staff nurse do?
   A. Give the NTG SL X 3 before administering the morphine
   B. Administer morphine 2 mg IV
   C. Inform the patient that he must wait 30 minutes until morphine can be given
   D. Discuss treatment options with the patient

1-60. You are planning care for a patient admitted with status asthmaticus. She has a history of severe asthma and multiple intubations. The goals of mechanical ventilation for this patient include
   A. Low tidal volumes and minimal PEEP
   B. High tidal volumes and low PEEP
   C. Low respiratory rate and high tidal volumes
   D. High PEEP and low FiO_2

1-61. After aortofemoral bypass surgery for acute arterial occlusion, the patient's CPK is elevated, and his serum potassium level is 5.9 mEq/L. Arterial blood gas values include PaO_2 90 mm Hg, P_aCO_2 24 mm Hg, and HCO_3 19 mm Hg. This patient is at risk for developing
   A. Dysrhythmias
   B. Graft occlusion
   C. Pulmonary embolus
   D. Heart failure

1-62. Mrs. Jones has been admitted to the ICU for upper gastrointestinal bleeding. She is alert and anxious on arrival but refuses to permit an assessment until she calls her daughter. The nurse reassures her that he will call the patient's daughter. The ICU nurse would like to assess the patient's understanding relative to her admitting diagnosis. Which of these questions would provide the nurse with information for understanding his patient's beliefs relative to her diagnosis?

A. When did you experience your first symptoms?

B. Does anyone else in your family have this bleeding problem?

C. Do you consume alcohol on a regular basis?

D. Why do you think you are sick?

1-63. A patient with long-standing history of COPD is admitted for worsening dyspnea and desaturation. She is on home oxygen therapy at 2 LPM. Her admission vital signs are: temperature 38.2°C HR 104/min; BP 130/60 mm Hg; RR 28/min; SaO_2 88%. For this patient, the nurse knows that increasing the FiO_2 should

A. Improve the patient's oxygenation

B. Only be done on the basis of ABG results

C. Be avoided because it may weaken the patient's respiratory drive

D. Only be used as a last resort because it may increase hypoxemic vasoconstriction

1-64. A respiratory arrest patient has arrived for admission to the ICU. He is receiving mechanical ventilation, and his admission diagnosis is acute pancreatitis. The critical care nurse assesses upper lip twitching, wheezing, and increased peak airway pressures. The patient is demonstrating an electrolyte imbalance. Which of these IV drug treatments will be ordered for administration?

A. Magnesium sulfate 25 mEq in 1000 mL D5W

B. Plicamycin 1050 mcg in 1000 mL NS

C. Vasopressin 100 units in 250 mL D5W

D. Calcium chloride 1000 mg in 1000 mL NS

1-65. A 33-year-old male is brought to the emergency department by a family member after vomiting blood at home. He had been drinking, and his alcohol history includes a six pack of beer on weekends. He also has a history of chronic back pain. He is admitted to the ICU with a diagnosis of upper gastrointestinal bleeding. His vital signs are BP 110/50 mm Hg; pulse 94 beats/min; respiratory rate 12 breaths/min. Initial results show a blood alcohol level of 0.10 mg/dL. After 30 minutes, the nurse notes that he is lethargic, pale, and diaphoretic: BP is now 94/60 mm Hg; heart rate 134 beats/min with thready pulses; respiratory rate 20 breaths/min; urine output 25 cc/hr. His abdomen is tender to palpation in the left upper quadrant, and bowel sounds are hyperactive. Which of these conditions is likely contributing to this patient's current findings?

A. Pulmonary embolism with hypoxemia

B. Erosive gastritis with 25% blood volume loss

C. Intracranial hypertension

D. Dehydration because of alcohol abuse

1-66. A firefighter has been burned over 60% of his body. He is being transported to the emergency room by police vehicle for immediate urgent care. You anticipate initiation of all of the following EXCEPT:

A. Immediate intubation with low-volume ventilation (5 mL/k–7 mL/k)

B. Aggressive IV fluid resuscitation (20–40 mL/k/percentage of body surface area burned) given over 8 hours

C. IV pain management

D. Large-bore peripheral IV placement

1-67. You are expecting a patient from the emergency room with a diagnosis of septic shock. Your patient in septic shock may present with a variety of clinical manifestations that may progress and worsen. Which of these physiologic symptoms will you most likely anticipate for the patient with worsening septic shock?

A. ↑ temperature and ↑ urine output

B. ↓ systemic vascular resistance (SVR) and ↓ cardiac output (CO)

C. ↑ mixed venous oxygen saturation (SVO_2) and ↑ heart rate (HR)

D. ↑ right atrial pressure (RAP) and ↑ respiratory rate (RR)

1-68. Recent research supports the provision of oral care to reduce hospital-associated pneumonia among ventilated patients. What would be the best approach for the nurse to use in implementing an oral care protocol on the unit?
   A. Place oral care kits at the bedside of every ventilated patient
   B. Establish a new multidisciplinary team for this purpose
   C. Hold a staff meeting to elicit colleagues' views on this issue
   D. Include "oral care every 2 hours" on the standing orders for ventilated patients

1-69. You have received report from the prior shift on Mrs. Jones. She is a heart failure patient receiving diuretics, beta blockers, and ACE inhibitors. Upon assessment, you notice that she is short of breath, has bibasilar crackles, and has had a weight gain of 2 kg since yesterday morning. Her current blood pressure is 100/60 mm Hg and heart rate 72 beats per minute. You call the ICU intern and suggest IV furosemide and which of the following?
   A. Discontinuing the beta blocker
   B. Decreasing the beta blocker dosage
   C. Administering an additional dose of beta blocker
   D. Administering an additional dose of ACE inhibitor

1-70. The physician orders a trial of noninvasive ventilation (NIV) for a COPD patient with worsening arterial blood gas results. The nurse knows that for this COPD patient, NIV
   A. Will require fairly heavy sedation to enable the patient to tolerate this therapy
   B. May be helpful in reducing the need for endotracheal intubation
   C. Needs to be used with caution because it increases the work of breathing
   D. Needs to be administered via nasal pillows rather than a full mask

1-71. A patient with a 15-year history of type 1 diabetes is admitted with diabetic ketoacidosis. His partner is at the bedside, and he has tears in his eyes. He asks you how his partner could have developed diabetic ketoacidosis when he has been so careful to manage his diabetes properly. Which of the following represents the best explanation the nurse could provide to this question?
   A. "Your partner must have been cheating on his diet or skipping insulin doses."
   B. "In times of stress, the body produces more cortisol than normal, and blood sugar increases."
   C. "Diabetic ketoacidosis is the result of a genetic abnormality affecting every other generation."
   D. "Your partner recently started a daily exercise routine without consulting his primary care provider."

1-72. A patient with severe dehydration is receiving fluid resuscitation for hypovolemic shock. Laboratory values are as follows: pH 7.28; PaO_2 80 mm Hg; $PaCO_2$ 24 mm Hg; and hematocrit 34%. Nursing management of this patient needs to include
   A. Administration of sodium bicarbonate
   B. Administration of 1 unit of packed red blood cells
   C. Administration of crystalloid 200 mL/hr
   D. Endotracheal intubation

1-73. A patient is admitted to the ICU after falling from a roof and sustaining fractures of the first three ribs on the right side. The patient is dyspneic and complains of hoarseness, and subcutaneous emphysema can be palpated. The patient is placed on 50% FiO_2 by facemask, and his oxygen saturation is 80%. The only notable findings on chest x-ray are the rib fractures and the presence of mediastinal subcutaneous emphysema. Auscultation reveals equal breath sounds bilaterally and a crunching sound during systole. Within a few minutes, the patient develops increasing respiratory distress. The next intervention the nurse should anticipate is
   A. Increasing the FiO_2 percentage to 80%
   B. Inserting a right chest tube
   C. Intubation and ventilator support
   D. Repeating the chest x-ray

1-74. You are providing end-of-life care for a patient. The best way for you to facilitate "a good death" for a patient would be
   A. Assign the same RN to care for the patient
   B. Allow unrestricted visiting for the patient.
   C. Encourage hope in the face of futile care
   D. Manage the patient's pain and discomfort

1-75. A patient is admitted with a diagnosis of pulmonary edema. The patient has a bounding carotid pulse, systolic ejection murmur, hypotension, and tachypnea. Chest x-ray shows cardiomegaly and interstitial pulmonary edema. ECG demonstrates bradycardia, left ventricular hypertrophy, and left bundle branch block. Which of the following is the most likely etiology of these findings?

A. Aortic regurgitation

B. Mitral valve stenosis

C. Tricuspid regurgitation

D. Pericardial effusion

1-76. John Doe was admitted to the ICU last night after he was found in an alley beaten and unconscious. He has not yet been identified, and his past medical history is unknown. He was intubated, treated prophylactically for TBI (traumatic brain injury) with anticonvulsants, and remains clinically stable on ventilator support with satisfactory laboratory and ABG results. During a midmorning assessment, the nurse notes that the patient demonstrates a rhythmic movement of his extremities and begins clenching his jaw on the endotracheal tube. He has not demonstrated this type of activity before. The nurse hypothesizes that the patient is most likely experiencing

A. Hypoxia

B. Delirium tremens

C. Substance withdrawal

D. Posttraumatic seizures

1-77. When caring for a patient admitted to the ICU after ingestion of 50 tablets of acetaminophen, the critical care nurse recognizes that hepatic encephalopathy with progressive symptoms occurs approximately 48 to 96 hours after ingestion and can develop an appropriate plan of care to prioritize patient management. What physiologic process contributes to the patient's progressive response to the toxic ingestion of acetaminophen?

A. Clearance

B. Absorption

C. Distribution

D. Chelation

1-78. A patient in the coronary care unit is supported with mechanical ventilation after experiencing a STEMI. He suddenly develops third-degree heart block with a rate of 38 beats/min. His blood pressure is 76/42 mm Hg. The most appropriate initial intervention for the nurse assigned to this patient would be to

A. Initiate transcutaneous pacing

B. Administer atropine 0.5 mg IV

C. Initiate an infusion of epinephrine at 5 mcg/min

D. Initiate an infusion of dopamine at 5 mcg/k/min

1-79. You are the preceptor orienting a new nurse in the ICU. You are tasked with evaluating her competency to provide the highest quality patient care. Which of the following clinical observations demonstrate that the new nurse is providing the highest level of caring practice?

A. Maintains a safe physical environment

B. Bases care on standards and protocols

C. Focuses on basic and routine needs of the patient

D. Patient and family needs determine caring practices

1-80. A patient is admitted to the ICU after a motor vehicle crash in which the air bag was deployed. The initial assessment of the patient reveals these findings: heart rate 120 beats/min; blood pressure 90/76 mm Hg; respiratory rate 28; SpO_2 94%. Breath sounds are equal bilaterally and shallow. The patient has bulging jugular veins, and heart tones are distant. Which of these interventions is most appropriate to relieve the patient's condition?

A. Prepare for chest tube insertion

B. Prepare for endotracheal intubation

C. Prepare for pericardiocentesis

D. Prepare for needle thoracostomy

1-81. A patient is admitted to the ICU with thoracic and facial bruises and abrasions sustained earlier that day in a motor vehicle crash. The patient was unrestrained in the car and indicates that he hit the steering wheel at the time of the incident. He complains of chest pain and has a respiratory rate of 33 breaths/min. His arterial blood gases on room air are pH 7.44; $PaCO_2$ 32 mm Hg; PaO_2 53 mm Hg; HCO_3 24 mEq/L. Which of these findings indicate a potentially life-threatening emergency for this patient?

A. Decreased breath sounds in both lung bases

B. Inspiratory wheezing that clears with coughing

C. Decreased breath sounds over right lung fields

D. Absent breath sounds over right lung fields

1-82. You are caring for an encephalopathic patient with decompensated cirrhosis. He has just arrived back from a CT scan that showed splenomegaly, ascites, and portal hypertension. You know that the patient is at high risk for sudden GI bleeding, so you send a stat type and crossmatch. What is the pathophysiology that puts this patient at risk for ruptured esophageal varices?

A. The development of right-sided heart failure

B. Excessive circulating blood volume associated with cirrhosis

C. Fibrotic nature of the hepatic tissue

D. Elevated pressure in esophageal veins

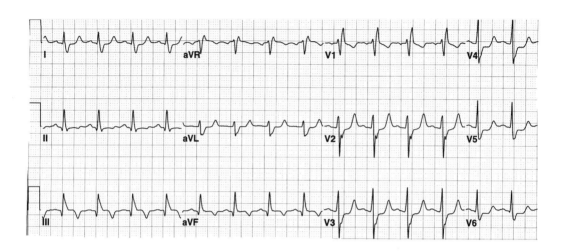

1-83. The 12-lead ECG shown above demonstrates which of the following?

A. Right bundle branch block

B. Left bundle branch block

C. Sinus tachycardia

D. Acute anterior wall myocardial infarction

1-84. What would be the physiologic benefit of optimal patient positioning post frontal craniotomy?

A. Maximizes jugular venous outflow

B. Decreases CPP

C. Facilitates the flow of CSF

D. Immobilizes the surgical site

1-85. Which of these findings indicates acute dissection of an aortic aneurysm?

A. Difference in systolic BP between left and right arms exceeding 10 mm Hg and facial edema

B. Visible pulsation in the abdomen and abdominal bruit

C. Sudden onset of back pain and syncope

D. Hypertension and renal insufficiency

1-86. The critical care nurse caring for a patient with an acute exacerbation of COPD can anticipate administering a variety of pharmacologic agents. Which of these combinations would be administered for this patient?

A. Bronchodilators and antiviral agents

B. Prostacyclin and oxygen

C. Mucolytic therapy and antibiotics

D. Glucocorticoids and cholinergic agents

1-87. A patient is admitted to the ICU with complaints of left arm pain and nausea. A 12-lead ECG shows sinus bradycardia with a heart rate of 40 beats/min and ST elevation in leads II, III, and AVF. Which of the following would be the best treatment for bradycardia in this patient?

A. Percutaneous coronary intervention

B. Temporary transvenous pacing

C. Transcutaneous pacing

D. Administration of atropine

1-88. A 45-year-old patient with stage 3 heart failure, a 1-month history of frequent episodes of ventricular tachycardia, and an ejection fraction less than 35% is returned from the OR after implantation of an ICD (implantable cardioverter-defibrillator). The patient was unsure about getting the device and hesitantly signed the consent form. For 3 hours after admission to the ICU, his vital signs are stable, and ECG monitoring shows normal sinus rhythm. The patient suddenly develops pulseless ventricular tachycardia, arrests, and receives 45 minutes of resuscitation efforts with no improvement. Given that the ICD did not operate during a sustained period of ventricular tachycardia, what step(s) should the nurse caring for this patient take now?

A. Document the resuscitation effort in detail because litigation will likely occur

B. Immediately call the risk management department

C. Complete an incident report and notify administration

D. Design an in-service on ICD malfunctions for the nursing staff

1-89. A 60-year-old patient is admitted to the ICU with a 3-day history of nausea, vomiting, and persistent diarrhea. Past medical history is significant for coronary artery disease and hypertension. Admitting vital signs reveal the following: temperature 38.9°C HR 110/min, sinus tachycardia; BP 90/40 mm Hg; RR 30/min. Laboratory values from the ER are as follows: WBC 20,000/mm³; hemoglobin 10.0 g/dL; BUN 80 mg/dL; creatinine 2.5 mg/dL; serum lactate 6 mmol/L. Cultures (blood, urine, sputum, and stool) have been sent, and antibiotic therapy has been initiated. The critical care nurse should expect the patient's immediate treatment to include

A. Inotropic support

B. IV fluid bolus

C. Blood transfusion

D. Beta-blocker therapy

1-90. You are the ICU nurse caring for a patient in cardiogenic shock. The patient is on IV norepinephrine, and he is supported by a left-sided percutaneous short term ventricular assist device. Which of these hemodynamic results indicate that the current therapy is appropriate?

A. HR 100 beats/min MAP 66 mm Hg, SVR 1200 dynes/sec/cm⁻⁵

B. HR 117 beats/min MAP 53 mm Hg, SVR 1900 dynes/sec/cm⁻⁵

C. HR 110 beats/min MAP 70 mm Hg, SVR 2800 dynes/sec/cm⁻⁵

D. HR 117 beats/min MAP 53 mm Hg, SVR 2400 dynes/sec/cm⁻⁵

1-91. A 50-year-old man is admitted to the ICU for treatment of cardiomyopathy. He had a cardiac biopsy 2 days before to rule out cardiac amyloidosis. The nurse knows that the result showed that the patient has amyloidosis. The patient asked the nurse if his test results are back. The nurse's best response would be:

A. "Do you want to receive this information when you are alone or with your family?"

B. "The physician will need to provide you with the results."

C. "Would you like to have the chaplain present when you get the results?"

D. "Your family should be present when we discuss the results."

1-92. A patient has been admitted for an exacerbation of COPD. When taking this patient's history, which of the following should the critical care nurse focus on as the most likely cause of moderate to severe exacerbations of COPD?

A. Inspissated secretions

B. Infectious processes

C. Inflammatory processes

D. Excessive sputum production

1-93. A postoperative cardiac surgical patient with increased chest tube output, a heart rate of 126 beats/min, blood pressure 80/68 mm Hg, and PAOP 5 mm Hg would benefit most from which intervention?

A. Administration of a 250-mL bolus of normal saline

B. Administration of one unit of packed cells

C. Initiation of a dopamine infusion at 10 mcg/kg/min

D. Vasopressin 40 units IV push

1-94. On postoperative day 3, a patient (status: post Roux-en-Y gastric bypass) is admitted to the ICU with a diagnosis of sepsis secondary to gastric perforation. On postoperative day 5, the patient's weight increases by 10 kg, urine output is less than 325 mL/day for the last 3 days, and there are crackles bilaterally on lung auscultation. The patient's BP is 94/40 mm Hg, HR 140 beats/min, RR 38/min, CVP 22 cm H2O, pulmonary wedge pressure 25 mm Hg. The patient's current laboratory values are Na 123 mEq/L; potassium 9.2 mEq/L; phosphorus 6.0 mg/dL; calcium 4.7 mg/dL; BUN 148 mg/dL; and creatinine 7.4 mg/dL. Based on these findings, nursing management of this patient will need to include

A. Continued administration of fluid boluses
B. Hemodialysis
C. Continuous renal replacement therapy
D. Peritoneal dialysis

1-95. A nurse is caring for a congestive heart failure patient who is recovering after an acute episode of pulmonary edema. The patient asks the nurse how he can avoid "ending up in the hospital again." The nurse should discuss the signs and symptoms that should be reported to his health care provider immediately. Which of the following is most important to reinforce?

A. Report a weight gain of greater than 3 lb over 3 days
B. Report fatigue and take an iron supplement to prevent anemia
C. Be compliant with all scheduled appointments
D. Limit your fluid intake to prevent shortness of breath

1-96. A patient is admitted to the ICU with syncope, hypotension, and shortness of breath. She has a history of lung cancer treated with chemotherapy and a left thoracotomy. Physical examination reveals HR 134/min, BP 80/66 mm Hg, sinus tachycardia, and RR 30 beats/min and shallow. Breath sounds are decreased on the side of previous thoracotomy but otherwise clear. A pericardial friction rub and JVD are present. An arterial line is inserted, and the waveform shows a decrease of 10 mm Hg with inspiration. Which of these conditions has this patient most likely developed?

A. Hypovolemia
B. Pericardial tamponade
C. Tension pneumothorax
D. Superior vena cava syndrome

1-97. A 40-year-old patient who presents with nausea, vomiting, jaundice, and severe abdominal pain is diagnosed with acute pancreatitis. In this disorder, autodigestion of the pancreas causes release of cytokines and kinins, which alter capillary wall permeability and vascular vasoactive properties. As the nurse anticipates potential complications that may result from these changes, which of these interventions is most important to institute at this point?

A. Monitoring of QT intervals and seizure precautions
B. Monitoring for Cullen's sign and measuring abdominal girth
C. Fluid restriction and pain control
D. Auscultation of bowel sounds and peripheral pulses

1-98. A patient is admitted to the ICU after surgery to repair a tracheoesophageal fistula. Her vitals are stable, and she is being mechanically ventilated via a low-pressure cuff airway. She is receiving enteral feeding via a nasally inserted postpyloric feeding tube. On postoperative day 2, the patient begins to cough up secretions resembling tube feeds. Which of the following is the highest priority nursing action?

A. Stop the tube feeding
B. Administer metoclopramide
C. Prepare the patient for bronchoscopy and/or endoscopy
D. Check placement of the feeding tube by auscultating an air bubble and aspirating residual

1-99. An patient was admitted to the ICU with a diagnosis of pulmonary edema. Her condition has stabilized, and she is resting comfortably. Which of these assessment findings would best indicate that therapy for acute pulmonary edema was effective?

A. Respiratory rate on BiPAP is less than 30 breaths/min
B. The patient has diuresed 3000 mL
C. Heart rate is sinus rhythm at a rate less than 100 beats/min
D. Systolic blood pressure is less than 150 mm Hg

1-100. In SIRS/MODS, cytokines are responsible for the massive inflammatory response that can lead to multiple organ dysfunction. The critical care nurse recognizes the hemodynamic response to cytokine production as evidenced by

A. SVR: 1500 dynes/sec/cm^{-5}; CVP: 16 mm Hg; SVO$_2$: 50%
B. SVR: 400 dynes/sec/cm^{-5}; CVP: 12 mm Hg; SVO$_2$: 70%
C. SVR: 500 dynes/sec/cm^{-5}; CVP: 4 mm Hg; SVO$_2$: 80%
D. SVR: 1350 dynes/sec/cm^{-5}; CVP: 2 mm Hg; SVO$_2$: 55%

1-101. A patient arrives in the ICU after coronary artery bypass graft surgery. Which of these findings best indicates that this patient may need to return to the operating room?
- A. Chest tube output greater than 200 mL per hour for 2 consecutive hours
- B. MAP 50 mm Hg for 2 hours despite norepinephrine infusion at 10 mcg/min
- C. Cardiac output 1.9 L/min
- D. PAOP 25 mm Hg

1-102. When orienting a new nurse to the ICU, the orientee's patient experiences cardiac arrest and requires resuscitation. The preceptor arrives and sees that the orientee has placed the patient in Trendelenburg position. Which of the following represents the best intervention by the preceptor to assist the facilitation of learning for this new nurse?
- A. Immediately begin chest compressions
- B. Initiate the unit's code blue response
- C. Reposition the patient supine
- D. Set up suction apparatus

1-103. A patient with hypertrophic cardiomyopathy is admitted to the hospital with shortness of breath. The critical care nurse would know that one of these medications may worsen the patient's heart failure. Which medication should not be given to the patient?
- A. Calcium channel blockers
- B. Beta blockers
- C. Nitroglycerin
- D. Amiodarone

1-104. A patient in the ICU has been diagnosed with disseminated intravascular coagulopathy (DIC). The medical team is at the bedside planning the patient's care. What is the primary goal of medical treatment for DIC?
- A. Accurately administer intravenous heparin infusion to prevent "using up" clotting factors
- B. Administer subcutaneous fibrinolytic to dissolve clots formed in the microvasculature
- C. Identify and treat the underlying conditions that lead to the development of DIC
- D. Provide supportive care as needed until the DIC subsides

1-105. A critically ill patient is admitted to the ICU with a diagnosis of septic shock. After insertion of a pulmonary artery catheter, the initial set of hemodynamic measurements are as follows: PAP 25/10 mm Hg; CVP 8 mm Hg; PAOP 12 mm Hg; CO 8 L/min; CI 3.0 L/min/cm^2; SVR 500 dynes/sec/cm^{-5}; DO$_2$ 600 mL/min; VO$_2$ 100 mL/min. These findings indicate that the patient is demonstrating which of these pathophysiologic effects of septic shock on the cardiovascular system?
- A. Vasoconstriction
- B. Maldistribution of blood flow
- C. Myocardial excitability
- D. Hypervolemia

1-106. A young patient is admitted to the ICU after a motorcycle accident involving the center median of the freeway in which she sustained blunt head and chest trauma. Within minutes of arrival on the unit, the patient complains of dysphagia and coughing. She develops upper airway obstruction unrelieved by oxygen, becomes cyanotic, and has palpable subcutaneous emphysema near the sternal notch. The nurse should prepare for which of these interventions?
- A. Intubation and mechanical ventilation
- B. Fiber optic bronchoscopy
- C. Emergent tracheostomy
- D. Initiation of cardiac compressions for CPR

1-107. An 80-year-old cachectic woman was found on the floor at home by her family. She has a past medical history of hypertension and atrial fibrillation, and she takes daily warfarin. She presents to the emergency room with left-sided paralysis and decreased level of consciousness. Her INR level is 6.7, and a head CT scan reveals a 2.5 × 2 cm deep, right hemispheric hemorrhage. Which of the following would be the most appropriate course of action?
- A. Urgent preparation for neurosurgery to evacuate the clot
- B. Aggressive correction of coagulopathy with vitamin K, fresh-frozen plasma, and recombinant factor VIIa
- C. Urgent brain MRI to rule out other potential etiologies for these findings
- D. Immediate infusion of EACA (Epsilon-aminocaproic acid) to correct coagulopathy

1-108. An 85-year-old man who had a cerebrovascular accident 2 years ago is cared for at home by his wife because of his limited functional ability. He is currently in the ICU on CPAP for community-acquired pneumonia. His wife states that she is unsure if she can take him back home this time because the workload of his care is increasingly draining her. She states that her preference would be to bring her husband home, but for now, thinks she must place him in a nursing home. What would be the nurse's best response to the wife's comment?

   A. "I will be glad to contact the ethics committee for you to help resolve this dilemma."
   B. "There are some health care resources available to help you provide care in your home."
   C. "You should feel hopeful because your husband is getting better."
   D. "You sound as though the future is uncertain."

1-109. A patient with acute coronary syndrome is scheduled for cardiac catherization and possible PCI within the hour. His morning laboratory work has resulted. Which of these laboratory results must be reported immediately to the interventional cardiologist?

   A. aPTT 65 sec
   B. Troponin 0.2 ng/mL
   C. Serum potassium 4.9 mEq/L
   D. Serum creatinine 2.3 mg/dL

1-110. A 36-year-old patient with type 1 diabetes is admitted with a 4-day history of nausea and vomiting. He reports that his children brought "the stomach flu" home, and all of the family had the virus. Three days ago, the patient stopped taking his routine dose of 45 units of Humulin 70/30, stating he was "not able to eat because of nausea and vomiting." He is admitted with DKA. On the day of admission, the patient's roommate reported that the patient was "sleeping too much and breathing really fast and deep." Available laboratory values are serum glucose 490 mg/dL; pH 7.25; PaO_2 98 mm Hg; $PaCO_2$ 15 mm Hg; bicarbonate 8.0 mEq/L. Which of these interventions should the nurse perform first?

   A. Administer the first infusion of antibiotics
   B. Administer 20 units of regular insulin via IV push
   C. Administer 100 mL of bicarbonate solution via IV push
   D. Administer 1000 mL of normal saline at 125 mL/hr

1-111. A nurse preceptor is working with an orientee who has just admitted a patient believed to have ventilator-associated pneumonia. In reviewing the various interventions that may be helpful in preventing this disorder, which should the preceptor emphasize as the most effective intervention for this purpose?

   A. Locating the tip of a nasogastric feeding tube in the postpyloric area
   B. Maintaining the head of the bed elevated at 30 to 45 degrees
   C. Suctioning the oropharynx and ET tube hourly
   D. Using hyperalimentation instead of enteral feedings

1-112. You have been assigned to care for a 49-year-old man post elective atrial fibrillation ablation. It is 0230 in the ICU, and your patient's monitor alarms. You assess his vital signs when he is sleeping and analyze the strip below. His heart rate is 53 beats/min; PR interval is 0.28 seconds; QRS is 0.12 seconds; and blood pressure is 100/60 mm Hg. Which of these actions would be most appropriate?

   A. Awaken the patient and obtain the BP with the patient awake
   B. Continue to monitor the patient when asleep
   C. Administer atropine 0.5 mg IV push
   D. Place the patient on oxygen by nasal cannula at 2 L/min

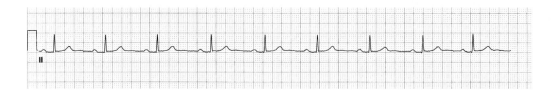

1-113. To improve resuscitation outcomes and reduce the incidence of multisystem organ failure for patients in shock, their serum lactate levels should be corrected in

A. Less than 24 hours
B. 24 to 48 hours
C. 49 to 72 hours
D. 73 to 96 hours

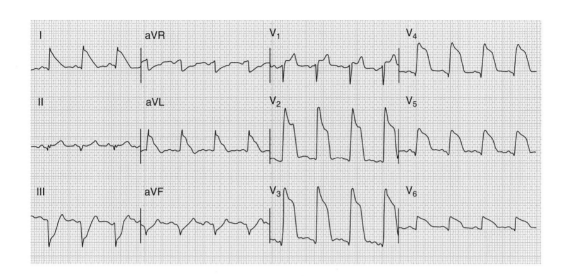

1-114. A patient has been admitted to the emergency room with chest pain. His ECG is posted above. Which of these findings would the nurse anticipate?
A. Sinus bradycardia with a rate of 40 beats/min
B. Hiccoughs and GI upset
C. Signs and symptoms of heart failure
D. JVD and peripheral edema

1-115. A patient is admitted to the ICU after a motor vehicle accident. Her blood alcohol level on admission was 0.18%. She has had two prior alcohol-related accidents earlier this year, and her driver's license was revoked. She is awake, alert, and oriented times three and she looks at you and smiles. How would you approach patient education with this particular patient?
A. Enter the room but avoid talking about the most recent incident
B. Discuss nonthreatening topics such as the weather to engage in conversation
C. Provide nonjudgmental encouragement aimed at reducing or ceasing alcohol consumption
D. Ask the patient if she would like to talk about what happened

1-116. A patient admitted with flash pulmonary edema secondary to noncompliance with his medication regimen is experiencing increased work of breathing. He has been on CPAP without improvement in his symptoms. He remains tachycardic and tachypneic, and he demonstrates accessory muscle use. However, he remains alert and oriented, and he follows all commands appropriately. The doctor explains to him that he will require intubation. He agrees to intubation but states, "I don't want to be tied up with those restraints." The patient has been intubated multiple times in the past, and he has a history of multiple self-extubations. What would be your most appropriate action?
A. Sedate the patient and then apply restraints
B. Call the patient's family to discuss restraining the patient
C. Obtain a physician's order to restrain the patient
D. Do not restrain the patient

1-117. A young woman is admitted to the unit after having ingested an unknown amount of amphetamines, barbiturates, and alcohol. She has three children who are currently with their grandparents and states that she has been out of work for over a month. The most effective approach for the nurse to provide for this patient's needs would be to

A. Contact the patient's family to ensure that the children are being cared for

B. Arrange for a social worker to conduct a comprehensive assessment of needs

C. Document that the patient is unemployed and may not be capable of providing for the children

D. Refer to Alcoholics Anonymous for drug and alcohol rehabilitation

1-118. When the nurse provides discharge teaching for a patient recovering from an acute exacerbation of asthma, which of the following should be emphasized as the best indicator for the patient to use to closely monitor this disease process?

A. Peak flow measurements

B. Pulse oximetry readings

C. Changes in the amount or quality of sputum

D. Experiences of dyspnea or breathlessness

1-119. A patient with chronic atrial fibrillation and heart failure has been admitted to the critical care unit for exacerbation of his heart failure. He is taking apixaban (Eliquis), beta blockers, and diuretics. The nurse recognizes that this patient is at highest risk for which of these preventable complications?

A. Stroke

B. Pulmonary embolism

C. Falling

D. Readmission

1-120. Patients in the ICU are at risk for developing ICU-related posttraumatic stress disorder (PTSD). By understanding risk factors for PTSD, nurses may be better prepared to identify and potentially mitigate some of these risk factors. PTSD can cause adverse health outcomes and worsen medical conditions. Adverse health outcomes associated with ICU-related PTSD include all of the following EXCEPT

A. Coronary heart disease

B. Metabolic syndrome

C. Stroke

D. Chronic hypotension

1-121. A patient admitted to the hospital has experienced an acute myocardial infarction treated with thrombolytic therapy. Which of these medications prevent early complications and mortality associated with this condition?

A. Calcium channel blockers

B. Magnesium sulfate

C. Lidocaine

D. Beta blockers

1-122. In a patient with cirrhosis and ascites who develops fever and generalized abdominal pain, the nurse needs to assess for additional evidence of

A. Acute appendicitis

B. Spontaneous bacterial peritonitis

C. Small bowel obstruction

D. Acute pancreatitis

1-123. A patient with newly diagnosed cancer was admitted for a pericardial effusion. She has had an indwelling pericardial catheter in place for 3 days. Which of these findings is the most reliable indicator that the catheter may now be removed?

A. Absence of pericardial drainage for 3 hours

B. Absence of symptoms of pericardial tamponade

C. Normal cardiac silhouette on chest x-ray

D. Bedside echocardiography demonstrates absence of pericardial effusion

1-124. A 91-year-old frail Vietnamese patient is in the ICU for treatment of severe shortness of breath, hypoxia, and persistent coughing with bloody sputum production. Currently, he is resting comfortably in bed surrounded by many family members. His biopsy and CT scan have confirmed a diagnosis of end stage lung cancer with metastasis to the brain and vital organs. The medical team determines that hospice care and a DNR status is the best option for treatment. The doctor is about to present the diagnosis to the patient, and he asks you to join the conversation. How would you proceed with this discussion?

A. Identify the head of the family and tell him the diagnosis

B. Identify the patient's wife and tell her the diagnosis

C. Gather the family in the patient's room and tell them the diagnosis

D. Ask the family to leave the room and tell the patient his diagnosis

1-125. A patient has survived a severe traumatic brain injury with a basilar skull fracture but has now developed an elevated temperature. Although the nurse's plan for managing fever in this patient population will be multifactorial, the most important aspect will center on identifying
   A. Deep vein thrombosis, a frequently neglected complication of immobility
   B. Meningitis, a potential complication of basilar skill fractures
   C. Hypothalamic dysfunction, or "storming," a potentially lethal febrile syndrome after head trauma
   D. Foreign bodies still embedded in the skull base, a common source of infection

1-126. The ICU nurse has received report from the emergency room on a patient admission. The patient has an acute gastric hemorrhage and hypotension. Laboratory values have just resulted and are Hct 30%; platelets 50,000/mm^3; INR 1.3. In addition to administering a fluid bolus of 250 mL of normal saline, the nurse anticipates administration of which of the following?
   A. 1 unit of packed red blood cells
   B. 6 units/300 mL of platelets
   C. Fresh-frozen plasma, 4 units/250 mL
   D. 50 mL of albumin 25%

1-127. A trauma patient is admitted to the unit with multiple injuries and a fractured pelvis. Trauma patients are at high risk for a number of potential complications. Which member of the health care team should be consulted by the ICU nurse within the first 24 hours in order to optimize the patient's potential for recovery?
   A. Psychiatrist
   B. Nutritionist
   C. Occupational therapist
   D. Physical therapist

1-128. All of these signs and symptoms were identified in a newly admitted patient with a history of severe asthma. Of these clinical findings, which poses the most significant concern to the nurse who suspects this patient may develop acute respiratory failure?
   A. Inability to readily speak a three-word sentence
   B. Wheezing audible without a stethoscope
   C. Respiratory rate of 38 breaths/min
   D. Inaudible breath sounds by auscultation

1-129. You are caring for a patient with chronic liver failure secondary to cocaine abuse. The patient is preparing for discharge in a few days, and her family will care for her at home. You are providing education to the patient and her family about complications of liver failure. What information will you provide to the family relative to immunosuppression?
   A. "You will be more susceptible to infection because of the medicines you take."
   B. "You have been experiencing malnutrition for a long time because of your substance abuse."
   C. "Because your liver does not process proteins properly, you no longer produce enough immune globulin to fight infection."
   D. "Because your liver is impaired, you will not have sufficient stores of fat-soluble vitamins and B$_{12}$ to protect against infection."

1-130. A patient who sustained traumatic brain injury after an assault 4 hours ago is admitted directly to the ICU from the emergency department. He is has an endotracheal tube and is mechanically ventilated. The nurse's admission neurologic examination findings are as follows: no response to voice or touch; when the patient's trapezius muscle is firmly squeezed, his eyes do not open, though he flexes his right arm and extends his left arm. This patient's total Glasgow Coma Scale score is
   A. 6
   B. 5
   C. 3
   D. 8

1-131. A 38-year-old man admitted to the ICU has been on hemodialysis for the past 6 months and is noncompliant with his diet and fluid restrictions. His laboratory work shows: K$^+$ 6.2 mEq/L; BUN 39; and creatinine 3.6 mg/dL. He also complains of severe fatigue and weakness. What is the best course of action for the nurse to take to understand this patient's noncompliance?
   A. Consult a nutritionist for dietary education
   B. Discuss his condition with his spouse
   C. Tell the patient that his nonadherence increases the risk of a stroke
   D. Ask the patient if he is interested in being placed on a transplant list

1-132. A patient arrives in the emergency room complaining of chest pain and shortness of breath. She has acute ST segment elevations in the anterior leads. The doctor orders a thrombolytic agent to be administered. Which of the following is an absolute contraindication to the administration of thrombolytics?
   A. Blood pressure 210/110 mm Hg
   B. Transient ischemic attack (TIA) 3 days prior
   C. Ischemic stroke 2 years prior
   D. Age 75 years

1-133. A chronic renal failure patient with a right arm arteriovenous fistula complains of pain, numbness, and tingling of the right hand. Nursing management of the patient's symptoms would include
   A. Elevating the arm on two pillows
   B. Applying warm compresses to the arm
   C. Keeping the arm flexed at 90 degrees
   D. Placing the arm in a sling

1-134. A nurse is precepting a new ICU nurse who is assigned to a recent postoperative abdominal surgical patient. The patient has bladder pressure measurements ordered. The new nurse has a measurement of 11 mm Hg but states that she does not understand how to interpret the results. As a preceptor for this new nurse, which of these points would represent a good starting place for instruction?
   A. Pressures between 15 and 30 mm Hg may be normal after abdominal surgery
   B. Pressures between 0 and 12 mm Hg may be normal after abdominal surgery
   C. Bladder pressures are not always accurate, so an average of three measures is needed
   D. Bladder pressures should only be done after the foley is clamped for 30 minutes

1-135. A patient admitted for a myocardial infarction is diagnosed with dilated cardiomyopathy. Which of these interventions would be most beneficial for the patient?
   A. Administration of ACE inhibitors
   B. Administration of diuretics
   C. Coronary artery bypass surgery
   D. Insertion of a permanent pacemaker

1-136. A patient who underwent a Roux-en-Y gastric bypass 7 days ago is now exhibiting fever higher than 38.6°C chills, tachycardia, nausea, malaise, and yellow-green drainage from the Jackson-Pratt drain. An increase in which of these laboratory values would support the nurse's suspicion that this patient has developed a complication associated with this surgical procedure?
   A. White blood cell count
   B. Potassium
   C. Platelets
   D. Lipase

1-137. A patient is recovering from a complicated case of *Klebsiella pneumoniae*. His morning assessment reveals diminished breath sounds at the right base; temperature 40°C HR 120/min; BP 90/40 mm Hg; RR 30/min; and SaO₂ 95% on 40% face mask. His chest x-ray reveals a right lower lobe fluid collection. The nurse should anticipate which of these interventions?
   A. Bronchoalveolar lavage (BAL) with a quantitative sputum culture
   B. Stat hematocrit and chest tube insertion
   C. Thoracentesis and antibiotic administration
   D. Aggressive bronchopulmonary hygiene with right lower lobe chest physiotherapy

1-138. A patient is sent to the hospital by her primary care physician after an ECG showed a new heart block. She has a past medical history of an ASD repair 2 years ago and pulmonary hypertension. Which of these heart blocks is most likely responsible for her hospitalization?
   A. Firstdegree heart block
   B. Second-degree heart block, type I
   C. Second-degree heart block, type II
   D. Complete heart block

1-139. A man with long-term alcoholism is admitted to the ICU for hypertensive crisis. He is homeless and malnourished. His admission diagnosis included Korsakoff psychosis secondary to thiamine deficiency. Which of these findings would the nurse anticipate with Korsakoff psychosis?
   A. Gait disturbances
   B. Paralysis of the eye muscles
   C. Impaired retrograde and anterograde memory
   D. Ataxia and vestibular dysfunction

1-140. An elderly woman is diagnosed with normoprogressive hydrocephalus and receives a ventricular-peritoneal shunt. During the postoperative period, she has a parietal stroke that leaves her with some blurred vision and expressive aphasia, which have impeded her recovery and caused her considerable frustration and anger. Her husband tells the nurse that he knows that she understands him, but he is distressed to see her get so upset every time she attempts to respond to his statements. He wonders if some type of activity would help his wife cope better. With which member of the health care team should the nurse consult for this problem?

A. Occupational therapist
B. Psychiatric social worker
C. Physical therapist
D. Speech therapist

1-141. A patient in the ICU has chosen to enter hospice care. The critical care nurse anticipates the process of end-of-life care. The five psychological stages of the dying process include all of the following EXCEPT

A. Depression
B. Rage
C. Despair
D. Bargaining

1-142. A middle-aged person is found unresponsive at a bus stop and is transported to the emergency department. The patient's capillary blood glucose measures 40 mg/dL and remains lower than normal limits after an initial IV push administration of 50 mL of 50% dextrose solution. What orders would the nurse expect to receive next for this obtunded patient?

A. Administer a serving of orange juice
B. Begin an infusion of 10% dextrose intravenously
C. Administer 1 mg of glucagon intravenously
D. Administer 10 units of insulin glargine subcutaneously

1-143. Sedation and analgesia for ICU patients is an important responsibility of the critical care nurse. Which level of sedation is defined as follows: "A drug-induced depression of consciousness in which the patient cannot be easily aroused but responds purposefully after repeated or painful stimulation"?

A. Minimal sedation
B. Moderate sedation
C. Deep sedation
D. Dissociative sedation

1-144. The patient experiencing renal transplantation has been having an unremarkable recovery over the previous 5 days. Which of these findings would the nurse need to report to the physician immediately?

A. Abdominal discomfort and bladder distention
B. Increasing urinary output with decreasing serum creatinine
C. Right upper quadrant tenderness with elevated serum bilirubin
D. Elevated serum glucose and decreasing level of consciousness

1-145. The critical care nurse is caring for a trauma patient who experienced a major crush injury to both lower extremities. The nurse notes that the patient's urine is dark and tea colored. In planning care for this patient, which assessment finding indicates the achievement of patient management goals?

A. Urine pH of 7.20
B. Serum sodium of 152 mEq/L
C. Urine output of 100 mL/hr
D. Serum pH of 7.37

1-146. A patient admitted with the diagnosis of acute coronary syndrome is in the intensive care unit on oxygen 2 L/min by nasal cannula and unfractionated heparin per protocol. The patient complains of upper abdominal pain, which is described as discomfort 1 of 10. The most appropriate initial intervention for the critical care nurse to perform would be to

A. Obtain serum troponin
B. Insert a nasogastric tube
C. Administer 1/150 nitroglycerin sublingual
D. Obtain a 12-lead ECG

1-147. A patient admitted to the emergency room has multiple stab wound to the chest and arms. He was diagnosed with a hemothorax, and a chest tube is in place. The nurse notes that the chest tube continues to drain 125 mL/hr of blood into the collection chamber of the drainage system. Which of these findings would the critical care nurse be most concerned about with this patient?

A. Fluctuation or tidaling in the water seal chamber
B. Discomfort at the chest tube insertion site
C. Sudden decrease or absence of drainage
D. Intermittent bubbling in the water seal chamber

1-148. A 72-year-old male patient with a history of a hospital admission last month for bacterial pneumonia is admitted to the ICU for treatment of symptomatic bradycardia. He has a large-bore peripheral IV and indwelling urinary catheter, and he is on mechanical ventilation. Which of the following is a risk factor for this patient to contract a hospital-acquired infection with methicillin-resistant *Staphylococcus aureus* (MRSA)?
   A. Recent pneumonia
   B. Age
   C. Gender
   D. Large-bore peripheral IV

1-149. The nurse's neurologic assessment reveals that her patient exhibits these clinical findings: right face, arm, and leg paralysis with sensory deficits; loss of half of the field of vision; left Horner syndrome; and aphasia. This set of neurologic findings indicates the need to plan and manage care tailored to a patient with stroke involving which of these vessels?

   A. Right middle cerebral artery
   B. Right vertebral artery
   C. Left anterior cerebral artery
   D. Left internal carotid artery

1-150. An 80-kg patient diagnosed with acute respiratory distress syndrome is on mechanical ventilation with these settings: continuous mandatory ventilation (CMV); tidal volume 400 mL, rate 12/min; PEEP 15 cm H_2O. Arterial blood gases on these settings are pH 7.28; PaO_2 75 mm Hg; $PaCO_2$ 62 mm Hg. Which of these interventions is most appropriate at this time?
   A. Increase the respiratory rate to decrease the $PaCO_2$
   B. Increase the tidal volume to increase the PaO_2
   C. Administer sodium bicarbonate to decrease the pH
   D. Continue to monitor the patient on these ventilator settings

Answers to Core Review Test 1

1-1. **(B)** Clinical signs of acute pulmonary edema include tachycardia, tachypnea, inspiratory crackles, and chest x-ray findings of Kerley B lines and peribronchial hilar enlargement. Enlargement of the cardiac silhouette reflects left ventricular enlargement because of left ventricular failure. Pericardial tamponade (Option A) would be associated with an enlarged cardiac silhouette and widened mediastinum from blood accumulation in the pericardial space, but it is not associated with adventitious breath sounds. Pneumonia would be associated with adventitious breath sounds, but consolidation would be present on the chest x-ray. Right ventricular failure would be associated with clear lung fields and breath sounds.

References: Storzer, D. N. (2018). Pulmonary system. In T. M. Hartjes (Ed.), *AACN core curriculum for high acuity, progressive, and critical care nursing* (7th ed.). St. Louis: Elsevier.

Efre, A., & Boling, B. (2018). Cardiovascular system. In T. M. Hartjes (Ed.), *AACN core curriculum for high acuity, progressive, and critical care nursing* (7th ed.). St. Louis: Elsevier.

1-2. **(C)** The nurse should intervene when informed consent for a research study has not been correctly provided. The nurse recognizes that informed consent in human subjects has not occurred with this patient. Informed consent must include the description and purpose of the research, procedures that are experimental, foreseeable risks, how confidentiality will be maintained, and a clear understanding that the subject can withdraw at any time. Option A is incorrect because it will delay correcting the problem. Option B is incorrect because the investigator may not be readily available, and informed consent should be corrected immediately. Option D is incorrect because, regardless of being a volunteer or paid employee, whoever is enrolling a subject in a study must ensure informed consent.

Reference: Dermenchyan, A. (2018). Professional caring and ethical practice. In T. M. Hartjes (Ed.), *AACN core curriculum for high acuity, progressive, and critical care nursing* (7th ed.). St. Louis: Elsevier.

1-3. **(C)** The administration of oxygen therapy is the key to relieving the hypoxia associated with a pulmonary embolism (PE). If there is severe cardiopulmonary compromise, intubation and mechanical ventilation will be necessary. A stat chest x-ray is an important diagnostic tool but neglects the need to significantly and rapidly improve this patient's cardiopulmonary status, particularly with signs of possible cerebral hypoxia, tachypnea, tachycardia, and declining cardiac output. In addition, chest x-ray findings vary from normal to abnormal and are of little value in confirming the presence of a PE.

In PE, early identification and intervention are key. The initiation of sequential compression devices is preventive, and at this stage, it is more important to initiate supportive therapy and improve oxygenation. Thrombolytic therapy would represent a secondary line of treatment that would be used only in patients in which cardiac failure is profound.

Reference: Storzer, D. N. (2018). Pulmonary system. In T. M. Hartjes (Ed.), *AACN core curriculum for high acuity, progressive, and critical care nursing* (7th ed.). St. Louis: Elsevier.

1-4. **(C)** Because this patient received thrombolytics and subsequently had the groin accessed for PCI, this patient is at great risk for hematoma at the groin insertion site. Hourly inspection of the site to determine whether a hematoma is present or expanding is essential to recognize and prevent permanent injury from this complication. The patient was alert and able to give consent to the physician, so an intracranial hemorrhage did not occur from the thrombolytics. Retroperitoneal bleeding would be suspected if signs of hypotension not associated with other obvious sources of bleeding were present. Grey Turner sign (flank bruising) is seen in retroperitoneal bleeding, but it is a relatively late sign. Bowel sounds are not anticipated early in the postoperative course and are a nonspecific indicator of GI bleeding. The NG tube aspirate would be a better indicator of GI bleeding.

References: Rutherford, R., Cronenwett, J., & Johnston, K. (2014). *Rutherford's vascular surgery*. Philadelphia: Elsevier Saunders.

Efre, A., & Boling, B. (2018). Cardiovascular system. In T. M. Hartjes (Ed.), *AACN core curriculum for high acuity, progressive, and critical care nursing* (7th ed.). St. Louis: Elsevier.

1-5. **(B)** The purpose of the primary and secondary trauma survey is to provide a consistent method of caring for individuals with multiple injuries and to keep the team focused on care priorities. The primary survey involves a continuous process of assessment, intervention, and reevaluation. Potentially life-threatening injuries can be identified during the primary survey and appropriate interventions instituted. The components of the primary trauma survey are A—airway; B—breathing; C—circulation; D—disability (neurologic deficits); and E—exposure and environmental control. Components of the secondary survey are F—full set of vital signs, facilitation of family presence, and five interventions (cardiac monitoring, nasogastric/orogastric tube, urinary catheter, laboratory tests, and pulse oximetry); G—give comfort measures; H—history and head-to-toe examination; and I—inspect the posterior surfaces.

Reference: Holleran, R. (2018). Multisystem: Multisystem trauma. In T. M. Hartjes (Ed.), *AACN core curriculum for high acuity, progressive, and critical care nursing* (7th ed.). St. Louis: Elsevier.

1-6. **(D)** Data suggest that leads III and V_3 should be used to perform ST segment monitoring in patients with acute coronary artery syndrome. Lead II (Option A) is useful for general cardiac monitoring, but it is not especially helpful for ST segment monitoring. Leads V_6 (Option B) and I (Option C) are helpful together for distinguishing ventricular aberration but not for ST segment monitoring.

References: Efre, A., & Boling, B. (2018). Cardiovascular system. In T. M. Hartjes (Ed.), *AACN core curriculum for high acuity, progressive, and critical care nursing* (7th ed.). St. Louis: Elsevier.

AACN Practice Alert. *ST segment monitoring.* Retrieved from www.aacn.org//AACN/practice Alert.nsf/Files/ECG%20ST%20Segment/.

1-7. **(B)** Norepinepherine is generally considered the first-line vasopressor for treating persistent hypotension in septic patients not responding to adequate resuscitation. Phenylephrine is a synthetic catecholamine that is a selective α-adrenergic agonist and is ideal in patients with tachycardia. However, the resulting increase in myocardial oxygen consumption, decrease in splanchnic blood flow, and decrease in cardiac output can be detrimental for patients with septic shock. Epinephrine, which is a potent α-, β1-, and β2-adrenergic agonist, increases peripheral arteriolar tone as well as cardiac contractility. It is the first-line agent for the treatment of anaphylactic shock and is used to support myocardial contractility after cardiac surgery. The positive chronotropic and inotropic effects of dopamine can lead to tachycardia and tachyarrhythmias; this effect frequently limits its dosing because the increased myocardial oxygen requirements promote the development of myocardial ischemia, especially in the presence of coronary artery disease.

Reference: Johnson, A. (2018). Multisystem: systemic inflammatory response syndrome and septic shock. In T. M. Hartjes (Ed.), *AACN core curriculum for high acuity, progressive, and critical care nursing* (7th ed.). St. Louis: Elsevier.

1-8. **(D)** Lung protective ventilation decreases pulmonary pressures by decreasing tidal volumes and preventing volutrauma. The patient's oxygenation is only minimally adequate and needs to be closely followed with the changes in tidal volume. Pressure support is not indicated with the clinical findings described. Although the patient is acidotic, increasing the ventilatory rate will not lessen the pressures, and lung protective strategies may include permissive hypercapnia.

References: Storzer, D. N. (2018). Pulmonary system. In T. M. Hartjes (Ed.), *AACN core curriculum for high acuity, progressive, and critical care nursing* (7th ed.). St. Louis: Elsevier.

Stacy, K. (2018). Shock, sepsis, and multiple organ dysfunction syndrome. In L. Urden, K. Stacy, & M. Lough (Eds.), *Critical care nursing: Diagnosis and management.* St. Louis, MO: Mosby/Elsevier.

1-9. **(C)** Common injuries resulting from blunt abdominal trauma can include injury to the liver, spleen, mesenteric vessels, pancreas, or kidneys. In a nonoperative approach to blunt abdominal trauma, observation and monitoring include serial hematocrits to evaluate for intraabdominal bleeding. The platelet count does not fluctuate unless there is a disease process (cirrhosis, leukemia) or significant blood loss. If there is significant blood loss, the platelet count is reduced along with total blood volume. Platelet levels are not good indicators for acute blood loss because they must be hand counted and may be influenced by medications and volume resuscitation. Protime (prothrombin time) is a monitor of coagulation status. The level can be prolonged without active bleeding. This is not an accurate measure of intraabdominal bleeding. Mean corpuscular volume measures the average volume or size of a single RBC and is used in classifying anemias. It is not a good measure of `intravascular blood volume in acute bleeding situations.

References: Radovich, P. (2018). Gastrointestinal system. In T. M. Hartjes (Ed.), *AACN core curriculum for high acuity, progressive, and critical care nursing* (7th ed.). St. Louis: Elsevier.

Marx, J., & Rosen, P. (2014). Blunt abdominal trauma. In J. Marx, R. Hockberger, & R. Walls (Eds.), *Rosen's emergency medicine: Concepts and clinical practice* (pp. 695–703). Philadelphia, PA: Elsevier/Saunders.

1-10. **(C)** The patient may have initially presented with the large nonreactive pupil and ptosis. A little bit of detective work through reviewing the patient's medical record can help the nurse distinguish whether the examination findings are old or new. Because the examination is otherwise nonfocal and the GCS is 15, no acute change in her condition is apparent, so notifying the neurosurgeon (Option A) is not indicated at this time. The findings are likely relatively old and do not warrant rushing the patient to the OR or a CT scanner (Option B). The patient's level of consciousness has not diminished, so intubation (Option D) is not indicated.

Reference: Blissitt, P. A. (2018). Neurologic system. In T. M. Hartjes (Ed.), *AACN core curriculum for high acuity, progressive, and critical care nursing* (7th ed.). St. Louis: Elsevier.

1-11. **(D)** The patient should be disconnected from the circuit and machine immediately because these findings suggest that the patient is experiencing a dialyzer or hemofilter reaction. Signs of this reaction include hypotension, pruritis, back pain, angioedema, and/or anaphylaxis. Once removed from the treatment, the patient is reassessed, and the symptoms are managed. At this time, administration of a fluid bolus may be used to manage hypotension. Assessment for bleeding at the access site is done routinely and with episodes of hypotension. The administration of diphenhydramine may occur if the patient continues to have pruritus, provided the patient is not hypotensive.

Reference: (2014). Type A reaction to new synthetic noncellulose membrane dialyzer. *American Journal of Kidney Diseases, 63*(5), n.p.

1-12. **(A)** The 12-lead ECG represents a narrow complex tachycardia. Immediate interventions for this stable tachycardia with an acceptable blood pressure include having the patient perform vagal maneuvers to slow conduction from the SA node to the

AV node. If this is ineffective in slowing or terminating the tachycardia, the next intervention would be to administer adenosine. Adenosine causes transient block in AV node conduction, which may cause asystole. If the patient is stable, administration of a medication that may cause asystole is contraindicated. Diltiazem is indicated for rate control in atrial fibrillation with a rapid ventricular rate. Synchronized cardioversion is indicated for unstable supraventricular tachycardias.

Reference: Efre, A., & Boling, B. (2018). Cardiovascular system. In T. M. Hartjes (Ed.), *AACN core curriculum for high acuity, progressive, and critical care nursing* (7th ed.). St. Louis: Elsevier.

1-13. **(D)** Two large-bore IV lines should be immediately inserted to enable fluid administration and vasopressor support. Laboratory studies for type and cross-match should be obtained for anticipated blood replacement. Surgery should not be delayed to complete a pericardiocentesis. Labetalol administration is contraindicated in hypotension. Norepinephrine administration is contraindicated in hypovolemia and will increase the force of contraction, which may cause the dissection to rupture.

References: Ankel, F. (2014). Aortic dissection. In J. A. Marx, R. S. Hockberger, R. M. Walls, J. Adams, & P. Rosen (Authors), *Rosen's emergency medicine: Concepts and clinical practice* (pp. 1124–1128). Philadelphia: Mosby/Elsevier.

Efre, A., & Boling, B. (2018). Cardiovascular system. In T. M. Hartjes (Ed.), *AACN core curriculum for high acuity, progressive, and critical care nursing* (7th ed.). St. Louis: Elsevier.

1-14. **(A)** Individuals with ICDs often fear that the device will shock them. Patients who received a shock from the ICD express anxiety about when the device may shock again, potential loss of independence, embarrassment about the reaction of others when the device shocked, fear of routine activities that may trigger the device, and fear of the pain associated with the shock. These patients do not report concerns about being awakened by the device or about the device being triggered by electronic interference, nor do they experience depression because of dependence on the ICD.

References: Efre, A., & Boling, B. (2018). Cardiovascular system. In T. M. Hartjes (Ed.), *AACN core curriculum for high acuity, progressive, and critical care nursing* (7th ed.). St. Louis: Elsevier.

Sears, S., Hauf, J., Kirian, K., Hazelton, G., & Conti, J. B. (2011). Posttraumatic stress and the implantable cardioverter-defibrillator patient: What the electrophysiologist needs to know. *Circulation: Arrhythmia and Electrophysiology, 4*(2), 242–250.

1-15. **(D)** The patient has likely suffered an aspiration. Cultures will need to be completed to determine the causative organism(s), and pulmonary hygiene will assist in clearing the lobar pneumonia. Administration of broad-spectrum antibiotics should await completion of the cultures. Bronchoalveolar lavage does not reach the distal airways, so it is not likely to help this patient. Steroid therapy is not indicated for this condition.

Reference: Storzer, D. N. (2018). Pulmonary system. In T. M. Hartjes (Ed.), *AACN core curriculum for high acuity, progressive, and critical care nursing* (7th ed.). St. Louis: Elsevier.

1-16. **(B)** The right direction and communication involves the delegating nurse providing a clear explanation of the task and the expected outcomes. The RN sets limits and expectations for the performance of the task. The right patient is communicated under "right person." The right time and the right location are covered under "right direction and communication."

Reference: Dermenchyan, A. (2018). Professional caring and ethical practice. In T. M. Hartjes (Ed.), *AACN core curriculum for high acuity, progressive, and critical care nursing* (7th ed.). St. Louis: Elsevier.

1-17. **(D)** MODS is characterized by the presence of progressive physiologic dysfunction of two or more organ systems after an acute threat to systemic homeostasis. SIRS is a systemic inflammatory response to a variety of severe clinical insults (such as pancreatitis, ischemia or reperfusion, multiple trauma and tissue injury, hemorrhagic shock, and immune-mediated organ injury) in the absence of infection. Septic shock is sepsis-induced shock with hypotension despite adequate fluid resuscitation, along with the presence of perfusion abnormalities. Bacteremia is the presence of viable bacteria in the blood.

Reference: Johnson, A. (2018). Multisystem: multiple organ dysfunction syndrome. In T. M. Hartjes (Ed.), *AACN core curriculum for high acuity, progressive, and critical care nursing* (7th ed.). St. Louis: Elsevier.

1-18. **(A)** The persistent air leak could suggest a bronchopleural fistula or other pulmonary parenchymal pathology. If the leak worsens, the patient could start losing tidal volume into the leak, which would be demonstrated by a discrepancy in his inspiratory and expiratory tidal volumes as well as adverse effects on his ABGs (Option A). The scenario does not suggest that this is an acute change, so STAT diagnostic tests are not warranted (Option B). Tracheal deviation is a late sign of a tension pneumothorax, which is unlikely as long as the chest tube drainage system is functioning properly (Option C). Placing the chest tube to water seal could place the patient at risk for accumulating a tension pneumothorax (Option D).

Reference: Storzer, D. N. (2018). Pulmonary system. In T. M. Hartjes (Ed.), *AACN core curriculum for high acuity, progressive, and critical care nursing* (7th ed.). St. Louis: Elsevier.

1-19. **(A)** A patient complaint of shoulder pain during peritoneal dialysis can result from the presence of air in the infusion tubing. To prevent this problem, the critical care nurse should ensure that all air is primed out of the infusion tubing. Once the problem has occurred, the nurse needs to drain the effluent with the patient in the knee-chest position. The knee-chest position facilitates the movement of air to the lower abdomen from where it may be expelled. Changing the patient to the right side-lying position will not move the air to the lower abdomen and is usually done to manage fluid obstruction. Failure to warm the infusion will cause severe abdominal cramping and hypothermia. Increasing the dwell time will affect the amount of fluid removed from the peritoneal capillaries; however, the increase is not proportional because of osmotic equilibrium.

References: Urden, L. (2018). Kidney alterations. In L. Urden, K. Stacy, & M. Lough (Eds.), *Critical care nursing: Diagnosis and management.* St. Louis, MO: Mosby/Elsevier.

Boling, B. (2018). Renal system. In T. M. Hartjes (Ed.), *AACN core curriculum for high acuity, progressive, and critical care nursing* (7th ed.). St. Louis: Elsevier.

1-20. **(B)** Diabetes insipidus may develop after trauma to the central nervous system. Criteria for this complication include urinary output of more than 500 mL/hr for 2 consecutive hours and low urine specific gravity. Failure to control diabetes insipidus may result in drastic shifts of fluids and electrolytes, which may evoke seizures; ventricular ectopy; circulatory collapse; and, eventually, death. Increases in abdominal girth measurement would be useful for detection of abdominal bleeding but cannot account for this patient's increased urine output. An elevated capillary glucose measurement may lead to polyuria; however, this is not as ominous a situation as a decrease in specific gravity, and polyuria will subside with treatment of hyperglycemia. The potassium level will change with polyuria, but discovering the source of the polyuria and treating the cause will limit the potential alteration in electrolyte balance.

Reference: MacDermott, J. (2018). Endocrine system. In T. M. Hartjes (Ed.), *AACN core curriculum for high acuity, progressive, and critical care nursing* (7th ed.). St. Louis: Elsevier.

1-21. **(C)** A normal BNP level is less than 100 pg/mL. Levels greater than 500 pg/mL are consistent with heart failure. A CPK-MB level of 5% and troponin level of 0.1 ng/mL do not support a diagnosis of acute myocardial infarction. Tricuspid valve insufficiency generally results in peripheral edema. ECG signs of pericarditis include diffuse ST segment elevation rather than depression.

Reference: Efre, A., & Boling, B. (2018). Cardiovascular system. In T. M. Hartjes (Ed.), *AACN core curriculum for high acuity, progressive, and critical care nursing* (7th ed.). St. Louis: Elsevier.

1-22. **(A)** Heparin-induced thrombocytopenia is the result of an antigen–antibody response to the drug heparin. The ELISA test establishes the presence of the antigen for heparin-induced thrombocytopenia, and a platelet count of 30% to 50% of baseline is the key indicator of this condition. Although international normalized ratio and partial thromboplastin time would help in understanding the degree of anticoagulation that has occurred with routine use of coumadin and heparin, respectively, they are not specific to heparin-induced thrombocytopenia. The complete blood count may be decreased for many different reasons, but the differential white blood cell count would not provide information needed to diagnose this autoimmune situation. Comparison of arterial with mixed venous gases provides information about gas exchange and oxygen use and would not be helpful in making this decision.

Reference: Dressler, D. (2018). Hematological and immunological systems. In T. M. Hartjes (Ed.), *AACN core curriculum for high acuity, progressive, and critical care nursing* (7th ed.). St. Louis: Elsevier.

1-23. **(A)** The patient needs to understand the possible causes of development of pancreatitis. If the patient's history does not include alcoholism, other possible etiologies associated with pancreatitis include gallstones and diet. Options B, C, and D are of a lesser concern for a diagnosis of pancreatitis. Option B does not apply because the patient scenario did not mention weight loss, and in any case, that finding is not true for all patients with pancreatitis. Determining food preferences (Option C) will become important if the pancreatitis is related to gallstones. Option D is inappropriate because nothing in the scenario suggests that the patient's prognosis is poor or terminal.

Reference: Radovich, P. (2018). Gastrointestinal system. In T. M. Hartjes (Ed.), *AACN core curriculum for high acuity, progressive, and critical care nursing* (7th ed.). St. Louis: Elsevier.

1-24. **(C)** Increased pulmonary capillary pressure (as measured by the PAOP) causes fluid to move out of the pulmonary capillaries into the pulmonary extravascular tissues and alveoli. Increased right atrial pressures cause fluid to accumulate in the venous system proximal to the lungs in the extremities. Decreased cardiac output may be a symptom of pulmonary edema related to redistribution of blood volume into lung tissue. Increased systemic blood pressure may precipitate pulmonary edema but only when lymphatic drainage is insufficient to compensate for fluid accumulation in lung tissue.

References: Hall, J., & Guyton, A. (2016) *Guyton and hall textbook of medical physiology* (pp. 509–516). Philadelphia: Elsevier.

Efre, A., & Boling, B. (2018). Cardiovascular system. In T. M. Hartjes (Ed.), *AACN core curriculum for high acuity, progressive, and critical care nursing* (7th ed.). St. Louis: Elsevier.

1-25. **(D)** In either pulmonary or fat embolism to the pulmonary vasculature, reduced preload results from obstruction to pulmonary blood flow, increased pulmonary resistance, and reduction in cardiac output (CO). The hypotension associated with a fall in CO then triggers release of catecholamines, prostaglandins, serotonin, and histamine, which attempt to restore CO by raising systemic vascular resistance via peripheral vasoconstriction. Then, increased afterload occurs as a compensatory response to the development of hypotension. The right heart dysfunction, rather than intravascular volume, elevates CVP. Cardiomyopathy may be caused by viral infections, coronary heart disease, congenital heart defects, vitamin deficiency, or alcoholism, but this patient does not show any risk factors for cardiomyopathy.

References: Efre, A., & Boling, B. (2018). Cardiovascular system. In T. M. Hartjes (Ed.), *AACN core curriculum for high acuity, progressive, and critical care nursing* (7th ed.). St. Louis: Elsevier.

Urden, L. (2018). Multisystem alterations. In L. Urden, K. Stacy, & M. Lough (Eds.), *Critical care nursing: Diagnosis and management*. St. Louis, MO: Mosby/Elsevier.

1-26. **(A)** Magnetic resonance angiogram (MRA) uses contrast to diagnose an abdominal aortic aneurysm and its relation to renal blood flow. During endovascular repair of AAA, fluoroscopy with angiography is used to determine that the position of the endograft is appropriate and does not occlude the renal artery. Blood losses are generally minimal with the endovascular approach unless retroperitoneal or endoleak bleeding is present. Fluoroscopic evidence of renal artery patency negates occlusion as a cause of diminished urine output. Absence of signs of bleeding, such as tachycardia, hypotension, and delayed capillary refill, indicate that hypovolemia and bleeding are not the cause of the decreased urinary output.

References: Efre, A., & Boling, B. (2018). Cardiovascular system. In T. M. Hartjes (Ed.), *AACN core curriculum for high acuity, progressive, and critical care nursing* (7th ed.). St. Louis: Elsevier.

Rutherford, R., Cronenwett, J., & Johnston, K. (2014). *Rutherford's vascular surgery* (pp. 1338–1356). Philadelphia: Elsevier Saunders.

1-27. **(D)** Dumping syndrome is a set of postprandial vasomotor and GI symptoms that occurs in some patients who have had gastric surgery or vagotomy that alters upper GI anatomy and neurologic innervation. When a volume of simple carbohydrates is consumed, accelerated gastric emptying causes hyperosmolar contents to be rapidly moved into the upper small intestine, causing bowel distention, abdominal fullness, and intestinal hypermotility that lead to osmotic fluid shifts from the intravascular compartment into the gut lumen, creating relative intravascular volume contraction and hemoconcentration. Compensatory changes lead to release of vasoactive GI hormones, which produce peripheral and splanchnic vasodilation and vasomotor symptoms such as tachycardia, weakness, fainting, dizziness, palpitations, diaphoresis, cramping, diarrhea, and reactive hypoglycemia. An acute MI may cause diaphoresis, nausea, and vomiting but would usually produce chest pain and ECG changes, which this patient does not exhibit. Pulmonary embolism can occur suddenly in a postsurgical patient, but this patient lacks common risk factors such as prolonged immobility and has experienced no chest pain or hemoptysis. Symptoms of hyperglycemia are polyuria, polydipsia, and blurred vision. This patient does not exhibit any of these symptoms.

References: Benefield, A. (2018). Critical care patients with special needs: Bariatric patients. In T. M. Hartjes (Ed.), *AACN core curriculum for high acuity, progressive, and critical care nursing* (7th ed.). St. Louis: Elsevier.

Berg, P., & McCallum, R. (2016). Dumping syndrome: a review of the current concepts of pathophysiology, diagnosis, and treatment. *Digestive Diseases & Sciences, 61*(1), 11–18. http://dx.doi.org/10.1007/s10620-015-3839-x.

1-28. **(A)** Advocating for the patient in this scenario means contacting the appropriate agency to file a report to start an investigation into the care of this older woman. The nurse recognized a finding that clearly constitutes evidence of neglect and failure by a caregiver to adequately meet the physical, social, or emotional needs of a dependent older person. Option B is an action that a nurse would take with any notable assessment finding and would not advocate for this patient's protection. Options C and D will delay an investigation of this incident started.

Reference: Dermenchyan, A. (2018). Professional caring and ethical practice. In T. M. Hartjes (Ed.), *AACN core curriculum for high acuity, progressive, and critical care nursing* (7th ed.). St. Louis: Elsevier.

1-29. **(B).** Hydralazine is a first line treatment for preeclampsia. It can be administered in 5- to 10-mg doses to a total max of 20 mg. Sodium nitroprusside (Nipride) is rarely used in the treatment of preeclampsia because of the risk of thiocyanate toxicity in the fetus. ACE inhibitors such as captopril should not be administered in the antepartum period because they have been shown to potentiate fetal abnormalities, cause fetal death in animals, and cause possible renal failure in neonates. Phentolamine (Regitine) is an alpha adrenergic blocker indicated in the treatment of acute hypertension related to cocaine or catecholamine-stimulating conditions such as pheochromocytoma.

Reference: Houston, J. F. (2018). Critical care patients with special needs: high-risk obstetric patients. In T. M. Hartjes (Ed.), *AACN core curriculum for high acuity, progressive, and critical care nursing* (7th ed.). St. Louis: Elsevier.

1-30. **(A)** The peak inspiratory pressure reflects airway resistance and compliance of lung tissue. The decrease in peak inspiratory pressure indicates that less pressure is necessary to deliver tidal volume and signifies improvement in compliance or distensibility of lung tissue. The decrease in $PaCO_2$ is not specific and may be related to the patient's respiratory rate rather than to any improvement. The increase in PaO_2 is minimal and may be related to factors such as suctioning, position change, or other laboratory factors. An increase in respiratory rate may be related to patient agitation, activity, or decrease in sedation.

Reference: Storzer, D. N. (2018). Pulmonary system. In T. M. Hartjes (Ed.), *AACN core curriculum for high acuity, progressive, and critical care nursing* (7th ed.). St. Louis: Elsevier.

1-31. **(A)** One of the most common sites of origin for bacteremia and sepsis is the respiratory tract. For patients who are intubated for an extended period of time (greater than 24 hr), the incidence of VAE increases significantly. Aspiration of oral and/or gastric fluids and colonization of the mouth are presumed to be precursors to the development of ventilator associated pneumonia. Patients in the supine position have an increased incidence of aspiration. Elevating the HOB to an angle of 30 to 45 degrees decreases that incidence. Oral care should be given every 2 to 4 hours for optimal outcomes; if care is delayed more than 4 hours, these benefits are lost. Research has shown that there is no increase in the incidence of VAE associated with prolonged use of ventilator circuits; thus, frequent changes of the circuit are not warranted. Saliva serves a protective function for the oral mucosa. Mechanical ventilation causes drying of the oral mucosa, affecting salivary flow and contributing to mucositis and gram-negative colonization. Mouth moisturizer should be applied with each cleansing.

Reference: Storzer, D. N. (2018). Pulmonary system. In T. M. Hartjes (Ed.), *AACN core curriculum for high acuity, progressive, and critical care nursing* (7th ed.). St. Louis: Elsevier.

1-32. **(B)** Hypertension after coronary artery bypass graft surgery should be treated promptly to prevent stress on graft sites and decrease bleeding. The nitroglycerin infusion should be increased to enhance vasodilation and decrease the blood pressure. Although the PAD and RAP are borderline low, the urine output indicates that the patient is not hypovolemic at this point, so a fluid bolus is not yet indicated. Increasing the pacing rate will increase the cardiac output, but CO of 3.5 L/min is acceptable immediately after surgery and does not require treatment. Beta-blocking medications are generally avoided in the early postoperative cardiac surgery period because of their negative inotropic effects during the period when myocardial stunning may be present.

Reference: Dellinger, P., Anthony, D., Diaz-Gomez, J., Bashour, C. A., & Johnson, R. (2014). Postoperative management of the cardiac surgery patient. In J. E. Parillo (Author), *Critical care medicine, 4th edition principles of diagnosis and management in the adult* (pp. 610–625). Elsevier Saunders.

1-33. **(D)** In a patient with longstanding asthma, respiratory acidosis and hypercarbia are signs of worsening gas exchange and a diminishing respiratory effort. These are generally considered ominous signs, so expeditious intubation is the best answer (Option D). Antiinflammatory agents such as steroids and leukotriene inhibitors (Options A and B) are administered in concert with bronchodilator therapy but should be added before the development of hypercarbia. Inhaled nitric oxide (Option C) via an endotracheal tube is used for the treatment of ARDS and pulmonary hypertension.

Reference: Urden, L. D. (2018). Pulmonary alterations. In L. Urden, K. Stacy, & M. Lough (Eds.), *Critical care nursing: Diagnosis and management.* St. Louis, MO: Mosby/Elsevier.

1-34. **(C)** This question illustrates the nurse's competency for systems thinking. Options A and B would diminish pneumonia incidence within the hospital but not to the extent afforded by Option C. Implementing a vaccination program for all patients age 65 years and older who come to the facility will have the farthest-reaching effect. DVT prophylaxis has not been associated with decreasing pneumonia. When choosing an intervention to improve outcomes, widereaching solutions should be considered over those with more limited effect.

Reference: Dermenchyan, A. (2018). Professional caring and ethical practice. In T. M. Hartjes (Ed.), *AACN core curriculum for high acuity, progressive, and critical care nursing* (7th ed.). St. Louis: Elsevier.

1-35. **(C)** Before administering interventions such as medications or food, the nurse should assess the patient. In this case, the capillary glucose level should be assessed because restlessness and irritability are classic signs of hypoglycemia, and this patient has an insulin drip. There is no indication for obtaining a stat ECG. Administration of an anxiolytic medication without first determining whether that medication is warranted could potentially be detrimental to a patient who needed glucose. Because irritability may also indicate hypoxemia, this would be an appropriate second area in which to assess this patient. Although providing milk and crackers for this patient will help to alleviate hypoglycemia over a long period of time, a person experiencing hypoglycemia initially needs a rapidly absorbed source of glucose after the assessment is completed.

References: MacDermott, J. (2018). Endocrine system. In T. M. Hartjes (Ed.), *AACN core curriculum for high acuity, progressive, and critical care nursing* (7th ed.). St. Louis: Elsevier.

Sudhakaran, S., & Salim, S. (2015). Guidelines for perioperative management of the diabetic patient. *Surgery Research and Practice*, 1–8.

1-36. **(A)** Allowing the patient to have things that make him or her feel more at home helps to reduce anxiety. Cats tend to carry many pathogens because of their bathing habits and litter box use, which could become opportunistic for this patient. School-aged children spend a large part of their days in a confined area with 20 to 30 other people, sharing many communicable diseases, and they may not be well-served by adult-sized masks, gowns, and gloves (used as barrier devices), so they pose potential sources of pathogens to the patient. Fresh foods may improve a patient's appetite and enhance a sense of well-being, but they carry the risk of transmitting bacteria and viruses from the fields in which they were grown, so commercially canned foods are preferable.

Reference: Dermenchyan, A. (2018). Professional caring and ethical practice. In T. M. Hartjes (Ed.), *AACN core curriculum for high acuity, progressive, and critical care nursing* (7th ed.). St. Louis: Elsevier.

1-37. **(C)** Unstable tachycardia should be treated with immediate synchronized cardioversion. Stable ventricular tachycardia, stable tachycardias of uncertain etiology, and atrial fibrillation with Wolff-Parkinson-White syndrome may be treated with amiodarone. Stable supraventricular tachycardia may be treated with adenosine. Defibrillation is indicated for pulseless ventricular tachycardia or ventricular fibrillation.

Reference: Efre, A., & Boling, B. (2018). Cardiovascular system. In T. M. Hartjes (Ed.), *AACN core curriculum for high acuity, progressive, and critical care nursing* (7th ed.). St. Louis: Elsevier.

1-38. **(A)** Using evidence-based protocols, policies, standards, and guidelines to improve patient care reflects the use of clinical inquiry. Option A indicates that the nurse needs to conduct a literature search for evidence-based practice for patients at high risk for SRMD and that the nurse's practice should be protocol driven. Although use of proton pump inhibitors (Option B) would be useful as an intervention for SRMD, not every patient needs prescribed a PPI, and prevention of SRMD is preferred over allowing the condition to develop. Option C turns the problem over to a medical committee, to which nurse input may not be included in development of the protocol. Option D adds needless delay to address the issue.

Reference: Dermenchyan, A. (2018). Professional caring and ethical practice. In T. M. Hartjes (Ed.), *AACN core curriculum for high acuity, progressive, and critical care nursing* (7th ed.). St. Louis: Elsevier.

1-39. **(A)** Pulsus paradoxus, a variation in pulse or blood pressure with respiration, is a sign of pericardial tamponade or hypovolemia. Pericardial tamponade may occur after PCI because of coronary artery dissection or perforation of the myocardium. Coronary artery spasm causes signs of myocardial ischemia such as chest pain and ECG changes but does not affect blood pressure. Dysrhythmias such as atrial fibrillation and premature ventricular contractions may cause irregularities in pulse pressure but do not cause pulsus paradoxus. Vasovagal reactions cause decreased blood pressure and bradycardia.

References: Efre, A., & Boling, B. (2018). Cardiovascular system. In T. M. Hartjes (Ed.), *AACN core curriculum for high acuity, progressive, and critical care nursing* (7th ed.). St. Louis: Elsevier.

Kern, M., Sorajja, P., & Lim, M. (2016). *Cardiac catheterization handbook*. Philadelphia: Elsevier.

1-40. **(B)** Morbid obesity contributes to immobility, one of the risk factors for deep vein thrombosis (DVT) and pulmonary embolism. Sudden onset of dyspnea and chest pain indicates an acute condition such as pneumothorax, aspiration, or pulmonary embolus. The chest x-ray findings of an enlarged, or prominent, pulmonary artery suggest that pulmonary obstruction is because of pulmonary embolism. There is no radiologic evidence of pneumothorax. Acute MI would be indicated by ST segment elevation. Aspiration pneumonia would not likely have acute onset unless the aspirate was large in volume (which would be demonstrated on x-ray) or acid in pH.

References: Benefield, A. (2018). Critical care patients with special needs: bariatric patients. In T. M. Hartjes. (Ed.), *AACN core curriculum for high acuity, progressive, and critical care nursing* (7th ed.). St. Louis: Elsevier.

Storzer, D. N. (2018). Pulmonary system. In T. M. Hartjes (Ed.), *AACN core curriculum for high acuity, progressive, and critical care nursing* (7th ed.). St. Louis: Elsevier.

1-41. **(C)** The patient is experiencing hyperphosphatemia and requires the administration of sevelamer. Calcium and phosphorus are regulated at the renal level by parathyroid hormone (PTH). PTH facilitates calcium reabsorption and phosphorus excretion in people with normal renal function. Patients with chronic renal failure require medications that bind with phosphorus so that phosphorus can be excreted via the stool. As the serum phosphorus level decreases, blood calcium levels increase. Administration of a potassium supplement will not correct the patient's hyperphosphatemia. Supplementing the patient with oral phosphates will worsen the problem. Sodium bicarbonate administration will not address the hyperphosphatemia.

References: Fink, M., Vincent J.-L., Abraham, E., Moore, F., & Kochanek, P. (2017). *Textbook of critical care*. Philadelphia: Elsevier.

Boling, B. (2018). Renal system. In T. M. Hartjes (Ed.), *AACN core curriculum for high acuity, progressive, and critical care nursing* (7th ed.). St. Louis: Elsevier.

1-42. **(B)** Inferior wall MI is caused by occlusion of the right coronary artery, which also supplies the right ventricle. ST segment elevation is present in II, III, and aVF, indicating inferior wall MI. In right ventricular MI, the right ventricle fails and requires higher volume to produce adequate cardiac filling and output, causing hypotension after administration of nitroglycerin. Although some drop in BP is expected after nitroglycerin administration, hypotension to this extent would not be anticipated in the supine position and, if hypersensitivity to nitroglycerin was the source, hypotension would likely have been accompanied by other findings such as nausea and vomiting. Papillary muscle rupture causes signs of left ventricular failure; symptoms would diminish after administration of nitroglycerin because of decreased afterload. Rupture of the ventricular free wall would cause symptoms of pericardial tamponade and shock.

References: Efre, A., & Boling, B. (2018). Cardiovascular system. In T. M. Hartjes (Ed.), *AACN core curriculum for high acuity, progressive, and critical care nursing* (7th ed.). St. Louis: Elsevier.

Schafer, A., & Goldman, L. (2016). *Goldman-Cecil medicine*. Philadelphia: Elsevier Health Sciences.

1-43. **(B)** The best reply is to provide the patient with an instructional rationale for holding fluids until it is safe for her or him to drink again. Option A is incorrect because the patient may be able to swallow and still not have a gag reflex. Option C ignores the patient's request and lacks any instructional value. Option D is incorrect because lunch cannot be given without verification that the patient has intact and fully functioning reflexes (gag, cough, and so on) and can safely ingest fluids and the assigned diet.

Reference: Dermenchyan, A. (2018). Professional caring and ethical practice. In T. M. Hartjes (Ed.), *AACN core curriculum for high acuity, progressive, and critical care nursing* (7th ed.). St. Louis: Elsevier.

1-44. **(B)** The goal of withdrawal of life-sustaining treatments is to remove treatments that are not beneficial and may be uncomfortable. Any treatment in this circumstance may be withheld or withdrawn. After the goal of comfort is chosen, each treatment should be evaluated to see if it is necessary or causes discomfort. Blood draws and blood glucose sticks cause discomfort. A daily chest x-ray is not necessary. In this case, the IV Lasix may keep the patient more comfortable by treating his congestive heart failure and preventing respiratory discomfort.

Reference: Wyckoff, M., & Hartjes, T. M. (2018). Critical care patients with special needs: Palliative and end-of life care in the ICU. In T. M. Hartjes (Ed.), *AACN core curriculum for high acuity, progressive, and critical care nursing* (7th ed.). St. Louis: Elsevier.

1-45. **(B)** A pacemaker magnet placed over the ICD generator will disable the ICD and prevent further inappropriate discharge. Transcutaneous pacing is indicated for symptomatic bradycardia. Medication administration will not prevent inappropriate shock delivery. Diltiazem will control the rate and amiodarone might convert the atrial fibrillation to sinus rhythm.

References: Efre, A., & Boling, B. (2018). Cardiovascular system. In T. M. Hartjes (Ed.), *AACN core curriculum for high acuity, progressive, and critical care nursing* (7th ed.). St. Louis: Elsevier.

Miller, R., & Cohen, N. (2015). *Miller's anesthesia.* Philadelphia: Elsevier/Saunders.

1-46. **(C)** Exogenous corticosteroid administration frequently results in a hyperglycemic state related to inhibition of gluconeogenesis and increased insulin resistance. Untreated, the serum glucose gradually climbs, but the presence of exogenous insulin prevents the development of diabetic ketoacidosis. In response to polyuria, the patient becomes hyperosmolar. Diabetes insipidus would cause hyperosmolarity but would not result in a serum glucose level of 624 mg/dL. In type 1 diabetes with such a high serum glucose level, ketoacidosis would have been evidenced in the laboratory work. Although the patient may develop polycythemia vera after years of poor oxygenation, that condition would not produce this serum glucose value.
References: MacDermott, J. (2018). Endocrine system. In T. M. Hartjes (Ed.), *AACN core curriculum for high acuity, progressive, and critical care nursing* (7th ed.). St. Louis: Elsevier.

Lebovitz, H. (2016). Hyperglycemia secondary to nondiabetic conditions and therapies. In J. Jameson (Ed.), *Endocrinology: Adult & pediatric* (pp. 747–751). Philadelphia: Elsevier-Saunders.

1-47. **(A)** The normal ejection fraction is 50% to 75%. Patients with diastolic dysfunction often have decreased early diastolic filling time and preserved ejection fraction. The left ventricular ejection time is reduced because of diminished left ventricular end-diastolic volume. Beta-blocking agents prolong the diastolic filling time, resulting in improved left ventricular contraction and decreased diastolic pressure.
References: Albert, N. (2012). Fluid management strategies in heart failure. *Critical Care Nurse, 32*(2). 20–32.

Efre, A., & Boling, B. (2018). Cardiovascular system. In T. M. Hartjes (Ed.), *AACN core curriculum for high acuity, progressive, and critical care nursing* (7th ed.). St. Louis: Elsevier.

1-48. **(B)** Researching the current ICD registries in use, the typical complications monitored, and the type of reporting required by the FDA should be the nurse's initial step in designing a program to monitor ICDs in the facility. When asked to develop a new program, current strategies should be researched to identify best practices. Option A would most likely provide information on that vendor's ICD but not other vendors' devices, and any vendor information would need to be considered for potential bias. Option C overlooks considering the complexity of the device and may therefore neglect appraisal of important features. Option D fails to demonstrate any competency in clinical inquiry.
Reference: Dermenchyan, A. (2018). Professional caring and ethical practice. In T. M. Hartjes (Ed.), *AACN core curriculum for high acuity, progressive, and critical care nursing* (7th ed.). St. Louis: Elsevier.

1-49. **(B)** The initial treatment is the restoration of adequate circulating blood volume to treat or prevent shock. Large-bore IV insertion is a priority in this patient so that initiation of fluid resuscitation can begin to ensure maintenance of a MAP of 60 mm Hg. The monitoring of coagulation studies will be of importance if there is prolonged bleeding or after the administration of blood products. These values adjust to reflect the patient's condition over time. An upright KUB (kidney, ureter, bladder) radiograph will assist in the determination if there is free air in the abdomen; however, stabilization of the patient's circulatory status is the initial focus for the nurse. Monitoring fluid balance and renal function is an ongoing intervention for this patient. It will be important to replace fluid losses and maintain intravascular volume, but this aspect of care is not the most immediate need of the patient.
References: Radovich, P. (2018). Gastrointestinal system. In T. M. Hartjes (Ed.), *AACN core curriculum for high acuity, progressive, and critical care nursing* (7th ed.). St. Louis: Elsevier.

Stacy, K. (2018). Gastrointestinal disorders and therapeutic management. In L. Urden, K. Stacy, & M. Lough (Eds.), *Critical care nursing: Diagnosis and management.* St. Louis, MO: Mosby/Elsevier.

1-50. **(C)** The most appropriate action for the nurse to take would be to inform the patient of the spouse's concerns and determine what his current wishes are. A trial period or a trial period with time limitations may be an option that the patient is willing to consider. An open atmosphere for both the patient and his spouse to express their desires and concerns should be encouraged. Although it is correct that the DPA is not in effect until the patient is no longer able to make decisions, informing the spouse of this fact may make the spouse feel that the nurse is not willing to listen to the spouse's concerns. A dyspneic patient is not likely to be able to carry on a discussion of this nature, and expectations that the patient would be physically able to discuss an emotional topic such as end-of-life decisions with his spouse are unrealistic under these circumstances.

Reference: Dermenchyan, A. (2018). Professional caring and ethical practice. In T. M. Hartjes (Ed.), AACN core curriculum for high acuity, progressive, and critical care nursing (7th ed.). St. Louis: Elsevier.

1-51. **(C)** High sticks are significantly linked with retroperitoneal hemorrhage resulting from the likelihood of puncturing the inferior epigastric artery. Low sticks can predispose patients to pseudoaneurysm, hematoma, and arteriovenous fistula. When the groin is accessed at or below the level of the femoral bifurcation, the femoral sheath is put into vessels that are smaller than the common femoral artery. Depending on the size of the sheath used, these vessels may not be large enough to accommodate the sheath. As a result, access below the femoral bifurcation is more likely to lead to a VASC (vascular access site complication). Low sticks are near the bifurcation to other blood vessels. Various vein branches that run along or anterior to the bifurcation may be accessed during arterial puncture, resulting in an arteriovenous fistula.

References: Efre, A., & Boling, B. (2018). Cardiovascular system. In T. M. Hartjes (Ed.), AACN core curriculum for high acuity, progressive, and critical care nursing (7th ed.). St. Louis: Elsevier.

Bhatt, D. (2015). Percutaneous coronary intervention. In D. Mann, & L. Mauri (Eds.), Braunwald's heart disease: A textbook of cardiovascular medicine (10th ed.) (pp. 1245–1268). Philadelphia: Elsevier Saunders.

1-52. **(A)** After surviving aneurysmal subarachnoid hemorrhage, patients are primarily at risk for developing any or all these three problems: (1) rebleed of the aneurysm if unsecured, (2) hydrocephalus because of problems with reabsorption of CSF, or (3) vasospasm. Blood in the subarachnoid space can block reabsorption of CSF by the arachnoid villi. This is a type of communicating hydrocephalus. A thrombus (Option B) could potentially cause an obstruction of CSF flow; however, hydrocephalus after SAH is generally communicating rather than obstructive in nature. Mass effect (Option C) can block CSF flow but would more likely be associated with a brain tumor than with SAH. This patient population is at risk of developing vasospasm (Option D), which can result in further stroke, but vasospasm directly affects blood flow, not CSF flow.

References: Blissitt, P. A. (2018). Neurologic system. In T. M. Hartjes (Ed.), AACN core curriculum for high acuity, progressive, and critical care nursing (7th ed.). St. Louis: Elsevier.

Stacy, K. (2018). Neurologic disorders and therapeutic management. In L. Urden, K. Stacy, & M. Lough (Eds.), Critical care nursing: Diagnosis and management. St. Louis, MO: Mosby/Elsevier.

1-53. **(C)** Decreased urine output may be the first indication that early compensatory mechanisms to prevent shock are occurring. When renal blood flow decreases, renin and angiotensin are released and produce vasoconstriction, which increases capillary refill time. Hypotension and tachycardia are later signs seen in a more advanced stage of shock.

Reference: Efre, A., & Boling, B. (2018). Cardiovascular system. In T. M. Hartjes (Ed.), AACN core curriculum for high acuity, progressive, and critical care nursing (7th ed.). St. Louis: Elsevier.

1-54. **(B)** Administration of oxygen is the first priority in this emergent situation. Monitoring the airway and breathing is the first priority. Although this patient likely has a pneumothorax, the physician will confirm that finding with a chest x-ray unless the patient is acutely decompensating. The patient may have pain, but administration of narcotics may decrease his respiratory drive and worsen hypoxia. Older patients with rib fractures often require 24 to 48 hours of observation in the ICU, but treatment of hypoxia takes priority at this time.

References: Storzer, D. N. (2018). Pulmonary system. In T. M. Hartjes (Ed.), *AACN core curriculum for high acuity, progressive, and critical care nursing* (7th ed.). St. Louis: Elsevier.

1-55. **(A)** Clinical inquiry is demonstrated when the nurse uses evidence-based information to make changes in nursing practice. Implementing a change in practice requires first identifying the key stakeholders for the change in order to introduce the proposed change. Research utilization and experiential knowledge can be applied to improve patient outcomes when others are part of the change process. Numerous studies have demonstrated the safety and accuracy of drawing blood from peripheral venous access devices (VADs) for PTTs. Option B is incorrect because the intended change has already been identified. Option C is incorrect because one does not implement a change without getting input from key stakeholders. Option D is incorrect because evaluation would not be performed until after the change had been implemented.

References: Dermenchyan, A. (2018). Professional caring and ethical practice. In T. M. Hartjes (Ed.), *AACN core curriculum for high acuity, progressive, and critical care nursing* (7th ed.). St. Louis: Elsevier.

Makic, M., Rauen, C., Jones, K., & Fisk, A. (2015). Continuing to challenge practice to be evidence based. *Critical Care Nurses, 35*(2), 39–50.

1-56. **(C)** Retained blood after cardiac surgery is common and significantly associated with higher in-hospital mortality and other postoperative complications. In cardiac tamponade, the patient becomes hypotensive because of inadequate cardiac filling. Right and left heart pressures equalize and the patient may develop jugular venous distention and tachycardia. Beck's triad is the classic presentation for cardiac tamponade and includes decreased systolic blood pressure, increased CVP/JVP, and muffled heart tones. Tachycardia may not be present in the early postoperative period of the open heart surgery patient because of myocardial stunning. Chest tube output is not a reliable indicator of whether pericardial tamponade is present because chest tube output may be decreased because of clot formation. No evidence of MI was presented in the case described.

References: Urden, L. (2018). Cardiovascular therapeutic management. In L. Urden, K. Stacy, & M. Lough (Eds.), *Critical care nursing: Diagnosis and management*. St. Louis, MO: Mosby/Elsevier.

Ley, S. (2015). Standards for resuscitation after cardiac surgery. *Critical Care Nurses, 35*(2), 30–38.

1-57. **(C)** Several recreational drugs and stimulants are associated with development of rhabdomyolysis, particularly agents that either mimic or stimulate the sympathetic nervous system. The appearance of discolored urine is indicative of large amounts of myoglobin in the urine and is often the initial clinical finding in rhabdomyolysis. The goal of treatment for rhabdomyolysis is to prevent renal failure. This is achieved by maintaining a urine output greater than 150 mL/hr with intravascular volume expansion using isotonic crystalloid and diuretics. Myoglobin is a dark red protein responsible for supplying oxygen to the myocytes. The breakdown of myoglobin produces a pigment-induced nephropathy with subsequent sloughing of the tubular epithelium. This exfoliate, together with large myoglobin molecules, results in the formation of brown casts that obstruct renal tubules. Low urinary pH facilitates the formation of casts and promotes the dissociation of myoglobin molecules into cytotoxic components. The addition of sodium bicarbonate to IV solutions alkalinizes urine to prevent dissociation of myoglobin into its nephrotoxic components. The goal for urinary pH is to maintain a level higher than 6.0. The purpose of insertion of an indwelling catheter and hemodynamic monitoring is to guide the bedside nurse in management and evaluation of the patients' response to fluid administration and diuretic therapy, not to prevent renal failure.

References: Boling, B. (2018). Renal system. In T. M. Hartjes (Ed.), *AACN core curriculum for high acuity, progressive, and critical care nursing* (7th ed.). St. Louis: Elsevier.

Adams, B., & Arbogast, C. (2013). Rhabdomyolysis. In J. Adams (Ed.), *Emergency medicine: Clinical essentials* (pp. 1429–1438). Philadelphia, PA: Elsevier Saunders.

1-58. **(B)** SPECT perfusion imaging is the most helpful in diagnosing myocardial ischemia in a patient with left bundle branch block.

LBBB may mask ST and T wave abnormalities during an exercise or Regadenoson stress test, making it difficult to determine whether ischemia is present. Perfusion defects are demonstrated during SPECT studies. Those that appear during exercise and disappear during rest indicate ischemia. In addition, a patient with severe peripheral vascular disease would not be able to perform an exercise stress test. MRI is useful in demonstrating structural defects of the heart, aorta, and pericardium but not the coronary arteries. MR angiography (MRA) may be useful to determine whether coronary grafts are patent.

References: Stević, M., & Vlajković, M. (2016). Increased accuracy of single photon emission computed tomography (SPECT) myocardial perfusion scintigraphy using iterative reconstruction of images. *Vojnosanitetski Pregled, 73*(5), 469–471.

Ben-Haim, S., & Israel, O. (2014). Vascular PET CT and SPECT CT. In R. Rutherford, J. Cronenwett, & K. Wayne (Eds.), *Rutherford's vascular surgery* (pp. 386–397). Philadelphia: Elsevier Saunders.

1-59. **(D)** The nurse in this situation should promote patient-centered decision making that honors the rights and interests of the patient even when the patient's choice is not what the nurse would chose. The patient has the right to have his reports of pain believed. Options A, B, and C do not involve the patient in the decision-making process. Giving the NTG before giving the morphine may be viewed by the patient as the nurse's not listening to his needs. Option B is incorrect because administering the morphine assumes that this is the drug the patient wants. Making the patient wait 30 minutes may imply to the patient that the nurse does not believe he is having pain and that his pain needs are not being met.

Reference: Dermenchyan, A. (2018). Professional caring and ethical practice. In T. M. Hartjes (Ed.), *AACN core curriculum for high acuity, progressive, and critical care nursing* (7th ed.). St. Louis: Elsevier.

1-60. **(A)** The optimal ventilation strategy for this patient includes use of low tidal volumes, minimizing potential barotrauma, and carefully monitoring respiratory rates. Patients in status asthmaticus are at great risk for air trapping and developing auto-PEEP because of airway constriction. As a result, high tidal volumes and high PEEP place the patient at risk for barotrauma (Options B, C, D).

References: Storzer, D. N. (2018). Pulmonary system. In T. M. Hartjes (Ed.), *AACN core curriculum for high acuity, progressive, and critical care nursing* (7th ed.). St. Louis: Elsevier.

Urden, L. (2018). Pulmonary disorders. In L. Urden, K. Stacy, & M. Lough (Eds.), *Critical care nursing: Diagnosis and management*. St. Louis, MO: Mosby/Elsevier.

1-61. **(A)** Revascularization may result in the release of products of anaerobic metabolism, lactic acid, and potassium into circulation. Acidosis and potassium imbalance place the patient at increased risk of dysrhythmias. Elevated CPK levels are expected after revascularization because of skeletal muscle ischemia. Graft occlusion may occur if hypotension or coagulopathy occur. Pulmonary embolus is a risk of surgery, but is usually associated with venous thrombus. Heart failure is a complication of fluids administered during surgery and the effects of anesthetics but is not indicated by an elevated potassium and metabolic acidosis.

Reference: Efre, A., & Boling, B. (2018). Cardiovascular system. In T. M. Hartjes (Ed.), *AACN core curriculum for high acuity, progressive, and critical care nursing* (7th ed.). St. Louis: Elsevier.

1-62. **(D)** The first three questions provide important information related to this patient's medical history, but only Option D poses a question that may solicit a belief or value rather than a fact. Nursing surveillance is a purposeful and ongoing acquisition, interpretation, and synthesis of patient data for clinical decision making. Inquiring about a patient's perception of their health status helps to link diagnosis with outcomes in the evaluation of care and services.

Reference: Dermenchyan, A. (2018). Professional caring and ethical practice. In T. M. Hartjes (Ed.), *AACN core curriculum for high acuity, progressive, and critical care nursing* (7th ed.). St. Louis: Elsevier.

1-63. **(A)** COPD is an umbrella term for a variety of pathologies such as emphysema and chronic bronchitis. Patients typically have components of both diseases, so they often benefit from carefully monitored increases in FiO_2. Although ABGs should be drawn to guide care of this patient, they should not be the sole determinant for clinical interventions.

Manipulations of oxygen should be done with careful monitoring of the patient's clinical response; however, hypoxia is a greater concern for this patient than respiratory drive. Hypoxemic vasoconstriction is a compensatory process that maximizes V/Q matching in this patient population. It does not create a diffusion defect.

References: Storzer, D. N. (2018). Pulmonary system. In T. M. Hartjes (Ed.), *AACN core curriculum for high acuity, progressive, and critical care nursing* (7th ed.). St. Louis: Elsevier.

Duncan, D. (2016). Chronic obstructive pulmonary disease: an overview. *British Journal of Nursing, 25*(7), 360–366.

1-64. **(D)** The initial therapy would be calcium chloride 1000 mg in 1000 mL NS (calcium gluconate might also be considered) because the patient is manifesting signs of hypocalcemia. In acute pancreatitis, calcium precipitates in the pancreas. Signs of hypocalcemia include positive Chvostek and Trousseau signs, tetany, seizures, respiratory arrest, bronchospasm, stridor, wheezing, paralytic ileus, and diarrhea. Magnesium sulfate would be used to manage hypomagnesemia. Plicamycin is used to treat hypercalcemia, and vasopressin is used for hyperosmolar disorders.

References: Boling, B. (2018). Renal system. In T. M. Hartjes (Ed.), *AACN core curriculum for high acuity, progressive, and critical care nursing* (7th ed.). St. Louis: Elsevier.

Hmed, A., Azim, A., Gurjar, M., & Baronia, A. K. (2016). Hypocalcemia in acute pancreatitis revisited. *Indian Journal of Critical Care Medicine, 20*(3), 173–177. http://dx.doi.org/10.4103/0972-5229.178182.

1-65. **(B)** The causes of erosive gastritis include drugs (especially NSAIDs), alcohol, and acute stress. When viewed with an endoscope, superficial erosions are seen that do not penetrate into the deeper layers of the stomach. They are frequently accompanied by some degree of hemorrhage. When gastritis is diffuse, the amount of blood loss can be extensive. A pulmonary embolism usually occurs in the setting of deep vein thrombosis. This patient has not been immobilized for a significant period of time. The signs and symptoms of a pulmonary embolism include acute chest pain, cough, and hemoptysis, which this patient is not exhibiting. Intracranial hypertension presents with widening pulse pressure and bradycardia,

findings inconsistent with this patient's presentation. Dehydration because of alcohol abuse may contribute to this patient's overall hydration status. Dehydration does not usually result in gastrointestinal bleeding.

Reference: Stacy, K. (2018). Gastrointestinal disorders and therapeutic management. In L. Urden, K. Stacy, & M. Lough (Eds.), *Critical care nursing: Diagnosis and management*. St. Louis, MO: Mosby/Elsevier.

1-66. **(B)** Formulas for fluid replacement or fluid resuscitation recommend 2 to 4 mL/k/percentage of body surface area burned—half given over the first 8 hours and half given over the next 16 hours. Overresuscitation can lead to pulmonary edema, compartment syndromes, and third spacing. Immediate intubation is required before edema potentially causes laryngeal obstruction. Low tidal volume ventilator management will prevent further lung injury from occurring. Immediate peripheral large bore IV placement permits rapid fluid resuscitation. Rapid IV pain management is required because of the severity of the burns.

Reference: Keiler, R. (2018). Multisystem: Burns. In T. M. Hartjes (Ed.), *AACN core curriculum for high acuity, progressive, and critical care nursing* (7th ed.). St. Louis: Elsevier.

1-67. **(C)** In septic shock, HR increases in response to stimulation of the sympathetic nervous system baroreceptors and release of epinephrine and norepinephrine by the adrenal gland. Mixed venous oxygen saturation (SVO_2) reflects the balance between O_2 delivery and O_2 consumption. A normal SVO_2 is 60% to 80%. Several factors can increase the SVO_2 such as an increase in oxygen saturation or an increase in cardiac output. In the patient with septic shock, a *decrease* in oxygen consumption occurs at the cellular level because of a reduced ability of the cells to use the oxygen and inadequate tissue perfusion related to vasoconstriction. The oxygen is not extracted from the blood at the tissue level, resulting in an abnormally elevated SVO_2. The patient's temperature is elevated in response to pyrogens released from invading microorganisms, immune mediator activation, and increased metabolic activity. Urine output declines because of decreased perfusion to the kidneys. Dilation of the arterial system causes SVR to fall, thereby reducing left ventricular afterload. If the patient is euvolemic, these compensatory changes help to produce a normal to high CO. Dilation of the venous system leads to a decrease in venous return to the heart, which results in decreased preload as evidenced by a decreased RAP. Ventilation and perfusion mismatching occurs in the lungs because of pulmonary vasoconstriction and the presence of pulmonary microemboli. Hypoxemia occurs, and the RR increases to compensate for the lack of oxygen.

Reference: Johnson, A. (2018). Multisystem: Systemic inflammatory response syndrome and septic shock. In T. M. Hartjes (Ed.), *AACN core curriculum for high acuity, progressive, and critical care nursing* (7th ed.). St. Louis: Elsevier.

1-68. **(B)** The best approach to establishing a comprehensive program of oral care should begin with forming a multidisciplinary team that can review supporting scientific literature and develop a policy or protocol, provide hospital-wide education, and measure outcomes of the intervention. Option A is incorrect because placing kits at the bedside does not ensure their use. Merely obtaining staff input does not designate any accountability for the project as Option B does. Option D is of very limited help because the nature of those oral care orders needs to coincide with a best-practices approach to care before outcomes could be expected to improve.

References: Dermenchyan, A. (2018). Professional caring and ethical practice. In T. M. Hartjes (Ed.), *AACN core curriculum for high acuity, progressive, and critical care nursing* (7th ed.). St. Louis: Elsevier.

Khan, R., Al-Dorzi, H., Al-Attas, K., Ahmed, F., Marini, A., Mundekkadan, S., Arabi, Y. et al. (2016). The impact of implementing multifaceted interventions on the prevention of ventilator-associated pneumonia. *American Journal of Infection Control, 44*(3), 320–326. http://dx.doi.org/10.1016/j.ajic.2015.09.025.

1-69. **(B)** The patient's blood pressure is adequate to give the beta blocker, but because of worsening symptoms of heart failure, a reduced dose is warranted. Abrupt discontinuation of beta blocker therapy can cause rebound hypertension and tachycardia. Tachycardia will worsen heart failure because it increases oxygen consumption and reduces ventricular filling time. Additional doses of beta blockers may worsen

symptoms. ACE inhibitor therapy reduces afterload and decreases sodium retention. ACE inhibitors have a mild diuretic effect and may be added to current therapy, but additional doses are not warranted to treat worsening symptoms.

References: Efre, A., & Boling, B. (2018). Cardiovascular system. In T. M. Hartjes (Ed.), *AACN core curriculum for high acuity, progressive, and critical care nursing* (7th ed.). St. Louis: Elsevier.

Ferri, F. (2017). *Ferri's clinical advisor: 5 books in 1* (pp. 542–549). Philadelphia: Elsevier.

1-70. **(B)** Noninvasive ventilation techniques (CPAP, BiPAP) are routinely used for COPD patients with moderate respiratory failure. NIV therapies improve respiratory mechanics by allowing the patient to take larger tidal volumes and preventing fatigue of respiratory muscles, which often precipitates a need for intubation. NIV is not an option for every patient, however, including those with significant cardiovascular compromise, arrhythmias with hypotension, or impaired consciousness (except O_2 induced) and those with significant risk of aspiration. Heavy sedation is contraindicated with NIV because this therapy requires that the patient be able to spontaneously ventilate and be sufficiently conscious to protect the airway. NIV reduces work of breathing in patients with COPD. Use of masks versus nasal pillows is a matter of patient preference and is not required for COPD patients.

Reference: Storzer, D. N. (2018). Pulmonary system. In T. M. Hartjes (Ed.), *AACN core curriculum for high acuity, progressive, and critical care nursing* (7th ed.). St. Louis: Elsevier.

1-71. **(B)** Breakdown of fat cells produces ketone bodies, which are acids. An increase in metabolic acids results in an increase of urinary output in an attempt to decrease serum glucose, diminish the concentration of acids, and rebalance electrolyte levels. The most common precipitating cause of DKA is infection. The patient may have faithfully adhered to his routine of managing his type 1 diabetes yet developed ketoacidosis when emotional or physical stress, such as a viral illness, led to increased release of cortisol. The next most likely cause of ketoacidosis is inadequate insulin in relation to caloric intake. Type 2 diabetes, not type 1, has been found to have a genetic predisposition.

Type 1 is currently believed to be autoimmune in origin. Increased levels of activity would result in hypoglycemia rather than hyperglycemia and ketoacidosis.

Reference: MacDermott, J. (2018). Endocrine system. In T. M. Hartjes (Ed.), *AACN core curriculum for high acuity, progressive, and critical care nursing* (7th ed.). St. Louis: Elsevier.

1-72. **(C)** This patient needs continued fluid resuscitation with crystalloids such as Ringer's lactate or normal saline. Continued administration of crystalloid will enable renal excretion of excess hydrogen ions and resolve acidosis. Administration of sodium bicarbonate may induce alkalosis and prevent oxygen release to tissues. The hematocrit is greater than 28%, so transfusion is not indicated. Endotracheal intubation is not indicated with a PaO_2 of 80 mm Hg and no evidence of hypercarbia.

References: Boling, B. (2018). Renal system. In T. M. Hartjes (Ed.), *AACN core curriculum for high acuity, progressive, and critical care nursing* (7th ed.). St. Louis: Elsevier.

Puyana, J. (2017). Resuscitation of hypovolemic shock. In J. L. Vincent, E. Abraham, F. A. Moore, P. Kochanek, & M. P. Fink (Authors), *Textbook of critical care* (pp. 1078–1080). Philadelphia, PA: Elsevier.

1-73. **(C)** Stabilization of the airway with endotracheal intubation is warranted given the patient's increasing respiratory distress. In patients with severe respiratory distress, increasing the FiO_2 is appropriate; however, it would be increased to 100% at least until airway intubation is completed. There is no radiologic evidence of a pneumothorax, so placement of a chest tube would not be appropriate, and there is no indication that a repeat chest x-ray is warranted at this time. Once intubation has been completed, the chest x-ray can be repeated to confirm correct placement of the endotracheal tube.

Reference: Holleran, R. (2018). Multisystem: Multisystem trauma. In T. M. Hartjes (Ed.), *AACN core curriculum for high acuity, progressive, and critical care nursing* (7th ed.). St. Louis: Elsevier.

1-74. **(D)** Controlling a dying patient's pain minimizes any suffering, a common fear related to end-of-life concerns. Option A is incorrect because there is no evidence that any staffing pattern will assure a "good death." Option B is incorrect because unrestricted visiting may be exhausting and undesired for the patient.

Encouraging hope when there is none represents a barrier to providing a good death.

Reference: Wyckoff, M., & Hartjes, T. M. (2018). Critical care patients with special needs: Palliative and end-of life care in the ICU. In T. M. Hartjes (Ed.), *AACN core curriculum for high acuity, progressive, and critical care cursing* (7th ed.). St. Louis: Elsevier.

1-75. **(A)** Aortic regurgitation may be caused by congenital or degenerative cardiac disease or by endocarditis. Symptoms of aortic regurgitation include systolic ejection murmur, bounding or water-hammer peripheral pulses, head bobbing with each heartbeat, dyspnea, syncope, and signs of left ventricular failure. Mitral valve stenosis may cause symptoms of right heart failure, atrial fibrillation, jugular venous distention (JVD), and a diastolic murmur. Tricuspid regurgitation causes a high-pitched holosystolic murmur and symptoms of right heart failure. Signs of pericardial effusion include JVD, tachycardia, and symptoms of decreased cardiac output. The ECG in pericardial effusion would typically demonstrate low voltage and tachycardia.

References: Efre, A., Boling, B. (2018). Cardiovascular system. In T. M. Hartjes (Ed.), *AACN core curriculum for high acuity, progressive, and critical care nursing* (7th ed.). St. Louis: Elsevier.

Yi, Z., Rongrong, S., Xianchi, L., Min, L., Shuang, C., & Peiying, Z. (2016). Pathophysiology of valvular heart disease. *Experimental & Therapeutic Medicine, 11*(4), 1184–1188. http://dx.doi.org/10.3892/etm.2016.3048.

1-76. **(C)** All of the options are possible reasons for seizures, but substance withdrawal is the most likely choice among these possibilities. Hypoxia (Option A) is less likely because the patient just started this activity of clenching on his endotracheal tube. Delirium tremens (Option B) is another possibility, but DTs usually occur 48 to 72 hours after cessation of alcohol intake. The patient received seizure prophylaxis for posttraumatic seizures (Option D), so although this is possible, it is a less likely cause.

References: Blissitt, P. A. (2018). Neurologic system. In T. M. Hartjes (Ed.), *AACN core curriculum for high acuity, progressive, and critical care nursing* (7th ed.). St. Louis: Elsevier.

Paur, R., Wallner, C., Hermann, P., Stöllberger, C., & Finsterer, F. (2016). Neurological abnormalities in opiate addicts with and without substitution therapy. *American Journal of Drug and Alcohol Abuse, 38*(3), 239–245.

1-77. **(B)** Absorption describes the process by which the chemical in the dosing solution or exposure medium moves across the biological membranes to get into systemic circulation. Factors affecting absorption include the route and the bioavailability of the particular substance. Clearance is the measurement of the body's ability to eliminate a substance from blood or plasma over time. Distribution is the way in which a substance disseminates throughout the body. Chelation describes one means by which toxic minerals, metals, or chemical substances may be removed from the body via chemical bonding with a chelating agent for elimination in urine and feces.

References: Berryman, L. (2018). Multisystem: Toxin exposure. In T. M. Hartjes (Ed.), *AACN core curriculum for high acuity, progressive, and critical care nursing* (7th ed.). St. Louis: Elsevier.

Krishnan, K., & White, P. (2013). Pharmacokinetics and toxicokinetics. In W. Haschek, C. Rousseaux, & M. Wallig (Eds.), *Haschek and Rousseaux's handbook of toxicologic pathology* (pp. 39–59). Amsterdam: Elsevier/Academic.

1-78. **(A)** The initial intervention should be to initiate transcutaneous pacing. Atropine IV may alter heart rate, with the predominant clinical effect being tachycardia. This increase in heart rate results in increased oxygen demand on the heart and can exacerbate myocardial ischemia (which could be the cause of the heart block). If the patient is symptomatic or hypotensive, transcutaneous or transvenous pacing is indicated. If these interventions fail, additional pharmacologic intervention includes dopamine (5–20 μg/kg/min IV); epinephrine (2–10 μg/min); and, potentially, isoproterenol. The latter, however, should be used with extreme caution and at low doses if at all because it can potentiate cardiac ischemia.

Reference: Efre, A., & Boling, B. (2018). Cardiovascular system. In T. M. Hartjes (Ed.), *AACN core curriculum for high acuity, progressive, and critical care nursing* (7th ed.). St. Louis: Elsevier.

1-79. **(D)** Caring practices are nursing activities that create a compassionate, supportive, and therapeutic environment for patients and staff, with the aim of promoting comfort and healing and preventing unnecessary suffering. These caring behaviors include but are not limited to vigilance, engagement, and responsiveness. At level 5 (the highest level), the nurse demonstrates that type of caring practice in which the patient's and family's needs determine caring practices. Maintaining a safe physical environment, basing care on standards and protocols, and focusing on basic and routine needs of the patient are level 1 practices.

Reference: Dermenchyan, A. (2018). Professional caring and ethical practice. In T. M. Hartjes (Ed.), *AACN core curriculum for high acuity, progressive, and critical care nursing* (7th ed.). St. Louis: Elsevier.

1-80. **(C)** Classic symptoms of cardiac tamponade include Beck's triad: hypotension, jugular venous distention and distant heart tones. Breath sounds are equal bilaterally, so pneumothorax requiring chest tube insertion or needle thoracostomy is not suspected. The SpO_2 is adequate, so intubation is not indicated.

Reference: Efre, A., & Boling, B. (2018). Cardiovascular system. In T. M. Hartjes (Ed.), *AACN core curriculum for high acuity, progressive, and critical care nursing* (7th ed.). St. Louis: Elsevier.

1-81. **(D)** The absence of breath sounds over all of the right lung fields strongly suggests a pneumothorax. If there is no penetrating trauma creating a sucking chest wound, these findings are significant for a tension pneumothorax. If the tension pneumothorax enlarges without relief, the patient can go into cardiopulmonary collapse within minutes. Inspiratory wheezing is indicative of narrowed airways; when wheezing clears with coughing, it indicates an intermittent and reversible concern. If the patient were receiving large volumes of IV fluids, frequent auscultation would be warranted. Decreased breath sounds in the bases or over the right lung fields may indicate areas of atelectasis, a collapsed lobe, or a hemothorax. Although these may be significant complications, they are not immediately life threatening.

References: Holleran, R. (2018). Multisystem: Multisystem trauma. In T. M. Hartjes (Ed.), *AACN core curriculum for high acuity, progressive, and critical care nursing* (7th ed.). St. Louis: Elsevier.

Storzer, D. N. (2018). Pulmonary system. In T. M. Hartjes (Ed.), *AACN core curriculum for high acuity, progressive, and critical care nursing* (7th ed.). St. Louis: Elsevier.

1-82. **(D)** Fifty percent of patients with cirrhosis develop esophageal varices. Variceal hemorrhage accounts for one third of deaths in patients with cirrhosis. The veins of the esophagus represent a high-flow but low-pressure system. When there is increased resistance to blood flow within the liver, the pressure within this system increases, resulting in portal hypertension and the development of esophageal varices. The varices are prone to rupture if they are not eliminated by endoscopy or if the pressure is not reduced by a beta blocker. Although portal hypertension can increase the risk of right-side heart failure, heart failure does not cause gastrointestinal bleeding. In cirrhosis, shunting and vasodilatation occur with elevated pressure in the venous portal system, but circulating blood volume does not increase. Normal liver tissues are not fibrotic. Damage to the liver causes hepatocyte necrosis, collapse of the healthy tissue, and replacement with fibrotic tissue. It is not until the liver becomes cirrhotic that portal hypertension leads to a risk of hemorrhage.

References: Radovich, P. (2018). Gastrointestinal system. In T. M. Hartjes (Ed.), *AACN core curriculum for high acuity, progressive, and critical care nursing* (7th ed.). St. Louis: Elsevier.

Garcia-Tsao, G. (2016). Cirrhosis and its sequelae. In A. Schafer, & L. Goldman (Eds.), *Goldman-Cecil Medicine* (pp. 1023–1031). Philadelphia: Elsevier Health Sciences.

1-83. **(A)** Right bundle branch block is demonstrated by an rSR′ pattern in leads V_1 or V_2 (the right chest leads), a slurred S wave in V_5 and V_6, and a QRS duration of greater than 0.12 seconds. LBBB would be demonstrated by a deep S wave in the right chest leads and a QRS greater than 0.12 seconds in leads V_5 and V_6. The heart rate is 99 BPM in this ECG, so it does not qualify as tachycardia. There is ST segment depression in the anterior leads (V_2 to V_5), which does not signify acute MI. Acute anterior wall MI would be demonstrated by ST segment elevation or Q waves in the anterior leads. This ECG demonstrates inferior wall MI with Q waves and ST segment elevation in II, III and a VF and reciprocal ST depression in V2 through V6.

Reference: Efre, A., & Boling, B. (2018). Cardiovascular system. In T. M. Hartjes (Ed.), *AACN core curriculum for high acuity, progressive, and critical care nursing* (7th ed.). St. Louis: Elsevier.

1-84. **(A)** Postoperative care basics are universal and include optimizing airway, breathing, circulation, pain management, wound care, and intake and output. In a neurosurgical patient, these universals also need to incorporate monitoring and optimizing cerebral perfusion and blood flow. Brain, blood, and CSF are the contents of the cranium. If blood flow—either arterial inflow or venous outflow—is altered, cerebral perfusion may be compromised. If jugular venous outflow is obstructed, cerebral blood volume increases. That volume directly corresponds to pressure, particularly because the cranium is fixed in size and cannot accommodate varying volumes or pressures. Not only would this affect intracranial pressure, but it may also influence postoperative bleeding. Generally, the nurse would not try to decrease CPP (Option B). The usual goal CPP in monitored patients with intracranial processes is 60 to 70 mm Hg. Positioning of a postoperative patient does not affect CSF flow (Option C) within the central nervous system. No physiologic benefits derive from immobilizing the surgical site or the head (Option D).

References: Blissitt, P. A. (2018). Neurologic system. In T. M. Hartjes (Ed.), *AACN core curriculum for high acuity, progressive, and critical care nursing* (7th ed.). St. Louis: Elsevier.

Pritchard, C., & Radcliffe, J. (2014). General principles of postoperative neurosurgical care. *Anaesthesia & Intensive Care Medicine, 15*(6), 267–272. http://dx.doi.org/10.1016/j.mpaic.2014.03.007.

1-85. **(C)** Sudden onset of back pain and neurologic changes such as syncope are classic findings in aortic dissection. BP differences and facial edema may be the initial indicators that a thoracic aortic aneurysm is present. Pressure differences greater than 20 mm Hg between the left and right arm may indicate the presence of an aortic aneurysm but do not signal that dissection is occurring unless they are accompanied by other findings. A pulsatile abdominal mass associated with a bruit is a sign that an abdominal aortic aneurysm is present and may be found on routine abdominal examination. These findings may be difficult to appreciate in an obese patient. Hypertension and renal insufficiency are frequently found in patients with abdominal aortic aneurysm because of decreased renal blood flow.

Reference: Efre, A., & Boling, B. (2018). Cardiovascular system. In T. M. Hartjes (Ed.), *AACN core curriculum for high acuity, progressive, and critical care nursing* (7th ed.). St. Louis: Elsevier.

1-86. **(C)** Bronchodilators, oxygen, mucolytic agents, antibiotics, and glucocorticoids are all commonly used to treat acute exacerbations of COPD. Although viral infections are a frequent cause of these exacerbations, antiviral therapy is not routinely administered to COPD patients. Inhaled prostacyclin is an option for maximizing V/Q matching in patients with ARDS; its intravenous administration is a common treatment for pulmonary hypertension, but it is not used in COPD. A recent review of evidence related to the efficacy of antibiotics in this patient population supports use of antibiotics for patients with COPD exacerbations who are moderately or severely ill with increased cough and colored sputum. Cholinergic agents would not be used in patients with COPD because they would intensify airway bronchoconstriction; COPD patients receive anticholinergic agents, which antagonize acetylcholine, thereby leading to bronchodilation.

Reference: Storzer, D. N. (2018). Pulmonary system. In T. M. Hartjes (Ed.), *AACN core curriculum for high acuity, progressive, and critical care nursing* (7th ed.). St. Louis: Elsevier.

1-87. **(A)** Percutaneous coronary intervention would eliminate the cause of the dysrhythmia, which is right coronary artery (RCA) occlusion. The RCA supplies the sinus node in most people, and patients with RCA occlusion and inferior wall myocardial infarction (IWMI) typically have bradycardia. ECG changes associated with RCA occlusion are ST segment elevation in leads II, III, and aVF. Temporary pacing and atropine will only temporarily treat the bradycardia associated with IWMI, and atropine may alter heart rate, with tachycardia as the predominant clinical effect. This increase in heart rate results in increased oxygen demand on the heart and can exacerbate myocardial ischemia.

References: Efre, A., & Boling, B. (2018). Cardiovascular system. In T. M. Hartjes (Ed.), *AACN core curriculum for high acuity, progressive, and critical care nursing* (7th ed.). St. Louis: Elsevier.

Rathod, S., Parmar, P., Rathod, G., & Parikh, A. (2014). Study of various cardiac arrhythmias in patients of acute myocardial infarction. *International Archives of Integrated Medicine, 1*(4), 32–41.

1-88. **(C)** This question illustrates the nurse's competency for systems thinking. Systems thinking is displayed as the nurse makes a connection between insertion of an ICD, its malfunction, regulatory requirements related to the incident, and effect on the facility. FDA regulations require manufacturers and hospitals to report all pacemaker and ICD malfunctions, especially those that result in death or surgery. Failure to communicate this device problem may lead to underreporting of their potential defects. Option A reflects an expanded concern that includes effects on the facility but does not approach the still wider repercussions of this scenario on the safety of numerous patients with ICDs. Immediate documentation of the event with an incident report and notification of management should be completed before the risk management department is notified. There is no evidence that indicates the staff needs instruction regarding ICD malfunctions, so that option is inappropriate at this time.

Reference: Dermenchyan, A. (2018). Professional caring and ethical practice. In T. M. Hartjes (Ed.), *AACN core curriculum for high acuity, progressive, and critical care nursing* (7th ed.). St. Louis: Elsevier.

1-89. **(B)** Administration of fluid (crystalloid) would be the most appropriate and *immediate* treatment at this time. The patient is hemodynamically compromised with hypotension and tachycardia. With the patient's history of nausea, vomiting, and diarrhea, intravascular volume deficit is the rationale for the patient's hemodynamic status. Fluid resuscitation is part of the initial sepsis bundle. Inotropic support would be detrimental to this patient until volume resuscitation is provided. The patient is slightly anemic and may need a blood transfusion, but it will require time to prepare the packed RBCs; therefore, this is not considered an *immediate* treatment. Beta blocker therapy to decrease the heart rate is not indicated for this patient in the presence of hypotension because the tachycardia is likely a compensatory change because of hypovolemia.

References: Johnson, A. (2018). Multisystem: Systemic inflammatory response syndrome and septic shock. In T. M. Hartjes (Ed.), *AACN core curriculum for high acuity, progressive, and critical care nursing* (7th ed.). St. Louis: Elsevier.

Rhodes, A., Evans, L. E., Alhazzani, W., et al. (2017). Surviving sepsis campaign: international guidelines for management of sepsis and septic shock: 2016. *Critical Care Medicine, 45*(3), 486–552. http://dx.doi.org/10.1097/CCM.0000000000002255.

1-90. **(A)** Therapeutic goals for the patient in cardiogenic shock include achieving a mean arterial pressure (MAP) sufficient to ensure central and peripheral perfusion. A MAP of 60 mm Hg will provide cerebral perfusion. Elevated systemic vascular resistance increases left ventricular work and the potential for decreased end organ perfusion. A heart rate nearing normal further indicates that myocardial work has decreased and oxygenation potentially improved.

Reference: Efre, A., & Boling, B. (2018). Cardiovascular system. In T. M. Hartjes (Ed.), *AACN core curriculum for high acuity, progressive, and critical care nursing* (7th ed.). St. Louis: Elsevier.

1-91. **(A)** The patient should have autonomy in deciding how the information will be shared and with whom. In the AACN synergy model for patient care, the patient needs to be given access to the resources (family) that he or she can bring to the situation. And the nurse needs to display the caring practices of following the patient and family lead. Option B completely avoids providing the patient with the information. Suggesting the chaplain's presence shrouds the reply in an undue, ominous tone that is inappropriate. Option D is inappropriate as it reflects a biased reply related to how the information should be conveyed.

References: Dermenchyan, A. (2018). Professional caring and ethical practice. In T. M. Hartjes (Ed.), *AACN core curriculum for high acuity, progressive, and critical care nursing* (7th ed.). St. Louis: Elsevier.

Monden, K., Gentry, L., & Cox, T. (2016). Delivering bad news to patients. *Baylor University Medical Center Proceedings, 29*(1), 101–102.

1-92. **(B)** More than 50% of COPD exacerbations are related to bacterial or viral infections. Patients with COPD typically experience considerable sputum production, but these secretions do not become inspissated in this disorder. Airway inflammation and sputum production typically occur as a result of the exacerbation rather than as its cause.

References: Storzer, D. N. (2018). Pulmonary system. In T. M. Hartjes (Ed.), *AACN core curriculum for high acuity, progressive, and critical care nursing* (7th ed.). St. Louis: Elsevier.

Niewoehner, D. (2015). Chronic obstructive pulmonary disease. In A. Schafter, & L. Goldman (Eds.), *Goldman-Cecil medicine* (pp. 555–562). Philadelphia: Elsevier Saunders.

1-93. **(B)** Hypotension and a low PAOP require volume replacement. Surgical blood loss that causes such a dramatic decrease in PAOP requires blood replacement. Packed cells would replenish intravascular blood volume, and the patient would benefit most from this intervention. Normal saline bolus would be a temporary volume replacement and may enter the extravascular space in several hours. Vasoconstricting agents such as dopamine and vasopressin should be withheld until volume status is corrected.

References: Efre, A., & Boling, B. (2018). Cardiovascular system. In T. M. Hartjes (Ed.), *AACN core curriculum for high acuity, progressive, and critical care nursing* (7th ed.). St. Louis: Elsevier.

Urden, L. (2018). Cardiovascular therapeutic management. In L. Urden, K. Stacy, & M. Lough (Eds.), *Critical care nursing: Diagnosis and management*. St. Louis, MO: Mosby/Elsevier.

1-94. **(C)** The patient is in acute renal failure. Given that the patient is fluid overloaded and hemodynamically unstable, continuous renal replacement therapy is the treatment modality of choice. Administering fluid boluses to a patient who is in the oliguric phase of ATN will worsen the fluid overload. Hemodialysis requires the patient to be hemodynamically stable. Peritoneal dialysis is not an option because of the patient's recent abdominal surgery.

Reference: Boling, B. (2018). Renal system. In T. M. Hartjes (Ed.), *AACN core curriculum for high acuity, progressive, and critical care nursing* (7th ed.). St. Louis: Elsevier.

1-95. **(A)** Weight gain is an early and reliable sign of fluid retention and potentially worsening heart failure, so these patients require instruction regarding daily weights and reinforcement that an increase in weight should be reported to health care providers to prevent a hospital readmission. Option B is incorrect in that not all heart failure patients have anemia. The literature reports that approximately 30% will experience fatigue and/or anemia. Option C is incorrect even though compliance with appointments might help to ensure early identification of problems by the health care provider. Fluid restriction is important and may eventually prevent a readmission; however, immediate intervention is needed when the patient identifies a weight gain.

Reference: Efre, A., & Boling, B. (2018). Cardiovascular system. In T. M. Hartjes (Ed.), *AACN core curriculum for high acuity, progressive, and critical care nursing* (7th ed.). St. Louis: Elsevier.

1-96. **(B)** Symptoms of pericardial tamponade include hypotension, narrowed pulse pressure, JVD, and pulsus paradoxus. Tamponade causes pulsus paradoxus because of cardiac compression and decreased stroke volume. Hypovolemia may cause tachycardia, hypotension, and decreased stroke volume, but it is not associated with JVD or a friction rub. Tension pneumothorax may cause hypotension and tachycardia but would be associated with severe dyspnea. Superior vena cava syndrome would cause enlargement of neck veins, edema of the face, shortness of breath, and altered mental status.

References: Efre, A., & Boling, B. (2018). Cardiovascular system. In T. M. Hartjes (Ed.), *AACN core curriculum for high acuity, progressive, and critical care nursing* (7th ed.). St. Louis: Elsevier.

Urden, L. (2018). Cardiovascular therapeutic management. In L. Urden, K. Stacy, & M. Lough (Eds.), *Critical care nursing: Diagnosis and management*. St. Louis, MO: Mosby/Elsevier.

1-97. **(A)** The protracted vomiting and abdominal fluid sequestration associated with acute pancreatitis may result in significant electrolyte imbalances, especially those of calcium, magnesium, and potassium. If severe hypocalcemia occurs, the QT intervals lengthen on the ECG, and seizures may occur. Cullen's sign, a bluish discoloration of the periumbilical skin typically associated with subcutaneous intraperitoneal hemorrhage, may or may not be observed in patients with acute pancreatitis, and measurements of abdominal girth are not typically warranted. Although

pain control is essential for patients with acute pancreatitis, fluids would not be restricted in patients with vomiting and diarrhea. These patients would be expected to have diminished bowel sounds because of fluid sequestration. Although vascular stasis and coagulopathies may eventually arise, peripheral pulses are not typically compromised.

References: Radovich, P. (2018). Gastrointestinal system. In T. M. Hartjes (Ed.), *AACN core curriculum for high acuity, progressive, and critical care nursing* (7th ed.). St. Louis: Elsevier.

Ahmed, A., Azim, A., Gurjar, M., & Baronia, A. (2016). Hypocalcemia in acute pancreatitis revisited. *Indian Journal of Critical Care Medicine, 20*(3), 173.

1-98. **(A)** The first nursing action is discontinuation of the tube feeding to remove the threat of aspiration and its associated complications such as aspiration pneumonia. Metoclopramide should be given after the tube feeding is stopped in order to promote gastrointestinal motility and stomach emptying, further diminishing the chance of aspiration of tube feedings. Checking feeding tube or endotracheal tube placement may be helpful to determine whether dislodgment of either tube is causing the aspiration rather than a reopening of the fistula, though auscultation of air through a feeding tube is often unreliable for assessing such dislodgment. Radiographic confirmation of the correct placement of the tube is recommended. Other diagnostic studies such as bronchoscopy or endoscopy may be indicated before continuing or resuming feedings.

References: Radovich, P. (2018). Gastrointestinal system. In T. M. Hartjes (Ed.), *AACN core curriculum for high acuity, progressive, and critical care nursing* (7th ed.). St. Louis: Elsevier.

Burns, S. (2014). *AACN essentials of critical care nursing*, 3rd ed. New York, NY: McGraw-Hill.

1-99. **(C)** Sinus rhythm at a rate of less than 100 beats/min indicates that the workload on the left ventricle has decreased effectively, and oxygenation has improved. The heart rate would be increased if hypoxia was present. Because respiratory effort may cause exhaustion, a slow respiratory rate may indicate fatigue and impending respiratory failure. The amount of diuresis is not a specific indicator that pulmonary fluid overload has resolved. Systolic blood pressure is influenced by multiple factors, including catecholamine release, blood volume, and vasodilation, making it a non-specific indicator for resolution of pulmonary edema.

References: Efre, A., & Boling, B. (2018). Cardiovascular system. In T. M. Hartjes (Ed.), *AACN core curriculum for high acuity, progressive, and critical care nursing* (7th ed.). St. Louis: Elsevier.

Urden, L. (2018). Cardiovascular disorders. In L. Urden, K. Stacy, & M. Lough (Eds.), *Critical care nursing: Diagnosis and management.* St. Louis, MO: Mosby/Elsevier.

1-100. **(C)** The response to cytokine release during sepsis results in: (1) systemic vasodilation with decreased afterload (↓ SVR) and hypotension; (2) increased capillary permeability with decreased preload (↓ CVP), third spacing, and interstitial edema; (3) relative hypovolemia; and (4) decreased tissue oxygen extraction (↑ SVO_2). The hemodynamic values in Option A are consistent with a patient in cardiogenic shock. The elevated SVR reflects the sympathetic nervous system response of vasoconstriction. The CVP is elevated because of pump dysfunction. The SVO_2 is decreased because of low cardiac output with increased oxygen extraction. Option B illustrates a patient with loss of vascular tone as seen in spinal cord injury. The patient has adequate preload and normal oxygen extraction at the tissue level. Option D describes a patient with hypovolemic shock. Again, the SVR is elevated as a compensatory response to low pressure with vasoconstriction. The low preload (↓ CVP) is consistent with decreased circulating volume. The SVO_2 is decreased due to the increased oxygen extraction from the low preload with resultant low cardiac output.

References: Johnson, A. (2018). Multisystem: Systemic inflammatory response syndrome and septic shock. In T. M. Hartjes (Ed.), *AACN core curriculum for high acuity, progressive, and critical care nursing* (7th ed.). St. Louis: Elsevier.

Bope, E. T., MD, & Kellerman, R. T., MD. (2017). The infectious diseases. In E. T. Bope, R. D. Kellerman, & H. F. Conn (Authors), *Conn's current therapy 2017* (pp. 479–635). Philadelphia, PA: Elsevier.

1-101. **(A)** Chest tube output greater than 200 mL for 2 consecutive hours indicates a need to return to the operating room to determine whether there is a correctable source of bleeding. Low MAP requires pharmacologic support and increasing the rate of norepinephrine infusion, adding therapy like epinephrine or vasopressin, and fluid bolus to increase blood pressure. Low cardiac output may indicate a need for vasopressor support, fluid administration, increased pacing rate, or cardiac assist device. Elevated PAOP should be treated with vasodilators or diuretics to decrease afterload.

References: Efre, A., & Boling, B. (2018). Cardiovascular system. In T. M. Hartjes (Ed.), *AACN core curriculum for high acuity, progressive, and critical care nursing* (7th ed.). St. Louis: Elsevier.

Ley, S. (2015). Standards for resuscitation after cardiac surgery. *Critical Care Nurse, 35*(2), 30–38.

1-102. **(C)** The patient must be repositioned because effective chest compressions need to be delivered with the patient in a supine position. Instructing the new nurse on use of the *2015 Guidelines for Cardiopulmonary Resuscitation and Emergency Cardiovascular Care* from the AHA provides current information on correct patient placement. Option A is incorrect because in order for chest compressions to be effective, the patient must first be positioned for optimal compression. Option B is a good response but not the best response. The nurse should begin CPR immediately, and then the preceptor can initiate the unit's code blue response. Option D is important, but suction should already be available at an ICU patient's bedside.

References: Dermenchyan, A. (2018). Professional caring and ethical practice. In T. M. Hartjes (Ed.), *AACN core curriculum for high acuity, progressive, and critical care nursing* (7th ed.). St. Louis: Elsevier.

American Heart Association. (2015). 2015 American Heart Association guidelines for CPR & ECC. *ECC Guidelines.* Web.

1-103. **(C)** In hypertrophic cardiomyopathy, treatment aims toward increasing afterload and/or increasing preload. Nitroglycerin decreases both preload and afterload, so when it is administered to patients with hypertrophic cardiomyopathy, both of these effects worsen the obstruction and intensify symptoms. Because hypertrophic cardiomyopathy is associated with diastolic dysfunction, medications (e beta blockers and calcium channel blockers) that slow the heart rate allow increased diastolic filling, which increases preload and promotes myocardial stretch with more efficient emptying of the ventricle. Amiodarone may be used in the treatment of hypertrophic cardiomyopathy to treat atrial or ventricular dysrhythmias.

References: Efre, A., & Boling, B. (2018). Cardiovascular system. In T. M. Hartjes (Ed.), *AACN core curriculum for high acuity, progressive, and critical care nursing* (7th ed.). St. Louis: Elsevier.

Hickey, K., & Rezzadeh, K. (2013). Hypertropic cardiomyopathy. *Nurse practitioner, 38*(5), 22–32. http://dx.doi.org/10.1097/01.NPR.0000428814.64880.f2.

1-104. **(C)** Regardless of the factors contributing to the development of disseminated intravascular coagulopathy, the definitive treatment is to eliminate the potential causes of this syndrome. Until this has been accomplished, the patient's situation will continue to deteriorate. Use of heparin may or may not be useful for the patient experiencing DIC, depending on the factors related to the etiology. Subcutaneous administration of any medication may lead to prolonged bleeding from the injection site and should be avoided, especially because the impairment of circulation would limit absorption. Although supportive care is necessary, unless the cause of the DIC is addressed, the patient will not survive.

References: Dressler, D. (2018). Hematological and immunological systems. In T. M. Hartjes (Ed.), *AACN core curriculum for high acuity, progressive, and critical care nursing* (7th ed.). St. Louis: Elsevier.

Urden, L. (2018). Hematologic disorders and oncologic emergencies. In L. Urden, K. Stacy, & M. Lough (Eds.), *Critical care nursing: Diagnosis and management*. St. Louis, MO: Mosby/Elsevier.

1-105. **(B)** Although septic shock is usually associated with vasodilation caused by the release of proinflammatory cytokines and prostaglandins, not all blood vessels dilate. The arterioles in the microcirculation remain vasoconstricted, leading to a maldistribution of blood flow and subsequent inadequate tissue perfusion. Inadequate tissue perfusion is evaluated by tissue oxygen indices, which include oxygen delivery (DO_2) and consumption (VO_2). Normal oxygen delivery is approximately 1000 mL/min, but normal oxygen consumption is estimated at 250 mL/min. In septic shock, the absolute intravascular volume may be normal, but because of acute vasodilation, a relative hypovolemia occurs. Myocardial depression can occur in patients with septic shock and is characterized by reversible biventricular dilation, decreased ejection fraction, altered myocardial compliance, and decreased contractile response to fluid resuscitation and catecholamines. It is caused primarily by myocardial depressant factors released as a result of sepsis and not by altered coronary perfusion or global ischemia. The patient's hemodynamic values indicate the patient has not received adequate volume resuscitation.

References: Johnson, A. (2018). Multisystem: Systemic inflammatory response syndrome and septic shock. In T. M. Hartjes (Ed.), *AACN core curriculum for high acuity, progressive, and critical care nursing* (7th ed.). St. Louis: Elsevier.

Saugel, B., Huber, W., Nierhaus, A., Kluge, S., Reuter, D. A., & Wagner, J. Y. (2016). Advanced hemodynamic management in patients with septic shock. *Biomed Research International*, 1–11. http://dx.doi.org/10.1155/2016/8268569.

1-106. **(C)** An emergent tracheotomy will provide immediate access to and maintenance of a patent airway so the patient can be ventilated and enable management of the pulmonary trauma that has resulted in the subcutaneous emphysema. The rapid onset of airway obstruction suggests that the obstruction is in the upper airways, so oral intubation will be ineffective to solve the problem. A fiberoptic bronchoscopy can only be used after the airway has been secured. There is no indication that cardiac compressions for initiation of cardiopulmonary resuscitation are warranted as the patient has not lost pulses.

Reference: Prokakis, C., Koletsis, E. N., Dedeilias, P., Fligou, F., Filos, K., & Dougenis, D. (2014). Airway trauma: a review on epidemiology, mechanisms of injury, diagnosis and treatment. *Journal of Cardiothoracic Surgery, 9*(1), 117. http://dx.doi.org/10.1186/1749-8090-9-117.

1-107. **(B)** Risk factors for intracerebral hemorrhage (ICH) include low weight (lower than 70 kg), hypertension, advanced age (older than 70 years), and thrombolytic therapy. Coagulopathies must be reversed as soon as possible. Warfarin should be reversed with vitamin K (three 10 mg IV doses) and fresh-frozen plasma to normalize prothrombin time. Factor IX concentrate can be used along with vitamin K. IV bolus dosing of recombinant factor VIIa can be administered within the first 3 to 4 hours after symptom onset or in patients at risk of additional bleeding, such as those with warfarin-related coagulopathies. It may limit hematoma enlargement and reduce morbidity and mortality after ICH. Surgery (Option A) for evacuation of a large deep hemispheric clot has been found ineffective in reducing mortality or disability. CT scan is appropriate for diagnostic evaluation in this case. MRI (Option C) may be considered in cases in which the clot morphology, location, or presentation is inconsistent with typical ICH. However, this patient does not present with any atypical findings. Epsilon-aminocaproic acid (EACA) (Option D) is indicated in patients who recently received a thrombolytic and are deteriorating. EACA can enhance hemostasis when fibrinolysis contributes to bleeding, but it can also cause excessive thrombosis and is generally not indicated in this scenario.

References: Blissitt, P. A. (2018). Neurologic system. In T. M. Hartjes (Ed.), *AACN core curriculum for high acuity, progressive, and critical care nursing* (7th ed.). St. Louis: Elsevier.

Solari, D., & Cavallo, L. (2014). Intracranial hemorrhage: how to return from the warfarin effect. *World Neurosurgery, 81*(1), 40–42.

1-108. **(B)** Identifying and locating resources for the patient's wife would help relieve the heavy burden of the husband's care. There is no basis for involving the ethics committee in this situation. Option C has a somewhat judgmental tone and is at odds with the wife's stated feelings and perspective on the situation. Option D may be supportive to some extent but fails to address the issues of greatest concern at the moment.

Reference: Dermenchyan, A. (2018). Professional caring and ethical practice. In T. M. Hartjes (Ed.), *AACN core curriculum for high acuity, progressive, and critical care nursing* (7th ed.). St. Louis: Elsevier.

1-109. **(D)** Renal insufficiency as demonstrated by elevated creatinine should be reported to the cardiologist as adjustments in the amount or type of contrast used for the catheterization may be necessary. Contrast dye is nephrotoxic and could precipitate renal failure. Heparin will be continued during catheterization and will be discontinued before sheath removal. A serum troponin level of 0.2 ng/dL is not indicative of myocardial ischemia. The potassium level is within normal limits. Contrast media frequently causes diuresis, which may decrease the serum potassium.

References: Boling, B. (2018). Renal system. In T. M. Hartjes (Ed.), *AACN core curriculum for high acuity, progressive, and critical care nursing* (7th ed.). St. Louis: Elsevier.

Honicker, T. (2016). Continuing nursing education. Contrast-induced acute kidney injury: comparison of preventative therapies. *Nephrology Nursing Journal, 43*(2), 109–117.

1-110. **(B)** Administration of insulin will begin to correct the patient's acid-base imbalances. This initial bolus should be followed up with an IV drip of regular insulin, which is fast acting and will stop the formation of ketone bodies, thereby correcting metabolic acidosis. Administration of antibiotics may not be an appropriate intervention because there is no indication the patient is febrile or producing purulent sputum or urine. The patient is compensating for his metabolic acidosis through an increase in the depth and rate of respirations (Kussmaul respirations), and bicarbonate level will likely return to a normal level as the cause of the metabolic acidosis is corrected. Normal saline is important for its hydrating effects; however, this rate of infusion would be inadequate to replace fluids lost over a 4-day period.

Reference: MacDermott, J. (2018). Endocrine system. In T. M. Hartjes (Ed.), *AACN core curriculum for high acuity, progressive, and critical care nursing* (7th ed.). St. Louis: Elsevier.

1-111. **(B)** Elevation of the head of the bed 30 to 45 degrees has been shown to decrease the rate and risk of aspiration and hospital-acquired pneumonia. Feeding tube placement does not decrease the risk of aspiration. No matter where the tip of a feeding tube is placed, residuals increase the risk of aspiration. To prevent tissue trauma and unwarranted oxygen desaturation, patients should be only suctioned when clinically indicated by the presence of secretions. Enteral feedings appropriately delivered have been shown to decrease mortality and morbidity compared with hyperalimentation.

References: Storzer, D. N. (2018). Pulmonary system. In T. M. Hartjes (Ed.), *AACN core curriculum for high acuity, progressive, and critical care nursing* (7th ed.). St. Louis: Elsevier.

Okgün Alcan, A., Korkmaz, D., & Uyar, M. (2016). Prevention of ventilator-associated pneumonia: use of the care bundle approach. *American Journal of Infection Control, 44*(10), e173–e176. http://dx.doi.org/10.1016/j.ajic.2016.04.237.

1-112. **(B)** The patient's rhythm strip indicates first-degree AV block with bradycardia, and the blood pressure is adequate; therefore, no immediate interventions are necessary. Bradycardia is common in healthy persons during sleep. If the automated blood pressure was lower than 90 mm Hg systolic, the nurse may awaken the patient to determine whether symptomatic bradycardia is present. If the patient had low blood pressure or symptoms of decreased perfusion, such as altered mental status, administration of atropine would be warranted. Administration of oxygen is indicated for symptomatic bradycardia.

References: Efre, A., & Boling, B. (2018). Cardiovascular system. In T. M. Hartjes (Ed.), *AACN core curriculum for high acuity, progressive, and critical care nursing* (7th ed.). St. Louis: Elsevier.
Mann, D. (2015). *Braunwald's heart disease: A textbook of cardiovascular medicine*, 10th ed. Philadelphia: Elsevier Saunders.

1-113. **(A)** The body uses oxygen to generate high energy phosphates via cellular metabolism. If oxygen delivery is not sufficient to meet cellular demands—as seen during periods of shock—the body must rely on anaerobic metabolism. The end product of anaerobic metabolism is lactate. Serum lactate can be used as an alternative parameter to measure the adequacy of oxygen delivery. Although initial serum lactate levels do not differ significantly between survivors and nonsurvivors, survival rates are highest in patients whose serum lactate levels return to normal within the first 24 hours. Thereafter, the longer it takes for lactate levels to clear, the higher the incidence of organ failure and mortality.

References: Johnson, A. (2018). Multisystem: Systemic inflammatory response syndrome and septic shock. In T. M. Hartjes (Ed.), *AACN core curriculum for high acuity, progressive, and critical care nursing* (7th ed.). St. Louis: Elsevier.
Bloos, F., Zhang, Z., & Boulain, T. (2016). Lactate-guided resuscitation saves lives: yes. *Intensive Care Medicine, 42*(3), 466–469. http://dx.doi.org/10.1007/s00134-015-4196-0.

1-114. **(C)** The ECG shows an anterior wall MI. The anterior wall is synonymous with the left ventricle. Acute myocardial infarction of the left ventricle is associated with left ventricular failure and signs of heart failure. Occlusion of the right coronary artery (inferior wall) is associated with SA and AV block and bradycardia. Hiccoughs and GI upset are also common with inferior wall MI. Right ventricular MI may cause right ventricular failure and related signs such as JVD and peripheral edema.

References: Efre, A., & Boling, B. (2018). Cardiovascular system. In T. M. Hartjes (Ed.), *AACN core curriculum for high acuity, progressive, and critical care nursing* (7th ed.). St. Louis: Elsevier.
Ibrahim, A., Riddell, T., & Devireddy, C. (2014). Acute myocardial infarction. *Critical Care Clinics, 30*(3), 341–364. http://dx.doi.org/10.1016/s0749-0704(0500079-5).

1-115. **(C)** Option C is the best because hospitalized patients are often highly motivated to change their lifestyles to improve their health, so hospitals are appropriate sites for prevention education. Option A does not facilitate communication. Options B and D avoid discussing an obvious and potentially life-threatening behavior problem.

Reference: O'Connor, P. (2015). Alcohol use disorders. In A. Schafer, & L. Goldman (Eds.), *Goldman-Cecil medicine* (pp. 149–156). Philadelphia, PA: Elsevier Health Sciences.

1-116. (D) The use of restraints in critical care has the potential to violate several principles and thus should be undertaken with caution. Informed consent must be obtained from the patient before the use of restraints. A patient with decision-making capacity should be able to refuse restraint. In addition, mechanical restraint can cause cognitive impairment, agitation, delirium, fear, withdrawal, emotional devastation, the perception of loss of dignity, soft tissue injury, and fractures. Sedating the patient and then applying restraints would disrespect the patient's wishes and could cause emotional harm. A physician's order does not override the patient's expressed refusal to be restrained. The patient is competent to make his own decisions. Calling the family to discuss restraints without the patient's consent is a violation of his privacy rights. The nurse can attempt less restrictive measures such as a bedside one to one monitor, appropriate sedation and analgesia, placing the patient in close view of the nursing station, and enhanced monitoring.

References: Dermenchyan, A. (2018). Professional caring and ethical practice. In T. M. Hartjes (Ed.), *AACN core curriculum for high acuity, progressive, and critical care nursing* (7th ed.). St. Louis: Elsevier.

March, P., & Schub, T. (2017). Restraint: minimizing use in acute, nonpsychiatric care. CINAHL Nursing Guide.

1-117. **(B)** This client requires referral to a social worker or psychiatric clinical nurse specialist who can conduct a comprehensive assessment of this patient's needs related to child care issues, financial and employment issues, and drug rehabilitation. Option A is not an immediate concern because the children are being cared for. Although the patient's employment status is a relevant point to document, the patient's competence to care for her children depends on numerous factors and cannot be assumed without further assessment. Referrals for drug and alcohol rehabilitation can be arranged by the social worker or CNS.

Reference: Chapa, D., Akintade, B. (2018). Psychosocial Aspects of Critical Care. In Hartjes, T.M. (ed.), *AACN Core Curriculum for High Acuity, Progressive, and Critical Care Nursing* (7th ed.). St. Louis: Elsevier.

1-118. **(A)** Asthma is primarily a disease of pulmonary mechanics and is best monitored by measuring ease of expiratory flow, which can be done using serial peak flow measurements. Hypoxia is usually a later sign during an exacerbation. Excessive mucous production is a common problem in COPD and exacerbations may be caused by infectious processes, but this will not track respiratory function. Patient reports of dyspnea are multifactorial and are not necessarily associated with an exacerbation.

Reference: Storzer, D. N. (2018). Pulmonary system. In T. M. Hartjes (Ed.), *AACN core curriculum for high acuity, progressive, and critical care nursing* (7th ed.). St. Louis: Elsevier.

1-119. **(C)** The patient is at highest risk of falling because of diuretic use. Concomitant use of anticoagulants places the patient at higher risk of bleeding complications at points of fall contact. Hematomas and cerebral bleeds will prolong this patient's hospital stay. The risk of stroke and pulmonary embolism is decreased because of anticoagulants. This patient is at high risk for readmission; however, he is currently at highest risk of an inpatient fall. With proper discharge teaching and follow up, his risk of readmission is reduced.

References: Ming-Huang, C., Hsin-Dai, L., Hei-Fen, H., & Shih-Chieh, W. (2015). Medication use and fall-risk assessment for falls in an acute care hospital. *Geriatrics & Gerontology International, 15*(7), 856–863. http://dx.doi.org/10.1111/ggi.12359.

Urden, L. (2018). Trauma. In L. Urden, K. Stacy, & M. Lough (Eds.), *Critical care nursing: Diagnosis and management*. St. Louis, MO: Mosby/Elsevier.

1-120. **(D)** Mechanisms that link PTSD with poor health outcomes are multifactorial. Alterations in the hypothalamic-pituitary-adrenal axis and the sympathetic adrenal medullary axis, as well as autoimmune dysfunction, are commonly linked to the pathophysiologic changes of PTSD. Cardiovascular complications caused by activation of the two axes lead to hypertension, tachycardia, diabetes, and endothelial dysfunction. If this upregulation of the stress response is prolonged, these cardiovascular changes cause endothelial damage to vessels and eventually atherosclerosis, which is associated with myocardial infarction and embolic stroke. In addition to cardiovascular disease, PTSD may also be linked with metabolic syndrome, a known cluster of cardiovascular signs and symptoms that puts a person at risk for coronary artery disease, stroke, and type 2 diabetes mellitus. PTSD can cause chronic hypertension, not hypotension.

Reference: Warlan, H., & Howland, L. (2015). Posttraumatic stress syndrome associated with stays in the intensive care unit: importance of nurses' involvement. *Critical Care Nurse, 35*(3), 44–52. http://dx.doi.org/10.4037/ccn2015758.

1-121. **(D)** Beta-blocking medications decrease the incidence of myocardial reinfarction as well as the incidence of ventricular and supraventricular dysrhythmias, reduce myocardial remodeling, and prevent sympathetic stress on the myocardium, making beta blockers useful in reducing mortality in acute MI. Calcium channel blocking agents do not prevent ventricular dysrhythmias and have not been shown to reduce mortality in acute MI. Magnesium prophylaxis does not reduce development of ventricular dysrhythmias in the setting of acute MI after thrombolytic therapy. Lidocaine decreases ventricular dysrhythmias, but side effects such as bradycardia, paresthesias, and altered mental status, which persist after the reperfusion dysrhythmias, make it a poor treatment choice.

References: Efre, A., & Boling, B. (2018). Cardiovascular system. In T. M. Hartjes (Ed.), *AACN core curriculum for high acuity, progressive, and critical care nursing* (7th ed.). St. Louis: Elsevier.

Goldberger, J., Bonow, R., Cuffe, M., et al. (2015). Effect of beta-blocker dose on survival after acute myocardial infarction. *Journal of the American College of Cardiology (JACC), 66*(13), 1431–1441. http://dx.doi.org/10.1016/j.jacc.2015.07.047.

1-122. **(B)** Spontaneous bacterial peritonitis is the infection of ascites fluid and is a common complication of decompensated cirrhosis. This should be suspected when a patient with cirrhosis and ascites also develops fever, abdominal pain, or deterioration in mental status. Although these clinical findings may be subtle, spontaneous bacterial peritonitis may precipitate septic shock, renal failure, and liver failure. Acute appendicitis typically manifests as a vague midline abdominal pain accompanied by nausea, vomiting, and a lack of appetite that slowly migrates to the right lower quadrant over 24 hours. A small bowel obstruction presents with nausea, vomiting, and severe cramping abdominal pain that often comes in waves at intervals every 5 to 15 minutes but does not include fever. Patients with acute pancreatitis present with severe upper abdominal pain, nausea, vomiting, and fever.

References: Radovich, P. (2018). Gastrointestinal system. In T. M. Hartjes (Ed.), *AACN core curriculum for high acuity, progressive, and critical care nursing* (7th ed.). St. Louis: Elsevier.

Jung Ho, K., Yong Duk, J., In Young, J., Mi Young, A., Hea Won, A., Jin Young, A., … Ku, N. S. (2016). Predictive factors of spontaneous bacterial peritonitis caused by gram-positive bacteria in patients with cirrhosis. *Medicine, 95*(17), 1–6. http://dx.doi.org/10.1097/MD.0000000000003489.

1-123. **(D)** Echocardiography best determines the absence of pericardial effusion and tamponade. Although the pericardial catheter is in place and functioning properly, the patient should demonstrate absence of symptoms of pericardial effusion and tamponade. A lack of drainage may signal catheter obstruction and does not necessarily indicate that pericardial effusion has resolved. Approximately 250 mL of pericardial fluid is necessary for the effusion to be visualized on chest x-ray as an enlarged cardiac silhouette or water bottle shape.

References: Efre, A., & Boling, B. (2018). Cardiovascular system. In T. M. Hartjes (Ed.), *AACN core curriculum for high acuity, progressive, and critical care nursing* (7th ed.). St. Louis: Elsevier.

Jneid, H., Maree, A., & Palacios, I. (2014). Pericardial tamponade: clinical presentation, diagnosis, and catheter-based therapies. In J. Parillo, & R. Dellinger (Eds.), *Critical care medicine: Principles of diagnosis and management in the adult* (pp. 82–89). Philadelphia: Elsevier/Saunders.

1-124. **(A)** The Vietnamese culture is very family oriented. The father or eldest son is the spokesperson and holds ultimate authority. Terminal illness discussion must first be presented to the head of family before it is discussed with any other family members, including the patient. Then the head of family will conduct a family discussion with extended family. A DNR status is a sensitive issue, and the decision must be made by the entire family.

References: Dermenchyan, A. (2018). Professional caring and ethical practice. In T. M. Hartjes (Ed.), *AACN core curriculum for high acuity, progressive, and critical care nursing* (7th ed.). St. Louis: Elsevier.

HealthCare Chaplaincy. (2013). Handbook of patients' spiritual and cultural values for healthcare professionals [Brochure].

1-125. **(B)** Meningitis is a potential complication of basilar skull fracture, and an elevated temperature is a key examination finding. Deep vein thrombosis (Option A) may present with an elevated white count and/or elevated temperature. Screening would include venous duplex of the extremities. However, infectious sources are a more likely cause of fever. Hypothalamic dysfunction or "storming" (Option C) characteristically presents with hypertension, tachycardia, and fever. The scenario presented does not include all of these key features. Although a retained foreign body (Option D) may eventually result in infection, the scenario described suggests a more common and likely source of infection for this patient.

References: Blissitt, P. A. (2018). Neurologic system. In T. M. Hartjes (Ed.), *AACN core curriculum for high acuity, progressive, and critical care nursing* (7th ed.). St. Louis: Elsevier.

Ratilal, B., Costa, J., Sampaio, C., et al. (2015). Antibiotic prophylaxis for preventing meningitis in patients with basilar skull fractures. *Cochrane Database of Systematic Reviews,* (4). http://dx.doi.org/10.1002/14651858.CD004884.pub4.

1-126. **(B)** The nurse would anticipate administration of platelets to decrease bleeding in this patient. The normal platelet count is 250,000 to 500,000/mm³. Packed RBCs are not indicated unless the hematocrit falls lower than 28%. Fresh-frozen plasma would be indicated to replace clotting factors if the INR was greater than 1.5. Salt poor albumin is used to replace volume in patients with low albumin or extravascular fluid overload.

Reference: Dressler, D. (2018). Hematological and immunological systems. In T. M. Hartjes (Ed.), *AACN core curriculum for high acuity, progressive, and critical care nursing* (7th ed.). St. Louis: Elsevier.

1-127. **(B)** Nutritional support is an essential component of the care of critically ill trauma patients. Within 24 to 48 hours after traumatic injury, a predictable hypermetabolic response occurs. Patients with trauma require prompt and effective nutritional support to optimize recovery. The metabolic response to injury mobilizes amino acids and accelerates protein synthesis to support wound healing and the immunologic response to invading organisms. A specialist should evaluate nutritional needs and begin feeding within 24 hours of admission. Nutrition is the key to ensuring adequate healing. Option A is not warranted unless the patient has an underlying psychiatric problem that needs to be addressed. Neither Option C nor Option D is required at this point in the patient's care.

Reference: Holleran, R. (2018). Multisystem: Multisystem trauma. In T. M. Hartjes (Ed.), *AACN core curriculum for high acuity, progressive, and critical care nursing* (7th ed.). St. Louis: Elsevier.

1-128. **(D)** A "silent chest" represented by inaudible breath sounds on auscultation is the most ominous sign of acute respiratory failure in the asthmatic patient because it reflects significantly diminished ventilation or movement of air into and out of the lungs. Poor ventilation may be because of respiratory muscle fatigue or bronchoconstriction. Wheezing indicates bronchoconstriction but also reflects the patient's ability to move sufficient air to produce the wheezing sounds. Although sentence length is a general indicator of severity of shortness of breath, it is not an indicator of respiratory failure. Tachypnea may lead to respiratory failure if its prolonged duration results in respiratory muscle fatigue.

References: Storzer, D. N. (2018). Pulmonary system. In T. M. Hartjes (Ed.), *AACN core curriculum for high acuity, progressive, and critical care nursing* (7th ed.). St. Louis: Elsevier.

Ferri, F. (2015). Asthma. In F. F. Ferri (Ed.), *2015 Ferri's clinical advisor: 5 books in 1* (pp. 152–161). Philadelphia: Elsevier Mosby.

1-129. **(C)** Hepatocytes are responsible for biosynthesis of 80% to 90% of innate immune protein. Kupffer cells, which account for 80% to 90% of the total population of fixed tissue macrophages, are a critical component of the mononuclear phagocytic system and are central to both the hepatic and the systemic responses to pathogens. When the liver loses its ability to break down and conjugate new proteins, immune globulins are produced in progressively smaller quantities. The pathophysiology of liver failure, not the patient's medications, is the cause of the patient's immune compromise. Adhering to the medication regimen will increase the patient's ability to ward off infection as laboratory values become more normal. Long-term malnutrition and impaired uptake of nutrients are not the primary reason for decreased immunity. Although it is true that fewer fat-soluble vitamins and vitamin B_{12} are stored, this is not the primary reason for immune compromise.

References: Radovich, P. (2018). Gastrointestinal system. In T. M. Hartjes (Ed.), *AACN core curriculum for high acuity, progressive, and critical care nursing* (7th ed.). St. Louis: Elsevier.

Foster, G., & O'Brien, A. (2017). Liver disease. In P. Kumar, & M. Clark (Eds.), *Kumar & Clark's clinical medicine* (pp. 437–488). Edinburgh: Elsevier.

1-130. **(B)** The highest Glasgow Coma Scale (GCS) score a patient can receive is 15, and the lowest is 3. For the eye score, the patient receives 1 point because his eyes do not open (even to noxious stimuli). His verbal score is 1 because he is intubated (although given his motor response, he is unlikely to make any better response). He flexes his right upper extremity (motor score of 3) and extends his left upper extremity (motor score of 2) to noxious stimuli. As the best motor score is used to calculate a patient's GCS score, his total GCS score is 5 (eye = 1, verbal = 1, motor = 3).

Reference: Blissitt, P. A. (2018). Neurologic system. In T. M. Hartjes (Ed.), *AACN core curriculum for high acuity, progressive, and critical care nursing* (7th ed.). St. Louis: Elsevier.

1-131. **(A)** Research shows that many (at least 50%) patients have difficulty with the dietary and fluid restrictions necessary when on hemodialysis. The best response is to have a nutritionist determine the need for additional education regarding renal diet and fluid restriction and provide any supplementation warranted. The nutritionist needs to design a dietary plan and work with the patient (and, if the patient wishes, with his spouse or other family members who assist with food shopping and cooking) to identify food selection and short-term goals. Option B would be implemented only at the patient's request. Option C may be a true statement, but attempts to improve compliance based on induced fear are not supported in the literature. Option D is a discussion he should have with his nephrologist and does not afford an immediate solution to his problem of diet and fluid protocol nonadherence.

Reference: Boling, B. (2018). Renal system. In T. M. Hartjes (Ed.), *AACN core curriculum for high acuity, progressive, and critical care nursing* (7th ed.). St. Louis: Elsevier.

1-132. **(A)** Uncontrolled hypertension is an absolute contraindication to the administration of thrombolytics. Blood pressure may be reduced with beta blockers or vasodilators to enable administration of thrombolytics to reduce the risk of intracerebral bleeding. Although TIA may increase the risk of stroke, it does not necessarily indicate that a thrombus is present, and the risk

of intracerebral bleed should be weighed against the benefit of thrombolytic administration. History of stroke is a relative contraindication to administration of thrombolytics. Remote stroke should not prevent administration of thrombolytics because intracerebral clots should be absorbed over time through normal processes. Age is also a relative contraindication. If percutaneous intervention (PCI) is available within 90 minutes for an elderly patient with acute myocardial infarction, PCI would be a better alternative. If PCI is not available, the patient should receive thrombolytic therapy.

References: Efre, A., & Boling, B. (2018). Cardiovascular system. In T. M. Hartjes (Ed.), *AACN core curriculum for high acuity, progressive, and critical care nursing* (7th ed.). St. Louis: Elsevier.

Thrombolytic therapy: Background, thrombolytic agents, thrombolytic therapy for acute myocardial infarction. (December 15, 2016). Retrieved March 14, 2017, from http://emedicine.medscape.com/article/811234-overview#a3.

1-133. **(B)** The patient is experiencing vascular steal syndrome. This syndrome occurs when blood is shunted away from tissues, causing tissue hypoperfusion. The incidence of vascular steal syndrome is higher in patients with grafts and/or upper arm accesses, in diabetics, and in the elderly; the incidence increases in extremities with previous access procedures. Management of the patient's symptoms includes comfort measures such as applying warm compresses and administering ordered analgesics that improve vascular supply to the hand. All other options would reduce blood flow and further exacerbate the patient's symptoms.

Reference: Harris, L. M. (2014). Hemodialysis access: nonthrombotic complications. In R. B. Rutherford, J. L. Cronenwett, & K. W. Johnston (Authors), *Rutherford's vascular surgery* (pp. 1135-1152). Philadelphia: Elsevier Saunders.

1-134. **(B)** Option B is the correct reply not only because it is factually correct but also because the easiest way to begin learning about a procedure such as this is by recognizing what constitutes a "normal" finding. Option A is factually incorrect. Both Option C and Option D are incorrect because these activities are not included in the procedures related to measuring bladder pressures.

Reference: Pande, R., & Khanna, P. (2016). Intraabdominal hypertension and abdominal compartment syndrome. *Critical Care, 516–520.* http://dx.doi.org/10.5005/jp/books/12670_64.

1-135. **(C)** If cardiomyopathy is a result of myocardial ischemia, the most definitive treatment is to restore coronary circulation by either percutaneous coronary intervention or coronary bypass surgery. ACE inhibitors can decrease pulmonary congestion and prevent ventricular remodeling, but they do not afford definitive benefit. Likewise, diuretics only temporarily relieve symptoms such as pulmonary congestion. Permanent pacing could be used to treat dysrhythmias or improve cardiac output caused by lack of AV synchrony.

References: Efre, A., & Boling, B. (2018). Cardiovascular system. In T. M. Hartjes (Ed.), *AACN core curriculum for high acuity, progressive, and critical care nursing* (7th ed.). St. Louis: Elsevier.

Huynh, K. (2016). Survival benefit of CABG surgery for ischemic cardiomyopathy. *Nature Reviews Cardiology, 13*(6), 312–313.

1-136. **(A)** Enteric leakage from anastomotic sites is a complication of the Roux-en-Y gastric bypass. In addition to an elevated WBC count, patients may have subtle signs of infection or have signs of sepsis and hemodynamic instability. In most cases of infection, the WBC count is elevated, and the platelet count remains unchanged. Potassium levels usually are reduced in patients with increased gastrointestinal drainage. Platelet counts are elevated in patients with hematologic disorders or in those who have undergone a splenectomy, neither of which pertain to this patient. Lipase is elevated in pancreatic disorders. This patient does not exhibit clinical evidence of pancreatic dysfunction.

Reference: Benefield, A. (2018). Critical care patients with special needs: Bariatric patients. In T. M. Hartjes (Ed.), *AACN core curriculum for high acuity, progressive, and critical care nursing* (7th ed.). St. Louis: Elsevier.

1-137. **(C)** Gram-negative pneumonia and persistent immunocompromise are both risk factors for developing a lung abscess or parapneumonic effusion. This patient's clinical and diagnostic test findings are consistent with those associated with these conditions and warrant manual thoracic drainage and antibiotic administration. Results from a BAL (bronchoalveolar lavage) would not reflect a process in the pleural space. Option B identifies interventions for hemothorax, a condition not evidenced in this patient's clinical presentation. Bronchial hygiene interventions will not affect an intrapleural process.

References: Storzer, D. N. (2018). Pulmonary system. In T. M. Hartjes (Ed.), *AACN core curriculum for high acuity, progressive, and critical care nursing* (7th ed.). St. Louis: Elsevier.

Parapneumonic pleural effusions and empyema thoracis. (January 06, 2017). Retrieved March 14, 2017, from http://emedicine.medscape.com/article/298485-overview.

1-138. **(D)** The patient has most likely developed complete heart block from scar formation subsequent to surgical repair of the atrial septal defect (ASD). Before the patient's surgery, the left-to-right atrial shunt associated with ASD caused pulmonary hypertension, which resulted in right ventricular and right atrial enlargement; RA and RV enlargement, in turn, may precipitate development of right bundle branch block (complete or incomplete) and delayed conduction from the SA to AV node evidenced by a prolonged PR interval. As a result, first- and second-degree AV block, type I, could have existed preoperatively with progression to complete AV block occurring gradually with scar tissue formation postoperatively.

Reference: Ferri, F. (2017). Atrial septal defect. In F. Ferri, *2017 Ferri's clinical advisor: 5 books in 1* (pp. 145–147). Philadelphia: Elsevier.

1-139. **(C)** Korsakoff syndrome is characterized by retrograde and anterograde memory impairment, decreased spontaneity, decreased initiative, and confabulation (filling in memory gaps with distorted facts). Gait disturbances, paralysis of the eye muscles, and ataxia and vestibular dysfunction are clinical manifestations of Wernicke encephalopathy. Both conditions are the result of chronic alcohol ingestion and a thiamine deficiency. Thiamine plays a key role in glucose metabolism. The major organ systems that are affected by a thiamine deficiency are those that depend on energy from metabolism of carbohydrates: the peripheral nerves, heart, and brain. Other symptoms of thiamine deficiency include peripheral neuropathy with myelin degeneration, hypertension, and cardiomyopathy.

Reference: Ferri, F. (2017). Korsakoff psychosis. In F. Ferri, *2017 Ferri's clinical advisor: 5 books in 1* (p. 705). Philadelphia: Elsevier.

1-140. **(D)** The immediate need of this patient is to alleviate her frustration by consulting a speech therapist who can assist the patient in regaining and improving her speech expression. Collaboration with the speech therapist will, in turn, help to alleviate the patient's vexation with her current limitations. Nothing in the scenario described supports this patient's need for either occupational or physical therapy. Although the patient's responses of anger and frustration might suggest the need for a psychiatric social worker, these are perfectly normal early behavioral responses to the patient's current physical challenges.

Reference: Dermenchyan, A. (2018). Professional caring and ethical practice. In T. M. Hartjes (Ed.), *AACN core curriculum for high acuity, progressive, and critical care nursing* (7th ed.). St. Louis: Elsevier.

1-141. **(C)** Kubler-Ross described the stages of the dying process as denial, anger and rage, bargaining, depression, and then acceptance. Each patient and family is heavily influenced by the circumstances surrounding the patient's death. Despair is a characteristic of Erikson's stages of development for the late adult.

Reference: Wyckoff, M., & Hartjes, T. M. (2018). Critical care patients with special needs: palliative and end-of life care in the ICU. In T. M. Hartjes (Ed.), *AACN core curriculum for high acuity, progressive, and critical care nursing* (7th ed.). St. Louis: Elsevier.

1-142. **(B)** 50% Dextrose injection is hypertonic and may cause phlebitis and thrombosis at the site of injection. A continuous infusion of 10% dextrose is less irritating to the peripheral veins than repeated doses of 50% dextrose and will allow correction of fluid and electrolyte imbalances to occur at a slower and more steady pace, helping to avoid seizure or dysrhythmia activity. Because the patient has a diminished level of consciousness, it would not be safe to administer any form of glucose as an oral fluid. After beginning the 10% dextrose infusion, glucagon may be administered intramuscularly, not

intravenously. Although glargine insulin produces a steady control of glucose, this patient is in an acute phase and reduction of glucose would not be desirable at this time.

Reference: MacDermott, J. (2018). Endocrine system. In T. M. Hartjes (Ed.), *AACN core curriculum for high acuity, progressive, and critical care nursing* (7th ed.). St. Louis: Elsevier.

1-143. **(C)** During deep sedation and analgesia, there is a drug-induced depression of consciousness during which the patient cannot be easily aroused. During minimal sedation, patients respond normally to verbal commands. With moderate sedation, the patient responds to verbal commands alone or with light tactile stimulation. Dissociative sedation is a drug-induced trance-like cataleptic state with significant analgesia and amnesia without compromise of protective airway reflexes.

Reference: Makic, M. (2018). Critical care patients with special needs: sedation in critically ill patients. In T. M. Hartjes (Ed.), *AACN core curriculum for high acuity, progressive, and critical care nursing* (7th ed.). St. Louis: Elsevier.

1-144. **(A)** Urinary tract complications occur in 3% to 10% of renal transplant recipients. Abdominal discomfort and bladder distention indicate urinary tract obstruction, which could progress to renal transplant graft failure. An increase in urinary output and decreasing serum creatinine indicate improved renal function. Right upper quadrant tenderness and elevation of liver enzymes and bilirubin are indicative of rejection of a transplanted liver. Elevation of serum glucose with symptoms of hyperglycemia is associated with pancreatic rejection and would appear days after signs and symptoms of renal rejection in the case of transplant of multiple organs.

Reference: Boling, B. (2018). Renal system. In T. M. Hartjes (Ed.), *AACN core curriculum for high acuity, progressive, and critical care nursing* (7th ed.). St. Louis: Elsevier.

1-145. **(D)** Patients with crush injuries are susceptible to the development of rhabdomyolysis with subsequent secondary kidney failure. Myoglobin (an intracellular substance) is released from muscle cell death and can cause renal failure. Dark, tea-colored urine suggests that the patient has myoglobinuria. After myoglobinuria is diagnosed, treatment is aimed at preventing subsequent renal failure. Aggressive administration of IV fluids increases renal blood flow and decreases the concentration of nephrotoxic pigments. Continuous infusion of mannitol and sodium bicarbonate will alkalinize the urine and prevent myoglobin crystallization in the renal tubules. Nursing management is aimed at achieving fluid and electrolyte balance. The patient needs to be assessed for hypernatremia, hyperosmolality, and volume overload. Patient management goals include maintaining a serum pH less than 7.5, serum Na of 135 to 145 mEq/L, urine output greater than or equal to 200 mL/hr, and urine pH of 6.0 to 7.0.

References: Holleran, R. (2018). Multisystem: Multisystem trauma. In T. M. Hartjes (Ed.), *AACN core curriculum for high acuity, progressive, and critical care nursing* (7th ed.). St. Louis: Elsevier.

Urden, L. (2018). Trauma. In L. Urden, K. Stacy, & M. Lough (Eds.), *Critical care nursing: Diagnosis and management*. St. Louis, MO: Mosby/Elsevier.

1-146. **(D)** Patients with inferior wall MI often complain of abdominal or gastrointestinal symptoms. A 12-lead ECG should be performed before administration of nitroglycerin to detect changes because of ischemia. NG decompression should be attempted with caution in a patient on heparin and is not indicated for this patient's symptoms. Troponin studies should be performed after the 12- lead ECG and nitroglycerin are administered.

Reference: Efre, A., & Boling, B. (2018). Cardiovascular system. In T. M. Hartjes (Ed.), *AACN core curriculum for high acuity, progressive, and critical care nursing* (7th ed.). St. Louis: Elsevier.

1-147. **(C)** A sudden decrease or absence of chest drainage may indicate an obstruction in the chest tube caused by tube kinking or the presence of a blood clot or tissue debris. Tube obstruction can interfere with the reexpansion of the lung after hemothorax or pneumothorax and contribute to hemodynamic compromise. Fluctuation or tidaling in the water seal chamber indicates a properly functioning chest tube. Discomfort at the chest tube insertion site can be relieved with analgesics. Intermittent bubbling in the water seal chamber may occur when the system is initially placed to suction and may continue until the patient's lung is re expanded.

References: Storzer, D. N. (2018). Pulmonary system. In T. M. Hartjes (Ed.), *AACN core curriculum for high acuity, progressive, and critical care nursing* (7th ed.). St. Louis: Elsevier.

Moore, S. M., Pieracci, F. M., & Jurkovich, G. J. (2017). Chest wall, pneumothorax, and hemothorax. In A. M. Cameron, & J. L. Cameron (Authors), *Current surgical therapy* (pp. 1151–1158). Philadelphia: Elsevier Saunders.

1-148. **(A)** The risk factors for hospital-acquired infection with methicillin-resistant *Staphylococcus* aureus (MRSA) include antibiotic treatment in the past 90 days, hospital stay of 5 or more days within the last 12 months, residence in a long-term facility, open skin wound or central intravenous catheter (including hemodialysis patients), recent major surgery, medical conditions that cause immunosuppression, and hospital stays at a health care facility with high rates of MRSA infection. A patient with recent bacterial pneumonia has received antibiotic treatment. Age, gender, and peripheral IV placement are not considered risk factors for the acquisition of MRSA.

Reference: Dressler, D. (2018). Hematological and immunological systems. In T. M. Hartjes (Ed.), *AACN core curriculum for high acuity, progressive, and critical care nursing* (7th ed.). St. Louis: Elsevier.

1-149. **(D)** In most people, the dominant internal carotid artery is on the left, so a stroke involving that artery would be expected to produce the clinical picture described. A right middle cerebral artery (Option A) stroke would produce left-side motor or sensory loss (greater in arm than leg), left-side motor loss in lower face, left-side visual field loss, and aphasia. A right vertebral artery (Option B) stroke would likely cause right facial weakness and numbness, facial and eye pain, clumsiness, ataxia, vertigo, nystagmus, hiccups, dysphagia, and dysarthria. Left anterior cerebral artery (Option C) stroke would typically result in confusion, personality changes, perseveration, incontinence, and right-sided motor or sensory loss (greater in the leg than the arm).

Reference: Blissitt, P. A. (2018). Neurologic system. In T. M. Hartjes (Ed.), *AACN core curriculum for high acuity, progressive, and critical care nursing* (7th ed.). St. Louis: Elsevier.

1-150. **(D)** The most appropriate nursing action is to continue to monitor the patient on the current ventilator settings. Permissive hypercapnia is used in ARDS to prevent volutrauma from large tidal volumes and high PEEP levels. The use of tidal volumes from 5 to 7 mL/kg decreases the risk of volutrauma in noncompliant lung tissue. Increased respiratory rates increase patient energy use and may also increase the risk of alveolar damage because of air trapping. Therapy goals in ARDS include maintaining the pH greater than 7.20. If the pH decreases to lower than 7.20, sodium bicarbonate may be used to raise the pH.

References: Storzer, D. N. (2018). Pulmonary system. In T. M. Hartjes (Ed.), *AACN core curriculum for high acuity, progressive, and critical care nursing* (7th ed.). St. Louis: Elsevier.

Stacy, K. (2018). Pulmonary disorders. In L. Urden, K. Stacy, & M. Lough (Eds.), *Critical care nursing: Diagnosis and management*. St. Louis, MO, Mosby/Elsevier.

2 Core Review Test 2

2-1. A patient with ARDS has a PaO_2 of 60% on mechanical ventilation with an FiO_2 of 0.8 and 20 cm H_2O of PEEP. Physical assessment findings include patient is unresponsive to pain; RR 14 breaths/min at ventilator setting of 12 breaths/min; temperature 38.6°C; BP 88/64 mm Hg; HR 112/min. Urine output is 20 mL for 2 hours. Chest x-ray shows complete opacification on left lung as well as right lower and middle lobes with radiolucence in right middle lobe. Which of these immediate interventions should the nurse now anticipate?
  A. Insertion of a chest tube to relieve pneumothorax
  B. Administration of furosemide (Lasix) 40 mg intravenous to stimulate diuresis
  C. Administration of norepinephrine (Levophed) to support systolic BP
  D. Obtaining a sputum culture before initiating antibiotics

2-2. An 89-year-old patient is in the ICU for 1 week with maximal medical therapy for a hemorrhagic stroke after warfarin overdose. Her Glasgow Coma Scale score is 3 since her admission to the hospital. Her pupils are equally nonreactive. She is being evaluated for brain death. Which of these neurologic deficits would the nurse correctly interpret as supporting a determination of brain death?
  A. Loss of vascular tone
  B. Loss of response to barbiturate infusion
  C. Loss of spinal reflex arc response
  D. Loss of spontaneous respiratory effort

2-3. The ICU nurse is receiving a patient from the emergency room. He was admitted with a 4-day history of chest pain, nausea, and vomiting. His cardiac workup is negative. The nurse suspects that the patient's complaints are related to electrolyte deficiencies. Which of these clinical findings support the nurse's suspicions?
  A. Hyperglycemia, peaked T waves, diarrhea
  B. Lethargy, confusion, bradycardia
  C. Headache, nausea, muscle weakness, orthostatic hypotension
  D. Tachycardia, abdominal cramps, increased reflexes

2-4. A pedestrian is hit by a truck when crossing the road. He is diagnosed with blunt thoracic trauma. Assessment of the patient reveals a flail chest with paradoxical chest wall motion. The critical care nurse notes that the unstable, injured segment of the chest moves
  A. Outward during inspiration, inward during expiration
  B. Outward during inspiration, outward during expiration
  C. Inward during inspiration, outward during expiration
  D. Inward during inspiration, inward during expiration

2-5. A patient with ARDS and severe acute respiratory failure is placed on ECMO (extracorporeal membrane oxygenation). The critical care nurse understands that for this patient, ECMO will
  A. Protect the lungs from barotrauma
  B. Remove CO_2 and add O_2 to the blood
  C. Reduce the risk of pulmonary embolism
  D. Decrease the risk of bacteremia

2-6. A patient has arrived to the ICU after having a reaction to peanuts. Her roommate was eating a peanut butter sandwich when the patient developed dyspnea, wheezing, chest tightness, pruritus, dizziness, and syncope. The ICU nurse anticipates which of the following hemodynamics?
  A. Increased systemic vascular resistance
  B. Increased cardiac output
  C. Increased cardiac index
  D. Decreased systemic vascular resistance

2-7. The nurse is providing patient teaching while administering immunosuppressive therapy to an organ transplant recipient. Which of these statements indicates that the patient has a correct understanding of his or her planned immunosuppressive regimen?
  A. "If I miss a dose of my immunosuppressive medication, I can just double the dose the next time to make up for it."
  B. "I can take my sirolimus and cyclosporine together before bed."
  C. "To reduce the chance of stomach ulcers, I will take my immunosuppressive medication with a meal."
  D. "My blood pressure will increase when I take my immunosuppressive medication, but this is normal."

2-8. A 62-year-old patient recently admitted with new onset of heart failure appears distressed regarding her health condition. During the admission assessment, the nurse should determine how this patient has viewed past successes in life as well as her health and satisfaction with life because considering these issues can
  A. Encourage patients to adapt to new challenges
  B. Explain their current health problems
  C. Enable patients to view their life within context
  D. Help patients confront their own mortality

2-9. During a code blue incident in an outpatient clinic, the patient was found to be hypoglycemic. Resuscitative efforts were successful after 50 mL of 50% dextrose was administered. When should the patient's capillary glucose measurement be repeated?
  A. 10 minutes after the patient's cardiac rhythm and pulse are restored
  B. 20 minutes after the dose of 50% dextrose was administered
  C. Upon admission to the ICU
  D. 30 minutes after the last capillary glucose measurement

2-10. A patient arrives at the emergency room with shortness of breath and rapid weight gain. This is the patient's third admission this month for CHF. The patient is known to be noncompliant with his medical regimen. Which of the following is a contributing factor to noncompliance?
  A. Employment status
  B. Advanced age
  C. Marital status
  D. Lack of family support

2-11. A patient has a central venous catheter, which was placed emergently during a cardiac arrest. Which of the following is indicated to help reduce the incidence of a catheter-related bloodstream infection?
  A. Use chlorhexidine gluconate solution for site care
  B. Change the intravenous tubing with crystalloid therapy every 48 hours
  C. Replace the transducer, flush device, flush solution, and tubing every 48 hours
  D. Collaborate with the physician to replace the catheter within 72 hours

2-12. Recommendations for monitoring patients thought to have carbon monoxide poisoning include obtaining carboxyhemoglobin levels and ABG samples to evaluate the SpO_2. In this patient population, the primary reason why pulse oximetry measurements (SpO_2) are considered unreliable and inaccurate for monitoring SpO2 is because the
  A. SpO_2 is often spurious in hemodynamically unstable patients
  B. Cherry red skin color changes associated with this disorder invalidate oximetry measurements

C. Patient must receive 100% oxygen

D. SpO_2 does not specifically reflect the percentage of hemoglobin saturated with oxygen

2-13. A postoperative CABG (coronary artery bypass graft) patient with a history of pulmonary hypertension is admitted to the ICU. He has a pulmonary artery catheter, and his mean pulmonary artery pressure is 30 mm Hg. He has signs of right ventricular failure and is unable to wean from the ventilator. Which of these therapies would be most appropriate?

A. Phlebotomy to maintain hematocrit at 48%

B. Fluid bolus to increase right ventricular output

C. Epoprostenol (Flolan) to dilate pulmonary arteries

D. Initiate IV anticoagulation

2-14. A morbidly obese patient is admitted to the unit after a laparoscopic cholecystectomy. The nurse knows that this patient is at risk for developing hospital-associated pneumonia because

A. His body habitus causes him to hypoventilate, leading to atelectasis

B. Obese patients are noncompliant with incentive spirometry

C. All patients with cholecystitis are at risk for developing pneumonia

D. Obese patients cannot get adequate pain management

2-15. A patient is in the critical care unit after emergency right hemicolectomy for a penetrating shotgun wound. Clinical findings include pulse 145 beats/min; temperature 38.9°C; abdominal distention; hypoactive bowel sounds; BP had been 140/86 mm Hg but is now 108/80 mm Hg; and extremities very warm to touch with bounding pulses. The physician orders rapid fluid administration, blood cultures, and antibiotics. What clinical finding would the nurse look for in this patient as evidence of an optimal clinical response to rapid IV fluid administration?

A. Central venous pressure of 4 mm Hg

B. Lactate level 3 mmol/L

C. Urine output less than 0.5 mL/Kg/h

D. Cool, dry skin

2-16. Which of these medications is administered to prevent sudden death associated with dilated cardiomyopathy?

A. Amiodarone (Cordarone)

B. Calcium channel blockers

C. Nitrates

D. Digoxin

2-17. A 78-year-old woman is admitted to the ICU for exacerbation of COPD and congestive heart failure. This is her third admission in the past 4 weeks. Her ejection fraction is less than 10%, and she is treated with home oxygen and milrinone therapy. The critical care nurse suggests that this patient would benefit from a palliative care consult. However, the critical care team refuses the suggestion. Which of these initiatives would be most beneficial to overcome the barriers to palliative care consultations?

A. Discuss palliative care with the patient and family

B. Notify the hospital ethics board

C. Develop unit-specific criteria for patient referral

D. Contact the nursing supervisor

2-18. A 54-year-old patient with end-stage renal disease (ESRD) is admitted to the ICU after falling down three flights of stairs. The patient's BP is 200/116 mm Hg, HR is 118/min, and RR is 32/min. The patient complains of fatigue, headache, lightheadedness, and palpitations; laboratory work reveals hemoglobin 7.6 g/dL and hematocrit 22.8%. The patient is currently receiving 3000 units of epoetin alfa (Epogen, Procrit) three times per week. Which of these interventions is the most warranted at this time?

A. Transfuse with one unit of packed red blood cells

B. Increase epoetin alfa by 1000 units

C. Continue to monitor the patient

D. Decrease epoetin alfa by 500 units

2-19. A patient is admitted to the ICU at a community hospital for complaints of chest pain, and he is currently chest pain free. Three hours after admission, the patient develops severe chest pain unrelieved by aspirin or nitroglycerin. A 12-lead ECG shows ST segment elevation in leads II, III, and aVF.

Which of these interventions would most benefit this patient?

A. Administration of thrombolytic therapy

B. Transfer to a facility that performs open heart surgery

C. Administration of heparin and G IIb/IIIa inhibitor

D. Immediate transfer to the cardiac catheterization suite for percutaneous coronary intervention

2-20. When planning nursing care for a suicidal patient, the ICU nurse is aware of characteristics of suicidal patients. Which of these statements about suicidal patients is false?

A. Directly asking a person about suicidal intent will not cause suicide

B. Suicidal behavior does not necessarily mean that the person has mental illness

C. Suicidal behavior is more prevalent in white men

D. Suicidal persons usually give clues about their intentions

2-21. A 26-year-old female is admitted to the ICU after a motor vehicle accident. She experienced a transient loss of consciousness at the scene of the accident but is currently alert and oriented. She is diagnosed with a linear left temporal skull fracture. Two hours after admission, the patient's neurologic status deteriorates. Which of these interventions would the critical care nurse anticipate?

A. Cerebral angiography and coil embolization

B. Ventriculostomy and cerebrospinal fluid drainage

C. Osmotic diuretic and corticosteroid therapy

D. Burr holes and clot evacuation

2-22. A 22-year-old female who received a renal transplant 1 year ago presents to the emergency room with complaints of urinary frequency and cloudy urine for the past 2 weeks. She is admitted to the ICU with pyelonephritis. Which of the following would be the nurse's best response to effectively address the patient's knowledge deficit and prevent delays in treatment of future infections?

A. "You need to restrict your physical activities to avoid complications."

B. "Avoid foods high in folic acid so your immunosuppressive therapy remains effective."

C. "Be sure to drink plenty of fluids to avoid becoming dehydrated."

D. "Report any unusual sensations you experience as they may be a sign of infection."

2-23. A 45-year-old homeless man is admitted to the ICU after he was found unresponsive in an alley. He is intubated on mechanical ventilation, and he is receiving a norepinephrine infusion at 2 mcg/min. A thorough assessment reveals stable vital signs, absence of cerebral motor reflexes, absence of brainstem reflexes, and absence of respiratory drive. The social service department is attempting to locate relatives for the patient. Which of the following interventions would be most important to perform next?

A. Contact the ethics department to initiate a DNR process

B. Consult care management for long-term care placement

C. Consult nutritional support

D. Notify the local organ procurement organization

2-24. A postoperative trauma patient in the ICU was admitted 2 days ago after a motor vehicle accident. On multidisciplinary rounds, which of the following should the nurse suggest to help prevent deep vein thrombosis in this patient?

A. Intermittent pneumatic compression devices and low molecular weight heparin

B. Venous foot pumps and low-molecular-weight heparin

C. Below-the-knee graded stockings and unfractionated heparin

D. Below-the-knee graded stockings and low-molecular-weight heparin

2-25. A patient with a high output enterocutaneous fistula is NPO on hyperalimentation at a rate of 80 mL/hr. The patient is listless but responds to commands appropriately. Heart rate is 124/min sinus tachycardia, and BP 88/50 mm Hg. Respiratory rate is 24/min on 40% face mask with a SpO_2 of 100%. Other assessment findings include 2+ edema in dependent areas and a capillary refill time of 4 seconds. Admission laboratory values include hematocrit 30%; serum sodium 150 mEq/L; glucose 90 mg/

dL; albumin 1.9 g/dL. The nurse antici-pates immediate administration of which of the following?

A. 1 unit of packed red blood cells
B. 25 mL of dextrose 50%
C. 250 mL of normal saline bolus
D. 250 mL of 5% albumin

2-26. A patient presents with flu-like symptoms, lymphadenopathy, a diffuse erythematous rash, and severe muscle weakness. The nurse admits the patient for close monitor-ing and further diagnostic workup to iden-tify the cause of these findings. The patient suddenly loses consciousness followed by a brief period of muscle rigidity and then rhythmic muscle jerking. The best immedi-ate course of action for the nurse is to

A. Obtain a serum laboratory specimen for STAT identification of a disease-specific antigen or antibody causing this syndrome
B. Observe, record, and report all details of these clinical events to the physician as soon as these muscular movements have subsided
C. Administer benzodiazepine per stand-ing order to stop the seizure activity
D. Quickly apply soft restraints to prevent injury

2-27. A multidisciplinary team has been formed to prevent pressure ulcers in the ICU. Criti-cally ill patients are at high risk for pres-sure ulcers and complications from pressure ulcers. Which of these statements about pressure ulcers is false?

A. Some pressure ulcers are unavoidable
B. Patients with an open chest and/or ECMO are usually too unstable to turn
C. A surgical bra can cause pressure ulcers
D. Tracheostomy related pressure ulcers can be caused by surgical techniques

2-28. A patient is admitted to the ICU with a diag-nosis of viral myocarditis. She complains of persistent chest pain. Which of these medication regimens would be most appro-priate to relieve chest pain associated with myocarditis?

A. Nitroglycerin 1/150 grains sublingual
B. Furosemide 40 mg IV
C. Ibuprofen 800 mg PO
D. Morphine sulfate 2 mg IV

2-29. The critical care nurse is assigned to care for a patient who presented an hour ago in the emergency room. The patient complains of malaise, fever, and jaundice. Her liver enzymes are markedly elevated. The criti-cal care nurse's primary concern would be to determine whether the patient manifests clinical features associated with

A. Intractable hypotension
B. Early stages of esophageal bleeding
C. Development of systemic infection
D. Diminished level of consciousness

2-30. A patient complains of substernal pressure and becomes diaphoretic. A 12-lead ECG obtained during chest pain demonstrates tall, broad R waves and ST segment depres-sion in leads V1 to V3. These findings sug-gest that the nurse now needs to

A. Continue monitoring the patient for unstable angina
B. Assess the patient for fever and other signs of pericarditis
C. Examine the patient for findings related to posterior wall MI
D. Prepare the patient for possible cardio-version for septal MI

2-31. You are caring for a 63-year-old patient with a left-side intracerebral hemorrhage. The next day, his level of conscious-ness deteriorates secondary to intracranial hypertension, which requires endotracheal intubation and mechanical ventilation. You initiate a mannitol infusion and notice a 2-cm area of blanched skin and edema that is cool to the touch at the IV site. Nursing interventions for this patient include all the following EXCEPT

A. Apply a warm pack to the site
B. Aspirating the residual medication from the IV with a 3-cc syringe
C. Elevate the extremity to prevent edema
D. Remove the IV catheter with minimal pressure applied for hemostasis

2-32. Mr. Jones is a 56-year-old patient admitted to the ICU for chest pain. His critical care team documents in the medical record that the patient has metabolic syndrome. The nurse knows that patient education has a critical influence on Mr. Jones' outcome.

What would be the most important concept to emphasize during patient education?

A. Eating low-fat foods will improve metabolic syndrome

B. Weight loss can prevent disease progression

C. Metabolic syndrome is associated with a higher risk of bone fractures

D. Metabolic syndrome always progresses to diabetes mellitus

2-33. A patient with chronic pulmonary disease is admitted to the ICU with worsening dyspnea and pulmonary mechanics. The patient's medical history includes chronic bronchitis that requires home oxygen, anxiety, and a 5-kg weight loss over the previous 4 weeks. In noting these findings, the critical care nurse will plan nursing care with the understanding that in this patient population, weight loss is typically associated with

A. Cor pulmonale

B. Increased mortality

C. Improved thoracic excursion

D. Dehydration

2-34. You are assigned to care for an ICU patient who is postoperative day 6 post gastric bypass surgery. He has failed to wean from the ventilator, and he remains intubated and sedated. After reviewing the chart, you suggest an intervention to improve this patient's survival. Which of these interventions would have the most effect on the patient's survival?

A. Consult with the wound and ostomy nurse to assess early signs of wound infection

B. Collaborate with the dietitian to carefully assess for nutritional deficiencies

C. Collaborate with the physician to start a bowel regimen

D. Consult with pharmacy regarding initiation of low-molecular-weight heparin

2-35. During sheath removal after percutaneous coronary intervention (PCI), a patient's heart rate decreases to 40 beats/min, BP decreases to 80/50 mm Hg, and the patient complains of nausea. Appropriate treatment for this patient would include which of the following?

A. Continue to monitor the patient, anticipating the heart rate and BP will return to baseline within 5 minutes

B. Administer atropine 0.5 mg intravenously to treat vasovagal reaction

C. Administer prochlorperazine (Compazine) 10 mg IV to reduce nausea

D. Notify the MD immediately of potential retroperitoneal bleeding

2-36. You are the preceptor for a new nurse on your unit. She is caring for a 45-year-old man diagnosed with pneumonia secondary to HIV. The new nurse asks you to assist her in choosing the best topic for patient education. Which would be the best choice of those listed below?

A. Sexual promiscuity

B. Methods to prevent infection

C. Pain management techniques

D. Avoid pneumococcal and influenza vaccines

2-37. A patient arrives in the emergency room with severe chest pain and shortness of breath. A bedside ECG reveals ST elevations in leads II, III, and aVF with reciprocal changes in I, aVL, V5, and V6. A right-side ECG shows ST elevation in V4R. The most appropriate treatment for this myocardial infarction includes which of the following?

A. Diuretics

B. Intravenous fluid bolus

C. Morphine

D. Nitroglycerin

2-38. During the neurologic assessment of a patient who was the driver involved in a head-on collision, the critical care nurse finds no evidence of motor function or ability to sense pain or temperature lower than the nipple line. These neurologic findings suggest that this patient will require nursing management for

A. Anterior cord syndrome

B. Central cord syndrome

C. Brown-Sequard syndrome

D. Posterior cord syndrome

2-39. An ICU patient is admitted for monitoring after she arrived to the ER reporting that her ICD had fired multiple times. Device interrogation demonstrated that the device was firing appropriately. Which of these assessments would be most appropriate at this time?

A. 12-lead ECG with magnet in place to identify intrinsic cardiac rhythm

B. Chest x-ray to determine whether lead fracture has occurred

C. Evaluation of serum electrolytes to identify source of dysrhythmia

D. Electrophysiology testing to determine the source of the dysrhythmia

2-40. The critical care nurse is caring for a patient who is recuperating from a stroke. The patient continues to demonstrate intermittent lethargy and expressive aphasia. As a result, the patient is being closely monitored for difficulty with coughing or swallowing. This patient is at high risk for aspiration. Which of these findings is an early indication that the patient may have aspirated?

A. Increased $PaCO_2$

B. Chest x-ray demonstrating bilateral infiltrates

C. Tachypnea and tachycardia

D. Coughing and positive sputum cultures

2-41. A patient is in the ICU for COPD exacerbation. He is intubated, sedated, and receiving IV steroids and antibiotic therapy. His morning blood glucose level is 465 mg/dL. As a result, he was administered 12 units of subcutaneous lispro insulin. After 4 hours, the repeat blood glucose level is 410 mg/dL. Which of these interventions would the critical care nurse anticipate?

A. Document the laboratory results and continue to monitor

B. Administer an additional 12 units of subcutaneous lispro insulin

C. Begin administration of intravenous insulin at 2 units/hr and repeat blood glucose hourly

D. Administer a bolus dose of 10 units of IV regular insulin

2-42. A patient is admitted with a diagnosis of hyperosmolar hyperglycemic syndrome. Which of these findings would not be expected for this patient?

A. Fever and elevated white blood cell count

B. High levels of urine ketones

C. Blood glucose greater than 600 mg/dL

D. Reversible hemiplegia, focal seizures

2-43. A nurse on the unit has expressed concerns that there have been many poor outcomes with the minimally invasive surgical patients. You have not observed this trend.

Which of the following would be the most appropriate suggestion that you could make to this colleague?

A. Start developing a list of patients admitted for minimally invasive surgery and document the outcomes for each over the next 6 months

B. Conduct a chart audit of all the minimally invasive surgical patients over the past 6 months

C. Discuss the observation with the cardiothoracic surgeon

D. Present the concern at the next staff meeting

2-44. A patient with supratentorial intracerebral hemorrhage is being transferred to the ICU from the emergency room. Which action would be most appropriate for this patient?

A. Aggressive reduction of blood pressure

B. STAT completion of cerebral angiography

C. Correction of coagulopathy

D. Surgical evacuation of the clot

2-45. An assault victim who was stabbed undergoes a right posterolateral thoracotomy for repair of a membranous tracheal tear located 4 cm higher than the carina, associated with pneumomediastinum and bilateral pneumothoraces. A few hours after the patient's return from surgery, a bronchoscopy is performed to clear secretions. Over the next few hours, it is important that the nurse monitors the chest drainage system to ensure

A. Bubbling in the water seal chamber

B. Adequate dependent loops in tubing

C. Positive pressure in the closed drainage system

D. Clamping of the chest tube

2-46. An elderly patient admitted for urosepsis is diagnosed with septic shock. The patient has received adequate crystalloid and colloid resuscitation; however, the current laboratory values show a high lactic acid level and SvO_2 of 84%. The critical care nurse anticipates initiating a vasopressor. Given the following vital signs and hemodynamic parameters, which vasopressor would be the best choice for this patient: HR 115/min, sinus tachycardia; BP 80/40 mm Hg; PAP

30/15 mm Hg; PCWP 14 mm Hg; CO 10.0 L/min; CI 5.2 L/min/cm^2; SVR 500 dynes/sec/cm^{-5}?

A. Dopamine
B. Epinephrine
C. Norepinephrine
D. Vasopressin

2-47. John Doe has arrived in the emergency room after a serious motorcycle accident. He will require massive blood and blood product transfusions and aggressive fluid resuscitation. Which of these interventions will prevent the greatest number of complications for this patient?

A. Use of warmed blood components and intravenous fluids
B. Vigilant monitoring of laboratory values
C. Premedication with antihistamines and antiinflammatory agents
D. Intramuscular administration of tetanus toxoid

2-48. A nurse in the ICU would like to change the unit's visitation policy to facilitate a family-centered care model that engages families to participate in patient care. Which of the following would be the best approach to initiate a change the visitation policy?

A. Ask the manager to provide unlimited visitation
B. Complete a literature search to identify different family-centered care models
C. Encourage colleagues to disregard the current visiting policy
D. Create a survey for patients and families to determine if they want the visitation policy changed

2-49. A patient with diabetes is admitted to the ICU with a diagnosis of hypertensive urgency 2 weeks after Roux-en-Y gastric bypass surgery. The patient says, "I don't understand how my blood pressure can still be so high. I thought that operation was going to fix my blood pressure problems." The most appropriate nursing response is

A. "I will ask the nutritionist to review your preoperative nutrition counseling materials with you. It might be from the food you are eating."
B. "An adjustable band was placed around the upper part of your stomach to create a small pouch. The band is adjustable

and can be tightened to allow feelings of being full longer. Your band may be a bit tight now, causing you stress."
C. "A leak is a common complication of your procedure and could potentially cause changes in blood pressure."
D. "Hypertensive patients taking antihypertensive medications have small blood pressure reductions after this surgery. It will take time for you to achieve the most blood pressure improvement."

2-50. Critical care nurses are at risk for experiencing aggression and violence in the ICU. Which of the following is an appropriate intervention to prevent the escalation of aggression in patients or family members?

A. Interrupt the patient or family member who is verbally ventilating to prevent escalation
B. Provide education for the patient and family about aggressive and violent behavior during episodes of escalation
C. Attempt to distract from the incident at hand
D. Place clear limits on what will or will not be tolerated and the subsequent consequences

2-51. Mrs. Jones is an 82-year-old 50-kg patient on the general medical floor with a diagnosis of failure to thrive. She is transferred to the ICU after the rapid response team was called for an acute change in mental status. Current assessment findings are as follows; GCS score 11, temperature 38.8°C; heart rate 114 beats/min, blood pressure 85/45 mm Hg, respiratory rate 32 breaths/minute, SpO$_2$ 93% on 4 L nasal cannula, and urine output of 10 mL/hr. The critical care prepares for which of the following **first** interventions?

A. Blood cultures and IV antibiotics
B. 0.9 % normal saline bolus followed by IV infusion at 500 mL/hr
C. Norepinephrine IV infusion
D. Goals of care discussion with the family

2-52. A patient is receiving a milrinone infusion for acute decompensated heart failure. Her ejection fraction is 15% secondary to ischemic cardiomyopathy. The critical care nurse notices increased ventricular ectopy on the heart monitor 8 hours after the infusion was initiated. The ectopy progresses to multiple runs of 3 to 6 beats of ventricular tachycardia. The critical care nurse anticipates which of these actions?

A. Discontinue the milrinone infusion
B. Obtain blood sample for electrolyte levels
C. Administer a 250-mL normal saline fluid bolus
D. Continue the milrinone infusion and administer 40 mg of furosemide (Lasix) intravenously

2-53. A patient admitted for a right lower lobectomy secondary to adenocarcinoma is admitted to the ICU. Two hours postoperatively, the patient is alert and oriented with stable vital signs and requires 4 L of oxygen via nasal cannula to maintain an O_2 saturation of 96%. During the night, his SpO_2 falls to 89%, his respiratory rate increases to 40 breaths/min, and he complains of increased pain in the right chest. His bilateral breath sounds are clear but diminished in both bases. What are the most appropriate initial nursing actions?

A. Place patient on a face mask at FiO_2 40% and obtain an ABG
B. Administer pain medication and encourage the patient to cough and use the incentive spirometer
C. Obtain an order for chest x-ray to evaluate for hemothorax and increase oxygen to 6 L/min
D. Administer a sedative and encourage use of deep breathing and relaxation techniques

2-54. In acute pancreatitis, acute respiratory distress syndrome (ARDS) represents a common complication caused by the release of pancreatic enzymes into the circulation. Which of these other possible complications of pancreatitis can then complicate management of ARDS?

A. Hypovolemia
B. Fistula formation
C. Pleural effusion
D. Severe pain

2-55. A patient admitted for symptomatic bradycardia will have an emergency bedside transvenous pacemaker placed. After insertion, the patient complains of chest pain. His blood pressure drops from 130/70 mm Hg to 96/78 mm Hg. JVD is visible, and his respirations become shallow and rapid, with clear equal breath sounds. The heart rate is 70 beats/min 100% paced. The most likely cause of these findings is

A. Hemothorax
B. Pneumothorax
C. Pericardial tamponade
D. Pacemaker lead infection

2-56. A new graduate is being precepted and is caring for a patient with neurologic impairment. The patient is intubated and sedated. The orientee inserts a nasogastric (NG) tube and is about to administer medication through the tube. When the preceptor asks how NG tube placement was verified, the orientee says that it was verified by auscultation of insufflated air at the gastric area. The preceptor's best initial response is to

A. Explain that observing for exhalation bubbles when the tube's hub is held under water is a more accurate method to verify tube placement
B. Verify the medication order before allowing the orientee to proceed
C. Observe the patient for the onset of respiratory symptoms (e.g., coughing, cyanosis, or dyspnea) for a few minutes before medication administration
D. Confirm placement with capnography, observation of gastric aspirate, and a chest radiograph before administering medication

2-57. The critical care nurse is at the bedside providing patient education for a 56-year-old male patient with acute renal failure. The nurse is reinforcing education about infection prevention and explains that the patient is at risk for infection as a result of which of the following?

A. Excessive carbohydrate intake
B. Fluid overload
C. Uremia
D. Fluid restriction

2-58. A patient with end-stage heart failure is admitted to the intensive care unit minimally responsive with a heart rate 86 beats/min BP 80/66 mm Hg, and RR 26/min on 60% BiPAP facemask. The patient has crackles at both lung bases. Home medications include

furosemide, atenolol, potassium, and captopril. Admitting labs include a serum albumin
level of 2.0 g/dL, HCT 52%, BUN 62 mg/dL,
and creatinine 3.0 mg/dL. The most appropriate initial treatment for this patient would be to
A. Initiate a dobutamine infusion
B. Initiate a norepinephrine (Levophed)
infusion
C. Administer a 250-mL bolus of normal
saline
D. Administer 40 mg of furosemide (Lasix)
IV

2-59. Patients with chronic COPD frequently
experience anxiety and depression as a psychological comorbidity. Which of these caring practices would be most supportive and
therapeutic for the COPD patient?
A. Administering more benzodiazepines
than for non-COPD patients
B. Restarting the patient's normal daily
medications before discharge
C. Having a psychology consultation
completed during their hospitalization
D. Continuing the patient's normal daily
routines and practices when hospitalized

2-60. You are precepting a new graduate registered nurse in the ICU and teaching her
about the role of spirituality in the ICU.
Which of these statements best explains the
role of spirituality?
A. Spirituality issues should be addressed
in the ICU after the patient has been
stabilized
B. Addressing spirituality is best reserved
for patients at end of life
C. Spirituality may influence understanding of illness in the ICU
D. Inquiring about spirituality preferences
does nothing to alleviate the stress
associated with an acute condition that
requires ICU admission

2-61. You are caring for a patient with cardiogenic shock. The patient has an intraaortic
balloon pump. A new RN is orienting on the
unit and asks you to explain counterpulsation. You explain that intraaortic balloon
counterpulsation is used to manage cardiogenic shock in order to increase
A. Coronary artery perfusion during systole
B. Myocardial oxygen supply
C. Left ventricular filling volume
D. Left ventricular systolic pressure

2-62. A patient in the ICU has been admitted for
seizures. The patient is accompanied by his
friend who reports that the patient ran out of
medication "a while ago" and has not refilled
it. The friend does not know the patient's
medications, but he reports that he knows the
patient has a history of epilepsy and "fainting spells" from a low heart rate. The patient
is stable now and responded well to IV benzodiazepines in the emergency room. His
current vital signs are: temperature 37.1°C;
HR 58 beats/min; RR 16 breaths/min; blood
pressure 110/62 mm Hg. The patient begins
to seize after arrival to the ICU. Which of
these medications would be contraindicated
to treat this patient's seizure?
A. Phenytoin (Dilantin)
B. Lorazepam (Ativan)
C. Valproic acid (Depakote)
D. Levetiracetam (Keppra)

2-63. The nurse is assigned an 82-year-old frail
woman who is being transferred from the
ICU to telemetry. She was admitted to the
ICU for syncope and was later found to
have taken her home medications incor-
rectly. The patient tells the nurse, "I just
can't read the label like I used to; the print-
ing is so faint." She lives alone and does
not have children or relatives nearby. What
intervention best demonstrates advocacy
and moral agency?
A. Contact her pharmacy to ask about pro-
visions for vision-impaired patients
B. Reevaluate her medications for possible drug interactions
C. Contact the case manager for assistance in long-term placement
D. Develop a plan of care that includes
side effects of medications

2-64. A patient diagnosed with Brugada syndrome
is admitted to the unit for monitoring. The
ICU nurse is planning to provide education
about treatment for the syndrome. Which
of these education topics best describes the
treatment plan?
A. Preparing for ablation
B. Pharmacologic treatment for Brugada
syndrome
C. Preparing for ICD (implantable cardioverter-defibrillator) placement
D. Preparing for permanent pacemaker
placement

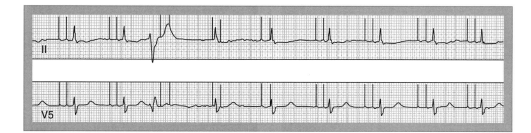

2-65. A patient with chronic COPD presents to the emergency room with worsening cardiac symptoms indicating cor pulmonale. Which of these manifestations describes the patient's symptoms?
- A. Fatigue and decreased CVP
- B. Distant heart sounds and jugular venous distention
- C. Exertional dyspnea and pedal edema
- D. Productive cough

2-66. A patient arrives in the emergency room complaining of severe "tearing" chest pain radiating to his back. His vital signs are temperature 37.0°C; HR 95 beats/min; RR 28 breaths/min; BP 164/92 mm Hg; pulse oxygen 99% on room air. A CT scan confirms aortic dissection. Which of these treatment regimens best describe initial treatment for this aortic dissection?
- A. IV morphine bolus and labetalol boluses and infusion titrated to a heart rate of 60 beats/min and systolic blood pressure 100 to 120 mm Hg
- B. IV hydromorphone bolus and sodium nitroprusside infusion titrated to a systolic blood pressure 100 to 120 Hg mm
- C. IV hydromorphone bolus and IV labetalol boluses and infusion titrated to a heart rate of 80 beats/min and systolic blood pressure 110 to 120 mm
- D. IV morphine bolus and sodium nitroprusside infusion titrated to a systolic blood pressure 90 to 100 mm Hg

2-67. A newly admitted patient with traumatic brain injury (TBI) is experiencing increased intracranial pressure (ICP). At this point in the patient's care, the nurse should maintain the patient's arterial $PaCO_2$ at a level
- A. Lower than 20 mm Hg
- B. Between 25 and 30 mm Hg
- C. Between 30 and 35 mm Hg
- D. Higher than 40 mm Hg

2-68. The permanent pacemaker rhythm strip above represents which of the following?
- A. Normal permanent pacemaker function
- B. Runaway pacemaker
- C. Failure to capture and undersensing
- D. Failure to capture and oversensing

2-69. An elderly woman presents to the emergency room with asymptomatic rapid atrial fibrillation and new onset urinary incontinence. The critical care nurse anticipates evaluating the patient for which of these reversible causes of urinary incontinence?
- A. Stool impaction
- B. Renal failure
- C. Dehydration
- D. Pregnancy

2-70. After a motor vehicle collision, a teenager is admitted with chest pain and an ineffective cough with hemoptysis. The admission chest x-ray reveals consolidation and pulmonary infiltration, likely evidence of a severe pulmonary contusion. The patient's respiratory rate is 23/min, and his arterial blood gases on room air are pH 7.42; $PaCO_2$ 30 mm Hg; PaO_2 54 mm Hg; HCO_3 24 mEq/L. Which of these pairs of interventions is most appropriate for this patient?
- A. Administer an analgesic and apply 100% O_2 by face mask
- B. Auscultate lung sounds and prepare for insertion of a chest tube
- C. Prepare for immediate intubation and mechanical ventilation
- D. Prepare for immediate thoracentesis and administer oxygen

2-71. A student nurse is working on the unit under your guidance. She has approached you about discontinuing a urinary catheter from her hospice patient. Her patient has a history of end-stage cardiomyopathy, and her diuretics cause urinary incontinence due to urgency and frequency. Which of these statements about catheter associated urinary tract infection prevention is most true?

A. "Daily meatal care prevents a UTI."
B. "The patient is on hospice care now, and it will improve comfort in the end of her life."
C. "The patient will develop UTI symptoms if she gets an infection."
D. "The family has demanded that the catheter remain."

2-72. A patient with hemorrhagic stroke has been on a ventilator for approximately 1 week and remains unresponsive. While he is receiving care, approximately 10 visitors from his church arrive and ask the nurse if they can have a prayer service in his room. The nurse agrees to give them time to be alone with the patient. After about 30 minutes, the nurse enters the room and finds that the patient's bed has been pulled away from the wall, and the 10 visitors have formed a circle around the bed and ventilator and are praying, chanting, and humming while the patient is resting quietly. The nurse's best response would be to

A. Interrupt the prayer session to continue providing supportive patient care
B. Quietly close the door and allow the group to finish their prayer
C. Move into the circle and join the prayer group
D. Stand against the wall and observe the group to ensure patient safety

2-73. The ICU nurse is caring for a patient with new-onset delirium. The patient is a 71-year-old male who has been in the ICU for 3 weeks for treatment of congestive heart failure. Which of these nursing interventions will have the most benefit for treating his delirium?

A. Administer additional diuretic
B. Encourage 24-hour visitation
C. Consult psychiatry to rule out dementia
D. Provide 6 hours of uninterrupted sleep at night

2-74. A patient is admitted to the ICU after ingestion of an unknown substance. The patient's arterial blood gas values are as follows: pH 7.50; $PaCO_2$ 22 mm Hg; PaO_2 120 mm Hg; HCO_3 15 mEq/L; anion gap greater than 20.

Based on these findings, the patient most likely ingested

A. Acetaminophen (Tylenol)
B. Salicylates (aspirin)
C. Nonsteroidal antiinflammatory medication (NSAID) (Advil)
D. Benzodiazepine (Valium)

2-75. A patient with medically refractory seizures is admitted to the unit. He has just arrived postoperatively after resection of a seizure focus. Which of these orders are inappropriate for this patient?

A. Neurologic examination hourly
B. Lorazepam 1 mg IV prn for seizures lasting longer than 10 minutes
C. Phenobarbital 10 to 20 mg/kg IV for refractory seizures
D. Postoperative brain MRI upon admission

2-76. Which of these vasopressors should the nurse anticipate using **first** for an end-stage cardiomyopathy patient with clinical evidence of pulmonary edema, signs and symptoms of shock, and systolic blood pressure less than 70 mm Hg?

A. Dopamine 10 mcg/kg/min
B. Dobutamine 10 mcg/kg/min
C. Nitroglycerin 20 mcg/min
D. Norepinephrine (Levophed) 5 mcg/min

2-77. A patient was admitted to the ICU yesterday after open heart surgery. Her husband inquires about the use of complementary therapies such as music to decrease pain. Which of these responses is the most appropriate?

A. "Use of music may reduce pain and tension."
B. "We will give your spouse as much pain medication as needed. Music therapy will not be necessary."
C. "Although use of music does not pose a safety concern, there are no studies to suggest that it will help manage postoperative pain."
D. "We can try it, but the portable radio or CD player will require approval by the biomedical department before it can be used, and headphones will be needed."

2-78. A patient in the emergency room complains of severe left lower extremity pain, especially during ambulation. He has a new

ulcer on his foot, and recently the extremity is painful even at rest. The critical care nurse anticipates transporting the patient to radiology for which of these tests?
- A. Lower extremity radiograph
- B. Magnetic resonance angiography
- C. Computed tomography angiography
- D. Ankle-brachial index

2-79. The critical care nurse has received report about a patient emergently transferring from a small community hospital. They are arriving for treatment of cardiogenic shock and papillary muscle rupture after a myocardial infarction. Which of these therapies would most benefit the patient upon arrival?
- A. Coronary artery bypass with mitral valve replacement
- B. PCI of occluded arteries and mitral valve replacement after the patient has stabilized
- C. Thrombolytic therapy to reperfuse occluded coronary arteries and mitral valve repair after the patient has stabilized
- D. Vasopressor support and intraaortic balloon pump counterpulsation

2-80. A young adult patient was found unconscious at home after missing an important family celebration. The patient had complained of nausea earlier in the day and had a dry, hacking cough for the previous 5 days. The following were found upon assessment and receipt of laboratory values: temperature 38.5°C; pulse 110/min; respirations 26/min; BP 92/64 mm Hg; capillary glucose 304 mg/dL; pH 7.32; PaO_2 98 mm Hg, $PaCO_2$ 32 mm Hg; and bicarbonate 18 mEq/L, with a urinary output of 20 mL in the previous hour. Which of the following should the nurse expect to administer at this time?
- A. 50 = mL bicarbonate intravenous push
- B. 100 units of glargine insulin subcutaneously
- C. 1000-mL normal saline via intravenous bolus
- D. 10 mEq of KCl in 100 mL of normal saline over 1 hour

2-81. You are caring for a patient with COPD who is intubated on mechanical ventilation. Her family is at the bedside, and they ask how the medical team will know when it is time to extubate. Which of the following is the best response to this question?
- A. Normal ABG values and chest x-ray findings
- B. Ability to wean pressure support to less than +10 cm H_2O
- C. Return to patient's baseline pulmonary function and ABG values
- D. Rapid shallow breathing index (RSBI) score

2-82. An 81-year-old patient with a history of severe heart failure, cardiomyopathy, and osteoarthritis is scheduled to receive physical therapy daily. The patient refuses PT due to severe arthritis pain. Which of the following is the most appropriate analgesic medication for this patient?
- A. A nonsteroidal antiinflammatory medication administered ½ to 1 hour before planned exercise
- B. Daily administration of corticosteroids to reduce inflammation
- C. Morphine sulfate 5 mg intravenously 10 minutes before planned exercise
- D. Acetaminophen 650 mg orally ½ to 1 hour before planned exercise

2-83. A 75-year-old patient was struck by a motor vehicle, sustaining a head injury. The patient is sedated, intubated, and on mechanical ventilation. Vital signs are mean arterial pressure 65 mm Hg; HR 84/min; RR 18/min; ICP 14 mm Hg. Which of the following is indicated at this time?
- A. Consult with the neurosurgeon regarding draining some fluid to decrease ICP
- B. Speak with the attending physician regarding administering a fluid bolus to increase MAP
- C. Call respiratory therapy to initiate hyperventilation to a $PaCO_2$ of 30 mm Hg
- D. No action is needed; these are acceptable values

2-84. A patient receiving chemotherapy for leukemia will be admitted to the ICU. She is expected to remain in the ICU for a prolonged duration. Which of the following nursing interventions will have the most impact on the patient's recovery?
- A. Encourage unlimited visitation from family and friends
- B. Provide frequent bathing, backrub, and oral care

C. Ask the family to bring in comfort articles from home like a pillow or blanket

D. Encourage family to bring the patient's cosmetics and comfortable clothing

2-85. Mr. Jones is admitted to the emergency room complaining of chest pain and shortness of breath. He has a history of hypertension, coronary artery disease, and ischemic cardiomyopathy. He informs the medical team that he ran out of his medications last week. His admission vital signs are temperature 37°C; HR 65 beats/min; RR 36 breaths/min; and BP 240/130 mm Hg. Mr. Jones has bibasilar rales, and his pulse oximetry reading is 85% on room air. Which of the following would be the most appropriate pharmacologic agent to lower the blood pressure in this patient?

A. Sodium nitroprusside (Nipride)

B. IV hydralazine (Apresoline)

C. Labetalol (Normodyne, Trandate)

D. Nicardipine (Cardene)

2-86. A 52-year-old healthy athlete is admitted to the ICU after complaining of progressive fatigue, loss of appetite, and a reduced tolerance for his exercise regimen. Upon examination, he has JVD, Kussmaul sign, edema, ascites, and a hepatojugular reflex. Tests are performed, and the cardiologist tells the patient that he has cardiomyopathy. The patient asks you how he can change his current lifestyle to prevent the progression of his cardiomyopathy. The best response of those listed below is

A. "If you control your blood pressure, the disease might not progress."

B. "There are no lifestyle changes you can make to prevent the progression of the disease."

C. "If you take a statin daily, have routine follow up with the cardiologist, and continue to exercise, the disease won't progress."

D. "If you stop drinking alcohol, the disease won't progress."

2-87. A chronic alcoholic is in the ICU with acute pancreatitis and congestive heart failure. She is receiving high-dose diuretics. Her ECG demonstrates flat T waves, ST segment depression, multifocal PVCs, and a prolonged QT interval. The initial management of this patient needs to include the administration of

A. Magnesium

B. Hypertonic saline

C. Sodium polystyrene sulfonate

D. Acetazolamide

2-88. A patient is admitted with a COPD exacerbation and worsening dyspnea. His admission vital signs are: temperature 38.1°C; HR 120/min; BP 180/80 mm Hg; SpO_2 90% on 2 L nasal cannula; RR 35/min and slightly labored. Initial ABGs are pH 7.3; $PaCO_2$ 57 mm Hg; PaO_2 61 mm Hg; SaO_2 87%; HCO_3 35 mEq/L. Which intervention should the nurse anticipate based on this assessment data?

A. Intubation related to the hypercarbia

B. Aggressive diuresis

C. Placing the patient on room air

D. Increasing O_2 to 4-L nasal cannula

2-89. A psychiatric patient with history of depression and suicide attempts arrives in the emergency room with severe agitation. She is accompanied by her spouse who reports that she has been very depressed lately, and this is different from her usual depression presentation. The patient is disoriented and complains of a headache. Which of the following would **not** be a first priority in her care?

A. Psychiatric evaluation

B. Pulse oximetry

C. Blood glucose level

D. Physical examination

2-90. Two hours after femoral-popliteal bypass graft surgery, a patient complains of pain unrelieved by ordered narcotics. Neurovascular examination of the affected extremity reveals skin staples that are dry and intact. Skin is warm, pale, and dry. Capillary refill time is 2 seconds, and the popliteal and dorsalis pedis pulses are 2+. Motor strength is slightly decreased from the previous hourly assessment. The gastrocnemius muscle appears slightly swollen and is "wood-like" to palpation. These findings indicate which of the following?

A. Compartment syndrome

B. Graft occlusion

C. Development of false aneurysm

D. Heparin-induced thrombocytopenia

2-91. A patient with chronic asthma and a severe cat allergy was admitted 3 hours ago in marked respiratory distress because of an acute exacerbation after spending the night at a friend's house who owns three cats. The patient's most recent ABGs while on 40% facemask are pH 7.28; $PaCO_2$ 62 mm Hg; PaO_2 58 mm Hg; and HCO_3 23 mEq/L. The patient is demonstrating increased work of breathing. Treatment has thus far included multiple doses of albuterol, ipratropium, and intubation with mechanical ventilation. New medical orders are now pending. Which of the following should the nurse question as inappropriate for this patient?
A. Inhaled bronchodilators
B. Intravenous magnesium sulfate
C. Administration of broad-spectrum antibiotics
D. IV corticosteroid

2-92. An 89-year-old woman is in the hospital for treatment of end-stage heart failure. The patient has a very supportive family, and her daughter has been at her bedside since admission. The cardiologist enters the room and advises both that he will be ordering a milrinone infusion for home therapy. The patient and daughter inform the physician that they do not want anything more done to prolong her life. Both the physician and the patient and her daughter continue to reiterate their opposing positions on this issue as the patient's nurse stands by observing this exchange. What is the nurse's best response upon entering this conversation?
A. "I have cared for her for the past week, and I know she would want everything done."
B. "It is only right and fair that everything be done for this wonderful lady."
C. "It seems that the physician's wishes are in conflict due to his own need to do good."
D. "It would probably be best for you and your daughter to listen to the physician."

2-93. A patient admitted to the ICU with a diagnosis of unstable angina is receiving these medications: low-molecular-weight heparin, aspirin, captopril, and continuous infusions of eptifibatide and nitroglycerin. Immediately after cardiac catheterization and percutaneous intervention, the patient is at high risk for which of the following?
A. Bleeding at groin access site
B. Coronary artery spasm
C. Restenosis
D. Heparin-induced thrombocytopenia

2-94. A patient is admitted to the hospital complaining of weakness, pallor, multiple bruises on all extremities, bleeding gums, and petechiae. She has a history of GERD, GI bleed, anemia, bleeding internal hemorrhoids, and antineoplastic therapy that she received 2 weeks ago for cancer. Her current platelet count is 38,000/mm³ and hematocrit is 24%. Along with a very thorough history, which intervention would be most appropriate?
A. Bone marrow biopsy
B. Spleen ultrasound
C. Endoscopy
D. Thrombopoietin administration

2-95. In caring for patients after coronary artery bypass surgery, the nurse knows the patient is most at risk for which of these dysrhythmias after surgery?
A. Atrial fibrillation
B. Supraventricular tachycardia
C. Atrial flutter
D. AV nodal reentrant tachycardia

2-96. Mary is a patient is admitted to the ICU with a diagnosis of syndrome of inappropriate secretion of antidiuretic hormone (SIADH). She is confused, disoriented, and agitated. Mary continues to yell, "I am thirsty, and they won't let me drink water." Her family arrives, and they ask why the patient can't have water to drink. The best response of those listed below is:
A. "Mary was already given water; she is confused and may not recall drinking it."
B. "We are keeping Mary nothing by mouth (NPO) because of her critical illness."
C. "Mary can have more water. I will bring her a water pitcher for the bedside if you will assist her."
D. "Mary is on a strict fluid restriction."

2-97. A 38-year-old woman had a cesarean section 4 days ago. She is admitted to the progressive care unit with abdominal pain, elevated white blood cell count, and a mild fever. An abdominal x-ray showed some free air in the abdomen and an ileus. Which of the following is the best treatment for her symptoms?

A. Enema administration
B. Emergency surgery
C. Abdominal CT scan
D. Nasogastric tube to suction

2-98. A trauma patient is in the emergency room after a severe motor vehicle accident. He receives 10 units of packed red blood cells for acute hemorrhagic shock. Which of these therapies is anticipated?

A. Fresh-frozen plasma and platelets
B. Acetaminophen and diphenhydramine (Benadryl)
C. Furosemide (Lasix) and calcium chloride
D. Normal saline at 200 mL/hr and 50 mL of salt poor albumin

2-99. Three days ago, a patient experienced a dominant hemisphere stroke after a motor vehicle collision that caused carotid artery dissection. The patient's GCS score is 3, and she has been declared brain dead. The patient's husband was informed of these findings, and he has consented to life support withdrawal. The critical care nurse talks with the husband, and he states, "I am leaving now; I don't want to watch this." The best response of those listed below is

A. "I would like to encourage you to reconsider; I will be here to support you."
B. "I can call clergy to stay with you at the bedside when this happens."
C. "I am here to support you. Would you like me to call you when she passes?"
D. "Why don't you want to be with your wife when she passes?"

2-100. A patient with a history of unstable angina receives his laboratory results after visiting with his cardiologist. Which of the following indicates that he is at risk for the development of an acute myocardial infarction?

A. BNP 150 pg/mL
B. C-reactive protein 5.0 mg/dL
C. Total cholesterol 180 mg/dL
D. HDL 60 mg/dL

2-101. Your hospital is initiating rotational therapy for patients experiencing respiratory failure. During the unit in-service, the critical care nurse learns that one important clinical implication related to rotational therapy is

A. Hemodynamic monitoring with a pulmonary artery catheter will be unreliable in both lateral and prone positions
B. Enteral feedings should not be administered because of a heightened risk of aspiration
C. A decrease in SpO_2 during lateral rotation will indicate the patient needs to be returned to the supine position
D. Hypotension and tachycardia that fail to return to baseline within 10 minutes of rotation will indicate the patient needs to be returned to the supine position

2-102. A 43-year-old patient with a BMI of 52 underwent bariatric surgery 2 months ago. He has not been taking his vitamin and mineral supplements. His vital signs are BP 133/87 mm Hg; pulse 78 beats/min; respirations 14 breaths/min. Which of these clinical findings would the nurse expect to see as manifestations of this patient's vitamin and mineral deficiencies?

A. Myelopathy, neuropathy, dementia, and short-term memory loss
B. Thirst, increased urination, diplopia, fatigue
C. Jaundice, dark urine, gnawing epigastric pain relieved by bending forward
D. Irritability, disorientation, asterixis, slowed mentation

2-103. A 72-year-old man is admitted to the CCU with shortness of breath, chest pain, diaphoresis, and tachycardia. His history includes myocardial infarction 5 years ago with two stents, anorexia, hypertension, fatigue, hypercholesterolemia, and arthritis. He is currently on amiodarone, metoprolol, captopril, lovastatin, aspirin, multivitamin, an herbal remedy called cat's claw, and nitroglycerin. For the past 4 days, all cardiac labs, 12-lead ECG, and cardiac catheterization have been normal, whereas FT_4 has been elevated and TSH low. The patient's tachycardia persisted until hospital day 4, when he developed a junctional rhythm. Now that numerous differential diagnoses have been ruled out, how could the health care team determine whether one of his medications is causing these symptoms?

A. Hold one medication each day to see if symptoms resolve

B. Review the literature for drug-induced thyroid dysfunction

C. Obtain a thyroxine-binding globulin level

D. Assess for a Wolff-Chaikoff effect

2-104. A patient is in the ICU after mitral valve replacement surgery. The patient has a right atrial pressure of 12 mm Hg and a pulmonary artery diastolic pressure of 6 mm Hg. Initial treatment for this patient would include administration of which of the following?

A. Normal 500-mL saline bolus

B. Furosemide 40 mg

C. Norepinephrine continuous infusion

D. Vasopressin 40 mg

2-105. A 67-year-old female presents to the emergency department after being found on the couch unresponsive. She has shallow, rapid respirations and dry mucous membranes. An admitting diagnosis of hyperglycemic, hyperosmolar, nonketotic coma was made. The nurse assigned to this patient anticipates her highest priority needs by preparing

A. Large amounts of intravenous normal saline for infusion

B. An insulin drip made with glargine insulin for infusion

C. Oxygen at 40% via mask

D. Padded side rails and a bite block

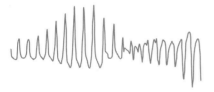

2-106. Pharmacologic therapy for the above rhythm would include

A. Amiodarone

B. Sotalol

C. Adenosine

D. Magnesium sulfate

2-107. The nurse admits a 50-year-old woman who complains of worsening dyspnea, a nonproductive cough, low-grade fever, malaise, fatigue, and a recent weight loss of approximately 10 lb. Her breath sounds reveal scattered inspiratory rales, and she quickly

desaturates to 85% off her nonrebreather. Initial labs reveal a normal WBC count with elevated sedimentation rate and C-reactive protein levels. Her chest x-ray shows diffuse, bilateral opacities. What interventions should the critical care nurse anticipate?

A. Blood, sputum, and urine cultures with the initiation of broad spectrum antibiotics as soon as possible

B. Blood, sputum, and urine cultures with the initiation of corticosteroid therapy

C. Initiating aggressive diuretic therapy and antibiotic therapy

D. Obtaining an echocardiogram and initiating inotropic therapy

2-108. The critical care nurse is caring for a 54-year-old patient who presents with complaints of cough and breathlessness on exertion. A chest CT scan shows honeycomb scarring in the periphery of the lung. Chest auscultation reveals bilateral crackles. The patient is given a diagnosis of pulmonary fibrosis and referred to a transplant center. Which of the following is not a contraindication for lung transplant?

A. Malignant squamous and basal cell tumors

B. Substance addiction, including alcohol, tobacco and narcotics, unless substance free for at least 6 months

C. Infection with HIV, hepatitis C, or hepatitis B

D. Uncorrectable coronary artery disease

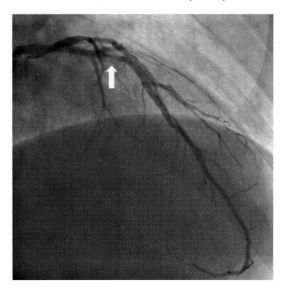

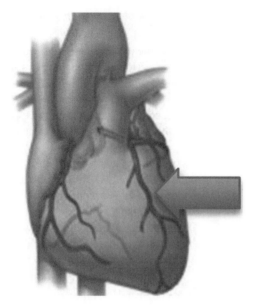

2-109. A patient arrives to the emergency room complaining of severe chest pain and shortness of breath. She is diagnosed with STEMI and emergently transported to the catheterization laboratory. Her catheterization image is pictured on the previous page, and the patient has a successful stent placement in the artery highlighted with an arrow in the illustration. The critical care nurse anticipates caring for a patient experiencing
   A. Acute inferior wall MI
   B. Acute lateral wall MI (high lateral wall)
   C. Acute anterior wall MI
   D. Acute posterior wall MI

2-110. A 66-year-old female is admitted post elective femoropopliteal bypass surgery. The critical care nurse anticipates that this patient is at high risk for multiple postoperative complications. The nurse anticipates monitoring for which of these complications?
   A. Pressure ulcer secondary to complete bedrest orders
   B. Pneumothorax
   C. Contrast dye–induced ATN
   D. Myocardial infarction

2-111. A patient has been referred to the emergency room by her primary care physician after the physician received her laboratory results. The patient has been complaining of cough, shortness of breath, nausea, muscle aches, and fatigue for the past 2 weeks. Her serum sodium level is 128 mEq/L, she appears euvolemic, and her urine sodium concentration is 55 mEq/L. Her admission vital signs are: temperature 38.1°C; HR 98/min; BP 160/80 mm Hg; SpO_2 89% on room air; RR 29/min. Her physical examination is unremarkable except for diffuse rhonchi and productive cough. Which of the following does the nurse anticipate as the next intervention?
   A. Rapid serum sodium correction
   B. Chest x-ray
   C. CT scan of the head
   D. IV steroid administration

2-112. An intubated patient with acute heart failure has been admitted to the ICU for treatment. The patient does not have a central line, pulmonary artery catheter, or arterial line. Which of these findings would best indicate adequate cardiac output?
   A. Ejection fraction greater than 50% on echocardiogram
   B. RR 20/min with SpO_2 of 94%
   C. Absence of peripheral edema
   D. The patient is alert with a serum creatinine of 1.0 mg/dL

2-113. A patient in the ICU was just admitted status post cardiac arrest. He is intubated and unresponsive. An immediate intervention for management of this patient should include
   A. Rapidly cooling the patient to 32° to 36°C based on hospital protocol
   B. Monitoring for signs and symptoms of hyperkalemia
   C. Titrating insulin infusion to maintain serum glucose level 120 to 150 mg/dL
   D. Assessing for elevations in white blood cell and platelet counts

2-114. A patient with a permanent pacemaker is in cardiac arrest. The monitor reveals sustained ventricular tachycardia, and the nurse prepares to place the defibrillation pads. Which of the following statements is true?
   A. A patient with a permanent pacemaker cannot be defibrillated
   B. A magnet must be placed over the pacemaker prior to defibrillation
   C. the defibrillator pads must be placed 1 to 2 inches away from the permanent pacemaker site on the chest
   D. The pacemaker will automatically defibrillate the patient

2-115. After experiencing multiple admissions with increasing frequency related to complications of his underlying condition, a 30-year-old patient experiencing extreme shortness of breath related to a sickle cell anemia crisis states that he no longer wishes to be intubated and that he is tired of so many resources being used to keep him alive when these funds could be used to benefit others. The best response of those listed below is
   A. "I am sure you won't feel that way after this exacerbation subsides."
   B. "Look at all that you contribute to your community. What will they do without you?"
   C. "Have you discussed this issue with your physician, friends, and family?"
   D. "When you get well, you can draft an advanced directive."

2-116. The progressive care nurse finds a patient lying in bed unresponsive. Her blood glucose is critically low. An injection of glucose is unsuccessful as the IV site is infiltrated. The nurse then administers glucagon. Which of these nursing interventions is the next most important?
   A. Recheck the capillary glucose level in 30 minutes
   B. Assess the patient's neurologic status
   C. Position the patient to avoid aspiration
   D. Prepare nourishments to administer over the next hour

2-117. The intensivist in the medical ICU wants to order a new bedside medication administration system. The current system is often bypassed as it is too time consuming for the bedside nurse because of frequent mechanical and battery failure. The intensivist wants to assemble a committee to evaluate and choose an appropriate system. The most appropriate initial action of the committee is to
   A. Send for all literature on the available bedside medication administration systems
   B. Include members of other units who may be using the new system
   C. Call other hospitals to determine their pros and cons for their medication administration systems
   D. Check for data on nationwide sentinel events involving all of the medication administration systems

2-118. The health care team is making rounds on a patient with status asthmaticus who was intubated and placed on mechanical ventilation earlier that shift. The patient's most recent ABG findings reveal persistent hypoxemia, and the team is now considering whether to use neuromuscular blocking agents (NMBs) to help this patient. When an orientee asks his preceptor to clarify use of NMBs in this situation, the preceptor's best explanation would be that in patients with status asthmaticus who are experiencing hypoxia despite mechanical ventilation, neuromuscular blocking agents should
   A. Never be administered when the patient is receiving steroids
   B. Be used routinely for paralysis to control airway pressures
   C. Be administered to augment smooth muscle relaxation
   D. Be used with caution if other options are ineffective

2-119. A postoperative patient is admitted to the unit after undergoing mitral valve replacement and maze procedure. The patient has a left atrial line. Which of the following is most likely the surgeon's rationale for using a left atrial line in this patient?
   A. To ensure accuracy of postoperative hemodynamic data
   B. To enable evacuation of a left atrial air embolus
   C. To provide a means of monitoring for cardiac tamponade more reliable than a PA line
   D. To ensure continuous monitoring of chamber pressures during valve replacement

2-120. A patient in septic shock evidences these hemodynamic parameters: HR 120/min; BP 80/40 (MAP 53) mm Hg; PAP 25/10 mm Hg; CVP 4 mm Hg; CO 4.0 L/min; CI 2.1 L/min/m^2; SVR 700 dynes/sec/cm^{-5}; SVO2 60%. Based on these hemodynamic values, which of these interventions would **most** likely result in improving the patient's hemodynamic status?
   A. Norepinephrine 10 mcg/kg/min
   B. Metoprolol 2.5 mg IVP slowly
   C. 500 mL bolus of 0.9% normal saline
   D. Dobutamine 5 mcg/kg/min

2-121. A 70-kg patient with acute respiratory distress syndrome (ARDS) is intubated and mechanically ventilated. The patient is currently on a continuous vecuronium infusion titrated to maintain "0" twitch. Peak inspiratory pressure is 55 cm H_2O. The patient currently has a PaO_2 of 60 mm Hg, and the physician orders these ventilator settings: TV 700 mL; rate 12/min; FiO_2 100%; PEEP 15 cm H_2O. The nurse knows that
   A. IV vecuronium should not be used with patients that have ARDS
   B. A tidal volume of 700 mL is inappropriate for this patient
   C. The PEEP should be increased to 20 cm H_2O to improve oxygenation
   D. The ordered ventilator settings are appropriate for this patient

2-122. A patient with a diagnosis of hypertensive crisis is admitted to the ICU. He is confused and mildly agitated. When prioritizing care, the critical care nurse's first concern is to prevent which of these complications?
   A. Stroke
   B. End-organ failure
   C. Seizures
   D. Left ventricular hypertrophy

2-123. The physician is at the bedside of a patient who needs to go to the operating room for a perforated bowel. The physician explains the procedure to the family, indicates it will last about 2 hours, and relates that the patient will then return to the ICU. The physician then presents the informed consent form to the patient and says there should be no problem with the surgery because she has performed this procedure many times. The patient asks if there are any risks to this surgery. The physician states that there are minimal risks and then prepares to leave the room. What is the nurse's best next response?
   A. Allow the physician to leave, documenting the physician's visit in the nurse's notes
   B. Ask the physician to discuss risks of the surgery with the patient
   C. Call clergy to request consultation for a high-risk surgery
   D. Obtain a patient education brochure on the procedure for the family

2-124. An 86-year-old female presents to the emergency room with acute rectal bleeding. She has a history of hypertension, diabetes, severe arthritis, cardiac stents, and atrial fibrillation. The critical care nurse anticipates that the cause of her bleeding is most likely caused by
   A. Intestinal polyps
   B. Crohn disease
   C. Ruptured diverticuli
   D. Angiodysplasia

2-125. Two days after abdominal aortic surgical repair, a patient develops hypotension, tachycardia, abdominal distention, diarrhea, and an elevated white blood cell count. The most likely cause of these findings is
   A. Postoperative graft infection
   B. Ischemic colitis
   C. Aortoenteric fistula
   D. Abdominal compartment syndrome

2-126. The critical care nurse is planning care for a critical trauma patient. The nurse is aware of the risk of multiple organ dysfunction syndrome (MODS) in a trauma patient. Which of these nursing interventions most likely has the highest effect on preventing MODS secondary to multiple trauma?
   A. Fall prevention
   B. DVT prevention
   C. Pressure ulcer prevention
   D. Infection prevention

2-127. A patient with acute pulmonary edema is receiving furosemide (Lasix) 40 mg BID, captopril (Capoten) 50 mg TID, and morphine sulfate 2 mg every 2 hours along with oxygen 70% by BiPAP mask. Current assessment data include HR 116/min, sinus rhythm with occasional PAC; BP 100/70 mm Hg; and RR 25 with SpO_2 97%. Which of these findings should alert the nurse to a need to change the current treatment plan?
   A. Serum creatinine 3.2 mg/dL
   B. Serum potassium 3.8 mg/dL
   C. SpO_2 95%
   D. HR 110/min with increasing premature atrial contractions

2-128. You are training a new nurse on the unit who informs you that she would like the opportunity to care for a patient who qualifies for a hybrid or minimally invasive procedure. Which of the following patients would not qualify for a minimally invasive or hybrid procedure?

- A. A patient with cardiogenic shock with a proximal RCA lesion and total LAD lesion
- B. A patient with multiple proximal and mid LAD lesions
- C. A 92-year-old woman with aortic stenosis
- D. A patient with mitral stenosis requiring repair

2-129. A postpartum patient is admitted to the ICU after an emergency cesarean section. She had experienced both pregnancy-induced hypertension and postpartum hemorrhage. The critical care nurse suspects that this patient is exhibiting clinical evidence of HELLP syndrome. Which of these laboratory values would support this suspicion?

- A. Elevated liver enzymes and a decreased platelet count
- B. Decreased hemoglobin and hematocrit
- C. Elevated serum magnesium and albuminuria
- D. Decreased blood urea nitrogen and increased serum creatinine

2-130. A patient with pulmonary edema has received 80 mg of furosemide (Lasix). Arterial blood gas values include pH 7.60; PaO_2 78 mm Hg; $PaCO_2$ 42 mm Hg. The nurse anticipates which of these interventions?

- A. Administration of acetazolamide (Diamox)
- B. Administration of additional furosemide (Lasix) 40 mg
- C. Endotracheal intubation
- D. Administration of hydrochlorothiazide

2-131. A patient has been admitted for treatment of diabetes insipidus. The critical care nurse anticipates the fluid management treatment for this patient. Which of the following describes the fluid management strategy?

- A. Electrolyte levels must be monitored to determine the correct IV fluids to administer
- B. If the diabetes insipidus is nephrogenic, vasopressin will need to be administered
- C. If the diabetes insipidus is neurogenic, only fluids will need replacement
- D. The patient's output must exceed his intake in order to prevent complications

2-132. A 58-year-old continuous ambulatory peritoneal dialysis (CAPD) patient is admitted to the ICU after a small bowel resection. The patient is hemodynamically stable and has a 3-L excess fluid balance. For these reasons, the critical care nurse anticipates the patient's end-stage renal disease (ESRD) will be managed using

- A. Peritoneal dialysis (PD)
- B. Slow continuous ultrafiltration (SCUF)
- C. Hemodialysis (HD)
- D. Continuous venovenous hemofiltration (CVVH)

2-133. An ICU patient is admitted after a severe motor vehicle accident. He is intubated and has both right and left chest tubes in place. The right chest tube has persistent bubbling during inspiration and expiration. His breath sounds are clear and equal with both chest tube systems draining properly. The goal of ventilator management for this patient is to

- A. Maximize PEEP
- B. Minimize airway pressures
- C. Minimize FiO_2
- D. Maximize tidal volumes

2-134. A nurse is caring for a patient admitted 2 days ago for septic shock. The patient has been intubated on mechanical ventilation and has not received nutrition since admission. The intensivist is concerned about initiating nutrition because the patient remains unstable. Which of the following would be the best choice for nutrition?

- A. Wait another 24 hours to initiate nutrition
- B. Hold nutrition until stable
- C. Initiate total parenteral nutrition (TPN)
- D. Initiate enteral nutrition

2-135. The nurse is caring for a Haitian immigrant. She has been admitted for an acute myocardial infarction and is scheduled for coronary artery bypass graft surgery the next day. The nurse is providing culturally competent care for the patient and her family. Which of these statements is not true?

- A. The patient's husband will decide if she will have surgery
- B. The nurse should make direct eye contact and touch the patient when providing care

C. The patient and family would prefer to read information about surgery (in Creole) rather than discuss the information

D. It can be difficult or impossible to get a family health history from the patient

2-136. A 60-year-old patient admitted 1 week ago for failure to thrive is transferred to the ICU with a new onset of fever, leukocytosis, and a cough productive of large amounts of rust-colored sputum. His vital signs are as follows: temperature 39.5°C; HR 120/min; RR 35/min; SpO₂ 90% on room air; BP 90/40 mm Hg. The critical care nurse knows that the highest priority interventions for this patient are to

A. Obtain sputum and blood cultures and start broad-spectrum antibiotics

B. Facilitate obtaining both a chest x-ray and a sputum culture

C. Administer acetaminophen and obtain a full set of cultures

D. Initiate administration of oxygen and IV fluids

2-137. A 28-year-old woman is in the ICU with a gunshot wound to the head. Surgery was performed to remove the bullet and stop bleeding. The patient has been in the ICU for 2 weeks and remains unresponsive. An EEG is flat, and the physician has declared the patient brain dead. The nurse is present with the physician when the diagnosis is shared with the patient's mother. One of the first issues that the nurse needs to anticipate at this point is

A. That the family may request a second opinion about brain death

B. The need to document this physician–family discussion

C. The need to initiate discussion related to organ donation

D. That the hospital ethics committee should be contacted

2-138. A patient in the emergency room is scheduled for emergency corrective surgery for an acute aortic dissection. Which of the following is the only circumstance in which a pericardiocentesis would be performed before transport to the operating room?

A. The patient has an elevated right atrial pressure

B. The patient demonstrates signs of cardiac tamponade with a stable blood pressure

C. The patient develops pulseless electrical activity (PEA)

D. Chest x-ray demonstrates indisputable evidence of mediastinal widening

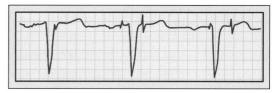

2-139. The strip above shows pacemaker activity. Which of the following best describes the pacemaker function?

A. Complete capture
B. Failure to capture
C. Failure to sense
D. Failure to pace

2-140. A patient admitted to the ICU with a diagnosis of sepsis and acute renal failure has these urinary laboratory results: specific gravity 1.028; osmolality 500 mOsm/kg; sodium 9 mEq/L; and FENa 0.8%. Based on these findings, the critical care nurse anticipates which of these actions?

A. Administration of normal saline fluid bolus

B. Fluid restriction of 1 L/24 hr

C. Administration of furosemide (Lasix) 40 mg IVP

D. Discontinued administration of cefazolin (Ancef)

2-141. A patient presents to the emergency room by ambulance after having a new-onset seizure. Diagnostic imaging reveals a 4-cm right frontal arteriovenous malformation. The nurse is planning the patient's care. Which of these conditions should the nurse anticipate?

A. Left-side weakness
B. Receptive aphasia
C. Left homonymous hemianopsia
D. Sensory deficits on the right face and arm

2-142. A patient was admitted with a history of blunt trauma to the head, chest, and abdomen related to a 30-foot fall. On admission, his vital signs were BP 148/82 mm Hg; pulse 120 beats/min; respirations 16 breaths/min. Over the past 45 minutes, the patient has become more agitated: his pulse has risen to 135 beats/min, his BP is now 100/60 mm Hg, and his skin is cool and clammy. The nurse's next interventions will be based on a high index of suspicion that the patient has sustained an acute

A. Increase in intracranial pressure
B. Myocardial infarction
C. Intraabdominal hemorrhage
D. Pulmonary embolism

2-143. A patient is admitted to the ICU after extensive surgical repair of a perforated colon. He received a 15-L resuscitation with fluids and blood products perioperatively and still requires intermittent fluid boluses. He is intubated, and his chest x-ray shows diffuse bilateral infiltrates suggestive of ARDS. Ventilator settings are SIMV mode with a set rate of 18; tidal volume of 5 mL/kg; PEEP + 10; and FiO_2 0.70. He is overbreathing to a rate of 30/min; his latest ABG is pH 7.28; $PaCO_2$ 45 mm Hg; and PaO_2 55 mm Hg. Pulmonary wheezes and crackles are audible bilaterally. He is grimacing and restless on the bed. In addition to having ventilator settings optimized, in what order does the nurse need to prioritize pharmacologic interventions?

A. IV steroids, sedation/analgesia, diuretic
B. Diuretic, bronchodilator, IV steroids
C. Bronchodilator, sedation, fluid bolus
D. Sedation/analgesia, bronchodilator, antibiotics

2-144. A patient with sickle cell disease is admitted for sickle cell crisis. This particular crisis has occurred because the microcirculation is occluded by sickled red blood cells. The patient is experiencing pain, and the nurse is monitoring closely for any signs of organ ischemia. These clinical manifestations best describe which of these sickle cell crises?

A. Hematologic crisis
B. Infectious crisis
C. Aplastic crisis
D. Vasoocclusive crisis

2-145. The preceptor for a new ICU nurse notices that the orientee is taking a noninvasive blood pressure measurement using the patient's forearm rather than her upper arm. When questioned about this cuff placement, the orientee states that he had heard that the cuff could be placed on the forearm. The preceptor has never heard of using the forearm for this purpose and has no information on this change from standard practice BP technique. Which of the following would be the best way to approach this change in practice?

A. Instruct the new nurse on the standard BP protocol of using the upper arm
B. Take the blood pressure in both the upper and lower arms and then compare readings
C. Design a research study to compare the relationship between upper and lower arm BP measurements
D. Review the current literature to identify evidence and recommendations related to this change in practice

2-146. A patient in the ICU is admitted for a lower gastrointestinal bleed. He is receiving a transfusion of packed red blood cells (PRBCs), and he rings his call bell to alert the nurse that he has developed sudden onset of chills. His temperature is 38.1°C. The initial nursing intervention for this patient would be to

A. Obtain a urine specimen
B. Administer antipyretics
C. Call the physician
D. Stop the transfusion

2-147. A patient arrives to the emergency room with complaint of flu-like symptoms. The patient's laboratory work reveals an elevated white blood cell count, elevated ALT and AST, and a positive hepatitis serologic marker. The patient's drug screen result is negative, and she is not sexually active. She reports eating sushi at a new restaurant 3 weeks ago. The nurse prepares to care for a patient with

A. Hepatitis A
B. Hepatitis B
C. Hepatitis C
D. Hepatitis D

2-148. A patient with a a history of chronic obstructive bronchitis is admitted to the ICU after a respiratory arrest. He was intubated and sedated prior to transfer to the ICU, and manually ventilated with 100% oxygen during transport. The patient is placed on mechanical ventilation with these settings: pressure-regulated volume control (PRVC); FiO_2 40%, respiratory rate 10/min. Arterial blood gases obtained 20 minutes after arrival are pH 7.54; PaO_2 76 mm Hg; $PaCO_2$ 45 mm Hg; oxygen saturation 91%. After reviewing these clinical findings and ventilatory settings, the nurse should conclude that the

A. Pressure ventilation is inappropriate for this COPD patient because it shortens expiratory time

B. Respiratory rate should be decreased to correct the pH

C. Fio_2 should be increased until the PaO_2 is at least 80%

D. Ordered ventilator settings are appropriate for this patient

2-149. A student nurse is shadowing the ICU nurse. A patient has been admitted with a diagnosis of diabetic ketoacidosis. The ICU nurse is providing aggressive fluid resuscitation. The student asks the ICU nurse why the fluids are administered so quickly. Which of these responses is not appropriate?

A. It lowers the blood glucose level

B. It increases the circulating blood volume to perfuse the body tissues

C. It decreases the ketone levels caused by the breakdown of fats

D. It helps to normalize blood pressure

2-150. Which of these patients is most at risk of developing heparin-induced thrombocytopenia after coronary revascularization?

A. A patient with unstable angina who received unfractionated heparin several days before coronary bypass surgery

B. A patient with diabetes, mild renal insufficiency, and multivessel coronary artery disease

C. A patient who has steroid-dependent asthma and RCA occlusion

D. An obese patient with hypertension and left ventricular hypertrophy

2 Answers to Core Review Test 2

2-1. **(A)** Pneumothorax appears as a frequent and potentially fatal complication in patients with ARDS, especially in those who need mechanical ventilation support. In patients with ARDS, pneumothorax is frequently related to the use of high PEEP and tidal volumes that are intended to promote oxygenation and is treated by insertion of a chest tube. Immediate treatment of pneumothorax is warranted to prevent further patient compromise. Although decreased urine output is of concern, improvement in oxygenation by relieving pneumothorax takes precedence. Although pneumonia may have contributed to sepsis, causing ARDS, sputum cultures would not be indicated for a patient with pneumothorax (indicated by the radiolucence in the right middle lobe). Administration of norepinephrine to increase blood pressure is not the immediate concern for this patient. Blood pressure may be improved by treatment of the pneumothorax.

References: Storzer, D. N. (2018). Pulmonary system. In T. M. Hartjes (Ed.), *AACN core curriculum for high acuity, progressive, and critical care nursing* (7th ed.). St. Louis: Elsevier.

Terzi, E., Zarogoulidis, K., Kougioumtzi, I., et al. (2014). Acute respiratory distress syndrome and pneumothorax. *Journal of Thoracic Disease, 6*(Suppl. 4), S435–S442. http://doi.org/10.3978/j.issn.2072-1439.2014.08.34.

2-2. **(D)** Signs of brain death include fixed pupils; no motor response to deep central pain, absent corneal reflexes; absent oculocephalic (doll's eyes) reflex; absent oculovestibular reflex (cold water calorics); positive apnea test result (no spontaneous breaths with $PaCO_2$ greater than 60 mm Hg and despite 100% FiO_2 ventilation 15 minutes prior). Loss of vascular tone (Option A) is not part of the diagnostic criteria for brain death, but hemodynamic instability can occur before or after diagnosis. Barbiturate infusion (Option B) is provided for refractory intracranial hypertension as a salvage measure. Lack of response to this treatment is not pathognomonic for brain death, but many patients have a poor outcome. Barbiturates are metabolized slowly, so it can take days before they are cleared to subtherapeutic values, a prerequisite before testing for brain death. All diagnoses should be made in the absence of hypothermia, metabolic, or drug cause; shock or anoxia; or immediately post resuscitation. Responses of the spinal reflex arc (Option C)—elicited with infliction of peripheral noxious stimuli such as nail bed pressure—are commonly present after brain death.

References: Wyckoff, M., & Hartjes, T. M. (2018). Critical care patients with special needs: palliative and end-of life care in the ICU. In T. M. Hartjes (Ed.), *AACN core curriculum for high acuity, progressive, and critical care nursing* (7th ed.). St. Louis: Elsevier.

Arbour, R. (2013). Brain death: assessment, controversy, and confounding factors. *Critical Care Nurse, 33*(6), 27–48. http://dx.doi.org/10.4037/ccn2013215.

2-3. **(C)** Hyponatremia and hypokalemia result from prolonged vomiting. Changes in serum sodium concentration usually reflect changes in water balance. The signs and symptoms of hyponatremia are often nonspecific, and most are related to the changes in serum osmolality and consequent fluid shifts in the central nervous system. These can include headache, lethargy, disorientation, seizures, muscle cramps, or weakness. Hypokalemia can develop as a result of intracellular shifts of potassium or as a result of increased loss of or decreased ingestion or administration of potassium. Clinical signs of hypokalemia include weakness, paralysis, respiratory compromise, rhabdomyolysis, ECG changes, cardiac dysrhythmias, and sudden death. Hyperglycemia may occur with extreme stress. Signs and symptoms of hyperkalemia in Option A (peaked T waves, diarrhea) are not associated with vomiting. These symptoms usually occur with ketoacidosis, tissue destruction, and renal failure and with certain medications such as beta-blockers. Lethargy, confusion, and bradycardia are caused by hypercalcemia (Option B). Serum calcium levels are increased by bone tumors: primary hypoparathyroidism caused by elevated PTF levels; excessive intake of supplemental calcium and vitamin D; hypomagnesemia; and as a complication of renal failure from decreased renal excretion of calcium. Hyperphosphatemia is described in Option D. Hyperphosphatemia is caused by renal failure and is not a result of protracted nausea and vomiting.

Reference: Boling, B. (2018). Renal system. In T. M. Hartjes (Ed.), *AACN core curriculum for high acuity, progressive, and critical care nursing* (7th ed.). St. Louis: Elsevier.

2-4. **(C)** Flail chest, caused by blunt trauma to the thoracic cavity, occurs when two or more adjacent ribs are fractured in two or more places. This flail segment moves independently from the rest of the thoracic cage and results in paradoxical chest wall movement during the respiratory cycle. Paradoxical motion refers to the movement of the flail segment in the direction *opposite* that of the intact chest wall. Instead of expanding outward with the rest of the thoracic wall during inspiration, the flail segment is drawn inward by the negative inspiratory pressure. Conversely, as this negative pressure falls during exhalation, the flail segment is pushed outward.

References: Storzer, D. N. (2018). Pulmonary system. In T. M. Hartjes (Ed.), *AACN core curriculum for high acuity, progressive, and critical care nursing* (7th ed.). St. Louis: Elsevier.

Holleran, R. (2018). Multisystem: Multisystem trauma. In T. M. Hartjes (Ed.), *AACN core curriculum for high acuity, progressive, and critical care nursing* (7th ed.). St. Louis: Elsevier.

2-5. **(B)** Patients with severe ARDS have significant impairment in their pulmonary gas exchange, which impairs the ability to oxygenate and decarboxylate the blood. Extracorporeal membrane oxygenation (ECMO) is a last-resort technique used in the treatment of severe ARDS. ECMO allows the lungs to rest by facilitating the removal of carbon dioxide and providing oxygen to the lungs. Mechanical ventilation during ECMO will continue to provide low tidal volume ventilation (LTVV), which reduces the damaging, excessive stretch of lung tissue and alveoli and prevents barotrauma. ECMO does not directly affect lung volumes or trauma. Systemic thromboembolism due to thrombus formation within the extracorporeal circuit is a common but devastating complication of ECMO. Aggressive anticoagulation is required to prevent thromboembolism and pulmonary embolism. Infective complications can be related to the indwelling lines, access sites, or comorbidities.

References: Storzer, D. N. (2018). Pulmonary system. In T. M. Hartjes (Ed.), *AACN core curriculum for high acuity, progressive, and critical care nursing* (7th ed.). St. Louis: Elsevier.

Moraca, R., & Magovern, G. (2014). Extracorporeal membrane oxygenation for respiratory failure in adults. In J. Cameron, & A. Cameron, *Current surgical therapy* (11th ed.) (pp. 1233–1238). Philadelphia: Elsevier Saunders.

2-6. **(D)** During anaphylactic shock, vasodilatation of the arterial system results in a decrease in the afterload as evidenced by a decreased SVR. Venous vasodilatation and massive volume loss lead to a decrease in preload, which causes a decline in the right atrial pressure and pulmonary occlusion pressure. Anaphylactic shock causes a decrease in the cardiac output, thus causing a decrease in the cardiac index

Reference: Dressler, D. (2018). Hematological and Immunological Systems. In T. M. Hartjes (Ed.), *AACN core curriculum for high acuity, progressive, and critical care nursing* (7th ed.). St. Louis: Elsevier.

2-7. **(C)** Gastric irritation is a frequent adverse effect of immunosuppressive agents, so taking this medication with food will help to prevent development of gastric ulcers. It is not safe to double the dose of immunosuppressive medications if a dose is missed because of the possibility of untoward effects. Resuming the normal dose as soon as possible will limit incidence of graft versus host disease. Sirolimus interacts with cyclosporine and must be taken 4 hours after cyclosporine. Elevated blood pressure represents a serious untoward effect of immunosuppressive agents and, if not monitored or reported to the primary health care provider, may lead to permanent neurologic deficits.

Reference: Lough, M. (2018). Organ donation and transplantation. In L. Urden, K. Stacy, & M. Lough (Eds.), *Critical care nursing: Diagnosis and management.* St. Louis, MO: Mosby/Elsevier.

2-8. **(A)** Option A is correct because encouraging patients to recall past successes or reflect on the past may support adaptation to life changes. Option B is incorrect because a patient's views on these issues would not explain the current diagnosis. Option C might be an informative and reflective experience but would not necessarily have health implications for the future. Option D is not appropriate because the scenario described does not suggest this patient needs to focus on their mortality at this time.

Reference: Dermenchyan, A. (2018). Professional caring and ethical practice. In T. M. Hartjes (Ed.), *AACN core curriculum for high acuity, progressive, and critical care nursing* (7th ed.). St. Louis: Elsevier.

2-9. **(B)** In cases of acute hypoglycemia, treatment should be administered, and then its effectiveness assessed through the use of capillary glucose measurement 15 minutes after administration of the glucose source. This time frame should be adhered to regardless of whether or when circulation is restored or the patient is transferred between units.

Reference: MacDermott, J. (2018). Endocrine system. In T. M. Hartjes (Ed.), *AACN core curriculum for high acuity, progressive, and critical care nursing* (7th ed.). St. Louis: Elsevier.

2-10. **(D)** Contributing factors to noncompliance are language barriers, lack of education, cultural or ethnic beliefs, financial constraints, lack of tools or supplies, and lack of family support. Noncompliance is an unwillingness to learn and does not necessarily mean that the patient is choosing not to participate in her or his care or follow medical instructions. A patient's employment status does not determine her or his willingness to learn. In addition, lack of employment does not necessarily cause financial constraint, especially if a spouse or parent is employed and has health insurance. Marital status does not determine the absence of healthy social relationships or lack of family support.

References: Dermenchyan, A. (2018). Professional caring and ethical practice. In T. M. Hartjes (Ed.), *AACN core curriculum for high acuity, progressive, and critical care nursing* (7th ed.). St. Louis: Elsevier.

Urden, L. (2018). Patient and family education. In L. Urden, K. Stacy, & M. Lough (Eds.), *Critical care nursing: Diagnosis and management.* St. Louis, MO: Mosby/Elsevier.

2-11. **(A)** Chlorhexidine gluconate solutions used for vascular catheter site care reduce catheter-related bloodstream infections and catheter colonization more effectively than povidone-iodine solutions. Data suggest that IV tubing containing crystalloids can be replaced every 72 to 96 hours, so Option B is not correct. Option C is not accurate because the transducer, tubing, flush device, and flush solution need to be replaced only every 96 hours. If aseptic technique during insertion cannot be ensured, the catheter should be replaced soon as possible but within 48 hours, not within 72 hours as Option D suggests.

Reference: Conley, S. B. (2016). Central line-associated bloodstream infection prevention: Standardizing practice focused on evidence-based guidelines. *Clinical Journal of Oncology Nursing, 20*(1), 23–26. http://dx.doi.org/10.1188/16.CJON.23-26.

2-12. **(D)** Pulse oximetry measures the percent of hemoglobin molecules that are saturated but does not distinguish whether that saturation is with oxyhemoglobin or carboxyhemoglobin. During the initial management of patients with CO poisoning, arterial blood gas studies need to be used to evaluate a patient's oxygenation status. Poor tissue perfusion because of hemodynamic instability leads to loss of pulsatile flow, signal failure, and unreliable readings. The cherry-red skin color is caused by the binding of hemoglobin and CO in the blood. SpO_2 readings in the presence of carboxyhemoglobin are falsely elevated. The amount of oxygen a patient receives has no bearing on the accuracy of pulse oximetry.

References: Keiler, R. (2018). Multisystem: Burns. In T. M. Hartjes (Ed.), *AACN core curriculum for high acuity, progressive, and critical care nursing* (7th ed.). St. Louis: Elsevier.

Williams, A., & Estrada, R. (2016). Carbon monoxide poisoning: The silent killer. *American Nurse Today, 11*(9), 7–9.

2-13. **(C)** The patient's pulmonary artery pressure is consistent with pulmonary hypertension. The administration of agents that dilate the pulmonary arteries such as epoprostenol or inhaled nitric oxide will, in some cases, reduce right ventricular work and improve pulmonary blood flow and oxygenation. Phlebotomy (Option A) may be considered in polycythemic patients with pulmonary hypertension when the hematocrit is greater than 60%. Fluid bolus (Option B) may reduce blood viscosity but would not improve the pulmonary hypertension. Anticoagulation is indicated for long-term management of pulmonary hypertension but is not indicated in the immediate postoperative period and will not improve pulmonary artery pressures..

References: Efre, A., & Boling, B. (2018). Cardiovascular system. In T. M. Hartjes (Ed.), *AACN core curriculum for high acuity, progressive, and critical care nursing* (7th ed.). St. Louis: Elsevier.

Miller, R., & Cohen, N. (2015). Nitric oxide and other inhaled pulmonary vasodilators. In R. Miller, & N. Cohen (Eds.), *Miller's anesthesia* (pp. 3084–3097). Philadelphia: Elsevier Saunders.

2-14. **(A)** The body habitus of morbidly obese patients predisposes them to hypoventilation and pneumonia, particularly when in the supine position. Limited diaphragmatic excursion leads to decreased vital capacity, functional residual capacity, and total lung capacity. There is decreased alveolar ventilation with atelectasis, and decreased thoracic and pulmonary compliance. Obesity does not predispose a patient to noncompliance with the medical regimen (Option B). Cholecystitis does not place a patient at risk for pneumonia (Option C). Postoperative pain management can be challenging in the bariatric patient but can be achieved (Option D).

References: Benefield, A. (2018). Critical care patients with special needs: Bariatric patients. In T. M. Hartjes (Ed.), *AACN core curriculum for high acuity, progressive, and critical care nursing* (7th ed.). St. Louis: Elsevier.

Berrios, L. (2016). The ABCDs of managing morbidly obese patients in intensive care units. *Critical Care Nurse, 36*(5), 17–26. http://dx.doi.org/10.4037/ccn2016671.

2-15. **(B)** The majority of postoperative complications in emergency hemicolectomy relate to infection, including sepsis, intraabdominal abscess, and wound infections. These complications are associated with increased morbidity and mortality. Using the sepsis bundle for early resuscitation, the intravascular volume needs to be reestablished, and the tissue beds need to be perfused to reduce tissue hypoxia. Lactate levels need to be kept less than 4 mmol/L. Normal central venous pressure is 5 to 8 mm Hg. A central venous pressure less than this indicates continued reduction in preload, which would not be an optimal response to the initiation of rapid fluid resuscitations. A normal urine output is more than 1 mL/kg/hr, a reduced urine output ranges from 0.5 to 1 mL/kg/hr, and a severely reduced urine output is less than 0.5 mL/kg/hr. During resuscitation, targeted therapy should additionally focus on improving or normalizing urine output. This would not be an optimal response to rapid fluid administration. Cool, dry skin could indicate that the patient is experiencing peripheral vasoconstriction, suggesting continued hypovolemia and the need for further fluid resuscitation.

Reference: Dressler, D. (2018). Hematological and Immunological Systems. In T. M. Hartjes (Ed.), *AACN core curriculum for high acuity, progressive, and critical care nursing* (7th ed.). St. Louis: Elsevier.

2-16. **(A)** Valvular heart disease, excess ethanol ingestion, hypertension, pregnancy, and infections are common underlying etiologic factors for dilated cardiomyopathy. A common feature of dilated cardiomyopathy regardless of the underlying cause is a propensity to ventricular arrhythmias and sudden death. Amiodarone significantly reduced the incidence of complex ventricular arrhythmias and sudden death among patients with dilated cardiomyopathy and ventricular tachycardia. Calcium channel blockers prevent supraventricular dysrhythmias, which are not common in dilated cardiomyopathy. Nitrates will improve coronary artery perfusion, but the primary defect in dilated cardiomyopathy is a structural defect in the ventricle that is not improved with administration of vasodilators. Digoxin improves contractility in cardiomyopathy but has no effect on the development of ventricular dysrhythmias, which may cause sudden death in this population.

Reference: Zipes, D., & Jalife, J. (2014). Ventricular tachycardia in patients with dilated cardiomyopathy. In D. Zipes, & J. Jalife (Eds.), *Cardiac electrophysiology: From the cell to bedside* (pp. 859–871). Philadelphia: Elsevier Saunders.

2-17. **(C)** To overcome barriers to palliative care consultation, critical care nurses need to be champions for palliative care. The advisory board of Improving Palliative Care in the ICU recommends using published criteria in conjunction with hospital-specific data to develop unit-specific criteria for a palliative care consult. Option A is incorrect because nurses should work with the palliative care team and other disciplines to ensure that a consistent message is conveyed. Patients and their families recall feeling supported when they were told by palliative care specialists **and** nurses that they would set goals for this part of their life together. Option B is incorrect as the medical team is not ethically bound to consult palliative care in this situation. Likewise, the nursing supervisor cannot compel the team to place a palliative care consult.

References: Wyckoff, M., & Hartjes, T. M. (2018). Critical care patients with special needs: Palliative and end-of life care in the ICU. In T. M. Hartjes (Ed.), *AACN core curriculum for high acuity, progressive, and critical care nursing* (7th ed.). St. Louis: Elsevier.

Ouimet Perrin, K., & Kazanowski, M. (2015). End-of-life care. Overcoming barriers to palliative care consultation. *Critical Care Nurse, 35*(5), 44–52. http://dx.doi.org/10.4037/ccn2015357.

2-18. **(A)** Transfusion of 1 unit of packed red blood cells should increase the hemoglobin by 1 g/dL and the hematocrit by 2% to 3% in this patient with symptomatic anemia. Patients with end-stage renal disease (ESRD) experience anemia secondary to a decrease in production of erythropoietin; as a result, there is diminished stimulation of the bone marrow to produce red blood cells. Acceptable hematocrit levels with epoetin alfa therapy are usually 33% to 36%. The patient is experiencing symptoms of anemia, including fatigue, headache, lightheadedness, and palpitations. Monitoring the patient without intervention does not provide treatment for these symptoms. Administration of epoetin alfa takes weeks to increase the hemoglobin and hematocrit and is contraindicated in patients with uncontrolled hypertension. Decreasing the dose of epoetin alfa will not address the problems of low hemoglobin and hematocrit.

References: Boling, B. (2018). Renal system. In T. M. Hartjes (Ed.), *AACN core curriculum for high acuity, progressive, and critical care nursing* (7th ed.). St. Louis: Elsevier.

Brugnara, C., & Eckardt, K. (2016). Hematologic Aspects of Kidney Disease. In K. Skorecki, G. M. Chertow, P. A. Marsden, B. M. Brenner, & F. C. Rector (Authors), *Brenner & Rectors the kidney* (pp. 1875-1911). Philadelphia (Pa.): Elsevier.

2-19. **(D)** An invasive strategy is preferred for persistent symptoms and signs of acute MI. The priority of care for acute MI is revascularization. Time to percutaneous coronary intervention (PCI) therapy must be minimized to increase survival and preserve myocardial tissue. Because the availability of open heart surgery as an intervention would cause further delay in treatment, PCI is the preferred therapy for this patient. Thrombolytic therapy is not used if PCI is available. The patient has evidence of STEMI. Heparin and G IIb/IIIa inhibitors are indicated for patients with acute coronary syndrome.

References: Efre, A., & Boling, B. (2018). Cardiovascular system. In T. M. Hartjes (Ed.), *AACN core curriculum for high acuity, progressive, and critical care nursing* (7th ed.). St. Louis: Elsevier.

Martin, L., Murphy, M., Scanlon, A., Naismith, C., Clark, D., & Farouque, O. (2014). Timely treatment for acute myocardial infarction and health outcomes: An integrative review of the literature. *Australian Critical Care, 27*(3), 111–118. http://dx.doi.org/10.1016/j.aucc.2013.11.005.

2-20. **(C)** An estimated 1 million adults (0.5% of the U.S. adult population) reported making a suicide attempt in the past year. Suicidal behavior has no racial, social, religious, cultural, or economic boundaries. Options A, B, and D are all true. Understanding the characteristics of suicidal patients helps the critical care nurse plan patient care.

Reference: Chapa, D., & Akintade, B. (2018). Psychosocial aspects of critical care. In T. M. Hartjes (Ed.), *AACN core curriculum for high acuity, progressive, and critical care nursing* (7th ed.). St. Louis: Elsevier.

2-21. **(D)** Linear fracture of the temporal bone leading to laceration of the middle meningeal artery is the most common cause of epidural hematoma. Classically, these patients present with a history of a brief loss of consciousness immediately after the injury with a subsequent period of lucidity. Subsequently, these patients often deteriorate because of the expanding arterial bleed. Epidural hematoma is a neurosurgical emergency. Urgent noncontrast head CT scan may be considered, but this patient's history would most likely result in immediate operative intervention for this surgical emergency. Cerebral angiography and coil embolization (Option A) would be indicated for a cerebral aneurysm not a traumatic brain injury (TBI). This patient was noted to have a linear left temporal skull fracture. After the likely underlying epidural hematoma is evacuated, the patient should significantly improve and is unlikely to need (Option B) ventriculostomy and CSF drainage. If there were additional intracranial findings, these actions may be indicated. Osmotic diuretic (Option C) may be given to patients with known head injury and focal neurologic deficits. However, corticosteroids are not indicated in traumatic brain injury.

References: Blissitt, P.A. (2018). Neurologic system. In T. M. Hartjes (Ed.), *AACN core curriculum for high acuity, progressive, and critical care nursing* (7th ed.). St. Louis: Elsevier.

Ferri, F. (2017). Epidural hematoma. In F. Ferri (Ed.), *2017 Ferri's clinical advisor: 5 books in 1* (pp. 441–442). Philadelphia: Elsevier.

2-22. **(D)** Sore throats, aching joints, and painful urination all signal activity of opportunistic bacterial and fungal growth associated with taking immunosuppressive medications to protect donor organs. Rapid recognition and intervention will help to avoid damage and potentially lethal infections. Neither restricted physical activity nor dietary restrictions will help avoid future infections. Drinking plenty of liquids will help avoid dehydration and infection, but this is not the best reply for avoiding delays in treatment.

Reference: Boling, B. (2018). Renal system. In T. M. Hartjes (Ed.), *AACN core curriculum for high acuity, progressive, and critical care nursing* (7th ed.). St. Louis: Elsevier.

2-23. **(D)** The patient meets the criteria for brain death. Organ transplantation is the only medical and surgical therapy that is regulated by law. These regulations ensure that organs are shared on an equitable basis. The critical care nurse is an essential member of the organ procurement team. The Centers for Medicare and Medicaid Services (CMS), The Joint Commission standards, and hospital policies require that patients meeting the criteria for imminent death and cardiac death be referred to an organ procurement agency in a timely manner. Nutrition support is important but will not change the outcome for this patient. Discharge planning will not be necessary for a patient who is declared brain dead. A DNR (do not resuscitate) status is not indicated at this time. If the patient can become an organ donor, full cardiopulmonary support is necessary.

References: Wyckoff, M., & Hartjes, T. M. (2018). Critical care patients with special needs: Palliative and end-of life care in the ICU. In T. M. Hartjes (Ed.), *AACN core curriculum for high acuity, progressive, and critical care nursing* (7th ed.). St. Louis: Elsevier.

Beal, E. (2013). U.S. organ donations: Nurses can make a difference. *American Journal of Nursing, 113*(9), 20-21. http://dx.doi.org/10.1097/01.NAJ.0000434167.46127.66.

2-24. **(B)** A systematic review was done to evaluate the efficacy of IPCDs (intermittent pneumatic compression devices) and VFPs (venous foot pumps) for DVT prevention in adult trauma patients, and the researchers reported that although both IPCDs and VFPs reduced the incidence of DVT, VFPs were more effective. A combination of mechanical prophylaxis and pharmacologic prophylaxis is thought to potentiate the overall efficacy of VTE prevention. In a meta-analysis done to evaluate VTE prophylaxis in trauma patients, researchers reported that patients who received both had a lower risk of DVT. Results of another meta-analysis done to examine VTE prevention in hospitalized patients also indicated that pharmacologic prophylaxis combined with IPC was more effective than IPC alone. Results of recent randomized controlled trials in critically ill patients also suggest that combination therapy is superior to either pharmacologic or mechanical prophylaxis alone.

References: Tocco, S., Martin, B., & Stacy, K. M. (2016). Preventing venous thromboembolism in adults. *Critical Care Nurse, 36*(5), e20–e23. http://dx.doi.org/10.4037/ccn2016638.

Arabi, Y. M., Alsolamy, S., Al-Dawood, A., et al. (2016). Thromboprophylaxis using combined intermittent pneumatic compression and pharmacologic prophylaxis versus pharmacologic prophylaxis alone in critically ill patients: study protocol for a randomized controlled trial. *Trials,* 171–178. http://dx.doi.org/10.1186/s13063-016-1520-0.

2-25. **(D)** Enterocutaneous fistulas can result in major fluid losses. The low serum albumin contributes to the development of edema and further increases intravascular fluid loss. Replacement of albumin is the most appropriate method to increase intravascular volume and blood pressure. The hematocrit is 30%, and blood replacement is not indicated until the hematocrit is decreased to 28% or less. The patient is on hyperalimentation, which contains glucose, and the serum glucose is low normal, so dextrose 50% is not indicated. Because the serum sodium is already elevated, fluid replacement with normal saline 0.9% would be controversial. Normal saline 0.45% may be preferred for fluid replacement in the hypernatremic patient.

References: Radovich, P. (2018). Gastrointestinal system. In T. M. Hartjes (Ed.), *AACN core curriculum for high acuity, progressive, and critical care nursing* (7th ed.). St. Louis: Elsevier.

Kate, V. (2016). *Enterocutaneous fistula clinical presentation.* Available from http://emedicine.medscape.com/article/1372132-clinical#b3.

2-26. **(C)** The patient is exhibiting findings characteristic of arthropod-borne encephalitis. CSF cultures would be most beneficial in identifying the causative organism. Although (Option A) serologic tests may be of help, the nurse would not obtain a specimen when the patient is experiencing a grand mal seizure. Also, the nurse would not wait to intervene until the seizure is completed (Option B) because prolonged seizure activity is life-threatening. If a standing order for a benzodiazepine is available for the patient, then the nurse would be able to quickly provide treatment to stop the seizure activity. If no order is available, the nurse should notify the physician to inform of the situation and obtain further orders. Although it is important to protect the patient from injury, restraints (Option D) are not appropriate in this circumstance. Padded side rails would be most appropriate.

Reference: Blissitt, P. A. (2018). Neurologic system. In T. M. Hartjes (Ed.), *AACN core curriculum for high acuity, progressive, and critical care nursing* (7th ed.). St. Louis: Elsevier.

2-27. **(B)** Occasionally, patients return from the operating room with delayed sternal closure or "open chest." Delayed sternal closure is used to manage reperfusion myocardial edema, hemodynamic instability, refractory bleeding, and malignant arrhythmias. This approach facilitates surgical reentry for bleeding control, clot evacuation, and cardiac massage. ECMO therapy can also complicate pressure ulcer prevention. If a patient is "too unstable to turn," it is a major indicator for pressure ulcer development. Labeling a patient "too unstable to turn" perpetuates the notion that turning will result in hemodynamic instability. Changes in heart rate and mixed venous oxygen saturation after lateral turning of intensive care patients is transient and expected, and most patients return to baseline within 5 minutes of completion of the repositioning. Option A is true. The 2010 consensus statement from the National Pressure Ulcer Advisory Panel established that some pressure ulcers are unavoidable in situations in which pressure cannot be relieved and perfusion cannot be improved. The 2014 consensus identified risk factors in specific situations that may lead to the development of unavoidable pressure ulcers. These include impaired tissue oxygenation or cardiovascular instability, hypovolemia, sepsis, anasarca, peripheral vascular disease: venous or arterial, sensory impairment, immobility, end-of-life skin failure, and multiorgan failure. Option C is true. A rare yet equally troublesome pressure ulcer occurs with the use of a postsurgical compression brassiere, which is reserved for female cardiac surgery patients who are larger in both chest circumference and breast size. Published reports are focused on the use of these garments for stabilization of the sternum, improved approximation of sternal wounds, and comfort. The bra can have fabric that does not stretch, and most important, edges that are abrasive, minimally elastic, and constrictive. Option D is true. Nursing standards of care related to tracheostomy management and pressure ulcer prevention are often impeded by surgical techniques. Providers often use sutures to secure the tracheostomy phalange to the patient's neck, with the intention of preventing potential dislodgment of the tracheostomy tube. However, sutures make it difficult for nurses to relieve pressure by preventing adequate barrier placement between the tracheostomy plate and the skin. This is especially a problem after fluid resuscitation or in patients with fluid volume overload. The combination of direct pressure on the skin, with potential additive effects of tracheal secretions, creates pressure ulcers that are often accompanied by maceration at the suture sites.

References: Dermenchyan, A. (2018). Professional caring and ethical practice. In T. M. Hartjes (Ed.), *AACN core curriculum for high acuity, progressive, and critical care nursing* (7th ed.). St. Louis: Elsevier.

Cooper, D., Jones, S., & Currie, L. (2015). Against all odds: Preventing pressure ulcers in high-risk cardiac surgery patients. *Critical Care Nurse, 35*(5), 76–82. http://dx.doi.org/10.4037/ccn2015434.

2-28. **(D)** Morphine sulfate is the most appropriate medication to relieve chest pain due to myocarditis. In myocarditis, pain is due to inflammation of the myocardium and is often related to autoimmune infiltration. Nitroglycerin is not effective in relieving the pain of myocarditis because the pain is not related to coronary blood flow. Diuretics may be effective to relieve symptoms of heart failure associated with myocarditis, but they would not relieve pain. Nonsteroidal antiinflammatory medications are contraindicated in chest pain associated with myocarditis because they may facilitate the disease process and increase mortality.

References: Efre, A., & Boling, B. (2018). Cardiovascular system. In T. M. Hartjes (Ed.), *AACN core curriculum for high acuity, progressive, and critical care nursing* (7th ed.). St. Louis: Elsevier.

Brock, A. (2018). Critical care patients with special needs: Pain in the critically ill patient. In T. M. Hartjes (Ed.), *AACN core curriculum for high acuity, progressive, and critical care nursing* (7th ed.). St. Louis: Elsevier.

2-29. **(D)** In patients with liver dysfunction, an altered level of consciousness occurs due to the development of hepatic encephalopathy, which occurs when the detoxification functions of the liver are lost, resulting in impairment of the central nervous system. Hepatic encephalopathy is a neuropsychiatric disorder associated with portal hypertension. In the patient with acute liver failure, the development of encephalopathy follows the development of jaundice and can present within 2 weeks of the onset of liver failure. An additional concern is that when patients develop encephalopathy, their ability to maintain a patent airway may become compromised. Hypotension is not a clinical feature of patients with hepatic dysfunction; hyperdynamic circulation is more likely with liver disorders. Although esophageal bleeding is a potential complication with liver failure, this patient evidences no indications of that problem. Although the patient has elevated liver enzymes, there are no findings that specifically reflect the presence of systemic infection.

Reference: Radovich, P. (2018). Gastrointestinal system. In T. M. Hartjes (Ed.), *AACN core curriculum for high acuity, progressive, and critical care nursing* (7th ed.). St. Louis: Elsevier.

2-30. **(C)** On the 12-lead ECG, posterior wall MI presents as tall, broad R waves and ST depression in leads V1 and V3. When reversed and rotated 180 degrees, these findings appear as deep Q waves and ST segment elevation. Unstable angina presents on the 12-lead ECG as transient ST depression and T wave inversion. Anterior septal MI presents with ST segment elevation in leads V1 to V3. Pericarditis would present on the 12-lead ECG as ST segment elevation in the anterior leads V1 and V6.

References: Efre, A., & Boling, B. (2018). Cardiovascular system. In T. M. Hartjes (Ed.), *AACN core curriculum for high acuity, progressive, and critical care nursing* (7th ed.). St. Louis: Elsevier.

Anderson, J. L. (2015). St segment elevation acute myocardial infarction and complications of myocardial infarction. In L. Goldman (Author), *Goldman-Cecil medicine* (pp. 441–456). Philadelphia: Elsevier Health Sciences.

2-31. **(A)** A warm pack should not be used for vesicant extravasation. A cold pack will provide a stimulus for vasoconstriction and extravasated drug reabsorption. Cold application is recommended for use with hyperosmolar fluids, such as mannitol. Cold packs should be applied for 15 to 20 minutes every 4 hours for 24 to 48 hours after the extravasation.

References: Vacca, V. M., Jr. (2013). Vesicant extravasation. *Nursing, 43*(9), 21–22. http://dx.doi.org/10.1097/01.NURSE.0000432917.59376.55.

Coyle, C., Griffie, J., & Czaplewski, L. (2015). Eliminating extravasation events: A multidisciplinary approach. *Journal of Infusion Nursing,* S43–S50. http://dx.doi.org/10.1097/NAN.0000000000000144.

2-32. **(B)** Metabolic syndrome is a multiplex risk factor that arises from insulin resistance accompanying abnormal adipose deposition and function. It is a risk factor for coronary heart disease, as well as for diabetes, fatty liver, and several cancers. The initial management of metabolic syndrome involves lifestyle modifications, including changes in diet and exercise habits. Weight loss can stop the progression of the disease. Option A is incorrect because low-fat foods are often high in sugar and carbohydrates. When the fat content is lowered by manufacturers, often sugar is substituted to improve the flavor of the products. As a result, these low-fat foods raise the triglycerides. The initial management of metabolic syndrome involves lifestyle modifications, including changes in diet and exercise habits. Option C is incorrect. Metabolic syndrome was associated with a lower risk of bone fractures in a meta-analysis. Studies demonstrate that Option D is incorrect. Evidence exists to support the notion that diet, exercise, and pharmacologic interventions may inhibit the progression of metabolic syndrome to diabetes mellitus.

Reference: Benefield, A. (2018). Critical Care Patients with Special Needs: Bariatric Patients. In T. M. Hartjes (Ed.), *AACN core curriculum for high acuity, progressive, and critical care nursing* (7th ed.). St. Louis: Elsevier.

2-33. **(B)** Anorexia or lack of appetite is common in chronic obstructive pulmonary disease (COPD) and may be caused or augmented by several symptoms affecting appetite and eating. Patients with long-standing COPD have difficulty maintaining adequate nutritional intake because of the caloric demands inflicted by increased work of breathing and by the great effort required to breathe and eat simultaneously. Poor nutrition negatively affects all body functions and can lead to additional health complications and increased mortality. Cor pulmonale presents as right heart failure and causes edema with weight gain. The weight loss may be associated with weaker thoracic excursion and diminished ventilation and is not usually related to dehydration.

References: Storzer, D. N. (2018). Pulmonary system. In T. M. Hartjes (Ed.), *AACN core curriculum for high acuity, progressive, and critical care nursing* (7th ed.). St. Louis: Elsevier.

Nordén, J., Grönberg, A., Bosaeus, I., et al. (2014). Nutrition impact symptoms and body composition in patients with COPD. *European Journal of Clinical Nutrition, 69*(2), 256–261. http://dx.doi.org/10.1038/ejcn.2014.76.

2-34. **(D)** Data support that pulmonary embolus, anastomotic leaks, and cardiac events account for almost of the deaths after bariatric surgery. Pulmonary embolism (30% to 40%) is the most common cause of death after bariatric surgery, followed by cardiac events (25%) and anastomotic leaks

(20%). These data need to be incorporated in the assessment and plan of care of these patients. Appropriate prophylaxis for venous thrombotic events usually includes low-molecular-weight heparin. Option A reflects some of the common short-term complications of bariatric surgery, which include wound infection, stomal stenosis, marginal ulceration, and constipation. Options B and C relate to some long-term complications of this surgery, including symptomatic cholelithiasis, dumping syndrome, persistent vomiting, and nutritional deficiencies.

Reference: Benefield, A. (2018). Critical care patients with special needs: Bariatric patients. In T. M. Hartjes (Ed.), *AACN core curriculum for high acuity, progressive, and critical care nursing* (7th ed.). St. Louis: Elsevier.

2-35. **(B)** Vasovagal reaction may occur during sheath removal. Atropine is used to block vagally induced slowing of the heart rate and hypotension. IV doses of 0.5 to 1.0 mg can be given immediately and reverse bradycardia and hypotension within 2 minutes. If decreased blood pressure occurs without bradycardia, a normal saline bolus may be administered. Nausea occurs due to decreased blood pressure. Prochlorperazine (Compazine) is associated with vasodilation and would cause a further decrease in blood pressure. Retroperitoneal bleeding generally becomes evident after sheath removal when the puncture site is no longer protected by the sheath.

Reference: Kern, M. (2015). Anticholinergics for vagal reaction. In M. Kern, P. Sorajja, & M. Lim (Eds.), *The cardiac catheterization handbook* (6th ed.) (pp. 1–53). Philadelphia: Elsevier.

2-36. **(B)** Overall disease prevention is of vital importance to persons with HIV infection. Immunizations are an important part of disease prevention in persons with HIV infection. Pneumococcal and influenza vaccine is recommended for all HIV-positive patients regardless of their CD4+ count. Opportunistic infections, which have been defined as infections that are more frequent or more severe because of immunosuppression in HIV-infected persons, are a principal cause of morbidity and mortality in the HIV population. Infection prevention techniques are critical to prevent opportunistic infections. In recent years, as many as 25% of HIV-positive patients may have otherwise unexplained arthralgia. Arthralgias and myalgias also form a part of the constitutional symptoms of HIV seroconversion. Patients with HIV are subject to HIV-associated arthritis, osteoporosis and osteopenia, avascular bone necrosis, and fibromyalgia. Pain management techniques will help patients with HIV cope with pain related to the disease progression (Option C). However, pain management techniques will not have the most benefit for this patient who was admitted with an infection. Sexual promiscuity is not an appropriate topic at this time.

Reference: Dressler, D. (2018). Hematological and immunological systems. In T. M. Hartjes (Ed.), *AACN core curriculum for high acuity, progressive, and critical care nursing* (7th ed.). St. Louis: Elsevier.

2-37. **(B)** Right ventricular infarction complicates up to 30% to 40% of inferior STE-MIs. Isolated RV infarction is extremely uncommon. In right ventricular myocardial infarction, the right ventricle (RV) is unable to maintain forward flow (due to poor RV contractility) to the lungs without adequate preload. Intravenous fluid administration increases right ventricular volume and promotes forward flow to the lungs. Diuretics would diminish circulating volume and preload and so would aggravate the problem. Nitroglycerin and morphine cause vasodilation that decreases preload and would diminish right ventricular filling and output, thus worsening myocardial ischemia.

References: Efre, A., & Boling, B. (2018). Cardiovascular system. In T. M. Hartjes (Ed.), *AACN core curriculum for high acuity, progressive, and critical care nursing* (7th ed.). St. Louis: Elsevier.

Abtahi, F., Farmanesh, M., Moaref, A., & Shekarforoush, S. (2016). Right ventricular involvement in either anterior or inferior myocardial infarction. *International Cardiovascular Research Journal, 10*(2), 67–71. http://dx.doi.org/10.17795/icrj-10(267).

2-38. **(A)** *Anterior cord syndrome* is commonly caused by flexion injuries as seen in head-on collisions or by acute herniation of an intervertebral disk. It is associated with injury to the anterior gray horn (motor) cells, the spinothalamic tracts (pain), the anterior spinothalamic tract (light touch), and the corticospinal tracts (temperature). This type of injury results in a loss of motor function and the ability to sense pain and temperature with intact position sense and sensation to pressure and vibration lower than the level of the injury. *Central cord syndrome* produces a motor and sensory deficit more pronounced in the upper extremities than in the lower extremities. *Brown-Sequard syndrome* presents as loss of voluntary motor movement on the same side as the injury with loss of pain, temperature, and sensation on the opposite side. *Posterior cord syndrome* results in loss of position sense, pressure, and vibration lower than the level of injury with intact motor function and sensation of pain and temperature.

References: Blissitt, P. A. (2018). Neurologic system. In T. M. Hartjes (Ed.), *AACN core curriculum for high acuity, progressive, and critical care nursing* (7th ed.). St. Louis: Elsevier.

Perron, A., & Huff, J. (2014). Spinal cord disorders. In J. Marx, P. Rosen, & H. Bessen (Eds.), *Rosen's emergency medicine: Concepts and clinical practice* (8th ed.) (pp. 1419–1427). Philadelphia: Elsevier.

2-39. **(C)** Electrical storm is the occurrence of either sustained VT (greater than 30 seconds) or greater than or equal to three distinct episodes of VT or VF in 24 hours that result in ICD therapy. An important step in evaluating this condition is to identify and reverse the causative factors of electrical storm. Specific precipitants include acute ischemia, worsening heart failure, hypokalemia, hypomagnesemia, arrhythmogenic drug therapy, hyperthyroidism, and infection or fever. Because the device functioned appropriately, lead fracture is not suspected. An ECG should be performed to rule out ischemia. However, a magnet is not required to perform the ECG. The magnet deactivates only the defibrillator function. EP testing would be indicated before device implant or if the dysrhythmia required ablation.

References: Efre, A., & Boling, B. (2018). Cardiovascular system. In T. M. Hartjes (Ed.), *AACN core curriculum for high acuity, progressive, and critical care nursing* (7th ed.). St. Louis: Elsevier.

Iftikhar, S., Mattu, A., & Brady, W. (2016). ED evaluation and management of implantable cardiac defibrillator electrical shocks. *American Journal of Emergency Medicine, 34*(6), 1140–1147. http://dx.doi.org/10.1016/j.ajem.2016.02.060.

2-40. **(C)** Dysphagia is a frequent occurrence after stroke. Swallowing problems are reported in 37% to 78 % of stroke patients. Findings of aspiration may include one or several of the following: dyspnea, tachypnea, low oxygen saturation (O_2 sat), putrid expectoration, malaise, and frequent coughing. The earliest indication that aspiration may have occurred would be the development of tachypnea and tachycardia. The $PaCO_2$ may decrease with tachypnea associated with aspiration, and the tachypnea associated with aspiration is generally the reason an arterial blood gas is obtained. Chest x-ray findings are later signs and may be seen in the right middle lobe because of the angle of the right mainstem bronchus, although infiltrates associated with aspiration may be located in any dependent lung field. This patient's cough reflex may be suppressed, and positive sputum cultures associated with bacterial infections may take up to 3 days to develop.

Reference: Storzer, D. N. (2018). Pulmonary system. In T. M. Hartjes (Ed.), *AACN core curriculum for high acuity, progressive, and critical care nursing* (7th ed.). St. Louis: Elsevier.

2-41. **(C)** Patients with hyperglycemia in the ICU have increased morbidity and mortality. Hyperglycemia is associated with immune dysfunction, increased systemic inflammation, and vascular insufficiency. Elevated blood glucose levels have been shown to worsen outcomes in medical patients who are in the ICU for more than 3 days. An hourly insulin infusion protocol provides tighter control over blood glucose management. Important considerations in the development of an insulin protocol include allowing 6 to 8 hours to safely lower glucose to target, reducing the risk of hypoglycemia, and accounting for patient insulin sensitivity and resistance. Simply documenting and monitoring the patient will not achieve desirable results, as the patient will continue to produce ketone bodies. In this acute phase, it is too early to move to subcutaneous insulin, which has a slower rate of absorption than the intravenous route. A bolus dose of IV regular insulin may lower the blood sugar too quickly or precipitate hypoglycemia. Patients experiencing hypoglycemia had higher Sequential Organ Failure Assessment scores, indicating more organ dysfunction. Hypoglycemia episodes are associated with increased morbidity and mortality in the ICU.

References: MacDermott, J. (2018). Endocrine system. In T. M. Hartjes (Ed.), *AACN core curriculum for high acuity, progressive, and critical care nursing* (7th ed.). St. Louis: Elsevier.

Schiffner, L. (2014). Glucose management in critically ill medical and surgical patients. *Dimensions of Critical Care Nursing, 33*(2), 70–77. http://dx.doi.org/10.1097/DCC.0000000000000025.

2-42. **(B)** Hyperosmolar hyperglycemic syndrome (HHS) is characterized by severe hyperglycemia without ketosis. In HHS, there may be enough insulin present to inhibit lipolysis or ketogenesis in the liver but not enough to control hyperglycemia. Urine ketones are either absent or "small." Infections cause up to 50% of cases (e.g., pneumonia, urinary tract infection, sepsis), so elevated WBC and fever can be expected. Infection, new diabetes diagnosis, noncompliance, and medications are some of the etiology that cause blood glucose levels higher 600 mg/dL. Reversible hemiplegia, focal seizures, neurologic changes, and coma are present in the clinical presentation of these patients.

Reference: MacDermott, J. (2018). Endocrine system. In T. M. Hartjes (Ed.), *AACN core curriculum for high acuity, progressive, and critical care nursing* (7th ed.). St. Louis: Elsevier.

2-43. **(B)** The most appropriate action is Option B because the most reliable source of information would be a chart audit to objectively quantify the number of cases and the specific outcome indicators for each. This option could also be accomplished quickly. Option A will delay securing data to determine the nature and extent of any problem for 6 months; if a problem were identified, its solution would be even further delayed, possibly compromising patient outcomes. Options C and D afford purely subjective discussions rather than the facts needed for future decision making at the organizational level.

Reference: Dermenchyan, A. (2018). Professional caring and ethical practice. In T. M. Hartjes (Ed.), *AACN core curriculum for high acuity, progressive, and critical care nursing* (7th ed.). St. Louis: Elsevier.

2-44. **(C)** The primary goals of emergency management of intracerebral hemorrhage (ICH) are to prevent subsequent damage from rebleeding, edema, or hypoxia and to identify the cause, site, and extent of the hemorrhage. If coagulopathies are present, these must be corrected in order to prevent further bleeding. In patients with ICH, blood pressure reduction (Option A) should be gradual and controlled because acute blood pressure normalization may reduce local cerebral perfusion pressure and cerebral blood flow to ischemic levels; in chronically hypertensive patients, it may shift the autoregulatory curve to higher pressures. Blood pressure treatment must be tailored to the needs of the individual patient. As a guide, for patients with a history of significant hypertension, the MAP should initially be maintained in the range of 120 mm Hg. In formerly nonhypertensive patients, lowering SBP to less than 160 mm Hg in the first hours after ICH may prevent additional bleeding. CT scan of the head is the primary imaging modality used for these patients, whereas cerebral angiography (Option B) is not commonly performed in this patient population. Size and location of an ICH are used to judge the usefulness of surgical interventions (Option D). Although surgical intervention may be beneficial for noncomatose patients with large or enlarging superficial clots, traditional craniotomy with evacuation of spontaneous supratentorial hematomas has been shown to be ineffective in reducing mortality or disability in this patient population as a whole. Infratentorial hematomas, which often present with signs of brainstem compression, are often treated with surgical evacuation and have significantly decreased mortality in this subgroup.

References: Blissitt, P. A. (2018). Neurologic system. In T. M. Hartjes (Ed.), *AACN core curriculum for high acuity, progressive, and critical care nursing* (7th ed.). St. Louis: Elsevier.

Le Roux, P., Pollack, C., Milan, M., & Schaefer, A. (2014). Race against the clock: Overcoming challenges in the management of anticoagulant-associated intracerebral hemorrhage. *Journal of Neurosurgery, 121*, 1–20.

2-45. **(A)** There should be bubbling in the water seal chamber when the patient exhales to indicate that air is escaping from the pleural space. A large amount of bubbling that does not coincide with the patient's phase of ventilation suggests a large air leak in the system. Bubbling in the water seal chamber will disappear slowly as the lung reexpands to fill the pleural space and air stops leaking. There should not be any dependent loops in the chest drainage tubing system, as these may inhibit drainage. The key is positioning drainage tubing to use physics principles and facilitate fluid drainage. Dependent loops containing fluid can completely block fluid drainage within 30 minutes and change pleural pressures from -18 cmH$_2$O to $+8$ cmH$_2$O, a change of 26 cm H$_2$O in pressure. If suction is ordered, it will be a negative pressure. Positive pressure is not applied to a closed drainage system. A chest tube is not to be clamped unless specifically ordered by the physician or unless unit procedure calls for clamping as part of replacing or changing the system.

References: Storzer, D. N. (2018). Pulmonary system. In T. M. Hartjes (Ed.), *AACN core curriculum for high acuity, progressive, and critical care nursing* (7th ed.). St. Louis: Elsevier.

Kane, C. J., York, N. L., & Minton, L. A. (2013). Chest tubes in the critically ill patient. *Dimensions of Critical Care Nursing, 32*(3), 111–117. http://dx.doi.org/10.1097/DCC.0b013e3182864721.

2-46. **(C)** Norepinephrine would be the vasopressor of choice in this particular patient. Norepinephrine is a positive inotrope and increases mean arterial pressure due to its vasoconstrictive effects, with little change in heart rate and less increase in stroke volume compared with dopamine. Because the patient is experiencing tachycardia with a heart rate of 110 beats/min, dopamine would not be the initial choice. Epinephrine also has strong positive chronotropic effects so would not be the preferred agent. Vasopressin is a direct vasoconstrictor and a negative inotrope. Use of vasopressin can lead to coronary artery and splanchnic ischemia, resulting in further compromise of a critically ill patient.

References: Morozowich, S. (2015). Vasopressors. In M. Murray (Ed.), *Faust's anesthesiology review*, 4th ed. (pp. 196–198). Philadelphia: Elsevier Saunders.

McFeely, J. (2017). 2016 Surviving Sepsis Guidelines Update. *Critical Care Alert, 25*(3), 1–3.

2-47. **(A)** Patients receiving a large volume of fluids and blood components are at high risk for dilutional coagulopathy, which is accentuated with hypothermia (temperature less than 36.5°C or 97.7° F); therefore, warming blood components and fluids will help control factors altering coagulopathy. Monitoring laboratory values alone will not prevent the development of complications. Antihistamine and antiinflammatory medication will help to decrease immune responses to blood transfusions, including febrile incidents and pruritus, but these are not life-threatening complications. In times of trauma and shock, intramuscular injections are poorly absorbed.

References: Holleran, R. (2018). Multisystem: Multisystem trauma. In T. M. Hartjes (Ed.), *AACN core curriculum for high acuity, progressive, and critical care nursing* (7th ed.). St. Louis: Elsevier.

Katrancha, E., & Gonzalez, L., III (2014). Trauma-induced coagulopathy. *Critical Care Nurse, 34*(4), 54–63. http://dx.doi.org/10.4037/ccn2014133.

2-48. **(B)** A literature review will provide resources for the identification of the many family-centered care models and their implementation. Family-centered care can include bedside rounds that are focused on informing, educating, and involving the patient's family. Other strategies have included team meetings and partnership to include the spouse and family members to improve patients' outcomes by improving care. A change in the visitation policy may be required to facilitate the family-centered care model that is implemented on this unit. Evidence-based practice found in the literature review will guide the specific visitation changes required to implement the new care model.

References: Dermenchyan, A. (2018). Professional caring and ethical practice. In T. M. Hartjes (Ed.), *AACN core curriculum for high acuity, progressive, and critical care nursing* (7th ed.). St. Louis: Elsevier.

Rosenberg, K. (2016). Easing ICU Visitation Restrictions Improves Family's Satisfaction. AJN, *American Journal of Nursing, 116*(4), 61. http://dx.doi:10.1097/01.naj.0000482146.06587.60.

2-49. **(D)** It was observed in studies that there is a hypertension resolution rate of 85.6% along with marked decrease in antihypertensive usage after Roux-en-Y gastric bypass. However, mean resolution time was 3.2 months. Option A does not answer the patient's question directly even though it illustrates the nurse's ability to collaborate with other members of the multidisciplinary team. Option B describes gastric banding, which is not the procedure the patient had. Gastric leakage does not necessarily cause a change in a patient's blood pressure.

References: Benefield, A. (2018). Critical care patients with special needs: Bariatric patients. In T. M. Hartjes (Ed.), *AACN core curriculum for high acuity, progressive, and critical care nursing* (7th ed.). St. Louis: Elsevier.

Bonfils, P. K., Taskiran, M., Damgaard, M., et al. (2015). Roux-en-Y gastric bypass alleviates hypertension and is associated with an increase in mid-regional pro-atrial natriuretic peptide in morbid obese patients. *Journal of Hypertension, 33*(6), 1215–1225. http://dx.doi.org/10.1097/HJH.0000000000000526.

2-50. **(D)** When a patient or family member becomes aggressive, the nurse should speak in a calm, soft, noncondescending manner. The patient and family should be permitted to ventilate verbally without interruption. The nurse should focus on the particular incident at hand. Clear limits should be placed on what will and will not be tolerated with the consequences for aggressive behavior clearly defined. The patient or family should not be educated on aggressive and violent behavior while the aggressive behavior is taking place.

Reference: Chapa, D., & Akintade, B. (2018). Psychosocial aspects of critical care. In T. M. Hartjes (Ed.), *AACN core curriculum for high acuity, progressive, and critical care nursing* (7th ed.). St. Louis: Elsevier.

2-51. **(B)** Mrs. Jones is admitted to the ICU for signs of septic shock, a medical emergency. The initial priority for this patient who is demonstration multi organ system compromise is to treat her low blood pressure. The Surviving Sepsis Campaign guidelines recommend the initiation of initial resuscitation with IV crystalloid solution ≥ 30 mL/Kg to target a MAP greater than 65 mm Hg. Antibiotic therapy should be initiated within one hour, after cultures are obtained. A norepinephrine infusion will be required if the patient does not respond to fluid resuscitation. A goals of care discussion would delay appropriate medical intervention and is not a first priority for this patient.

Reference: Johnson, A. (2018). Multisystem: Systemic inflammatory response syndrome and septic shock. In T. M. Hartjes (Ed.), *AACN core curriculum for high acuity, progressive, and critical care nursing* (7th ed.). St. Louis: Elsevier.

2-52. **(B)** Milrinone is FDA approved for the short-term IV treatment of patients with acute, decompensated heart failure. The use of IV milrinone has been associated with an increased frequency of ventricular arrhythmias, including nonsustained ventricular tachycardia. Ventricular arrhythmias are the most frequent adverse reactions that occur during milrinone therapy. Improved cardiac function after administration of milrinone can induce diuresis, predisposing the patient to hypokalemia and arrhythmias. In addition, concurrent use of IV diuretics for heart failure can lead to electrolyte imbalance. Correction of underlying electrolyte imbalances will minimize proarrhythmic potential during milrinone administration. A fluid bolus will not improve the electrolyte levels and may worsen heart failure. Additional diuretics can worsen hypokalemia.

References: Efre, A., & Boling, B. (2018). Cardiovascular system. In T. M. Hartjes (Ed.), *AACN core curriculum for high acuity, progressive, and critical care nursing* (7th ed.). St. Louis: Elsevier.

Milrinone. (2016). In J. Aronson (Ed.), *Meyler's side effects of drugs* (16th ed.), (pp. 1038–1040). Elsevier Science.

2-53. **(B)** Alleviation of postoperative pain will allow the patient to perform breathing exercises focused on prevention of atelectasis. Although the patient may require increased oxygen, the breathing exercises will likely restore his oxygen saturation to acceptable levels. There is no clinical evidence of hemothorax; breath sounds are diminished because of lobe removal on the right and atelectasis on the left. Anxiety management alone would be insufficient to improve this patient's pulmonary status, and a sedative may cause somnolence and decreased participation in pulmonary toilette.

Reference: Storzer, D. N. (2018). Pulmonary system. In T. M. Hartjes (Ed.), *AACN core curriculum for high acuity, progressive, and critical care nursing* (7th ed.). St. Louis: Elsevier.

2-54. **(C)** Pleural effusion is a complication of pancreatitis that can negatively affect management of ARDS. Pancreatic enzymes released into the circulation damage pulmonary vasculature and stimulate inflammation, leading to intrapulmonary shunt and hypoxemia. Exudates may then cross the diaphragm and enter the pleural space through lymphatic channels, causing pleural effusions. Pleural effusions can reduce pulmonary compliance and limit lung expansion. The hypovolemia experienced by patients with acute peritonitis secondary to pancreatitis is typically a relative form because of third spacing of fluids within the abdomen and can be managed with fluids to optimize preload and circulating volume. Autodigestion of body tissues by pancreatic enzymes can lead to fistula formation and impaired skin integrity, but these problems do not significantly affect pulmonary function. The pain associated with acute pancreatitis is often characterized as "the worst ever" and could compromise pulmonary function through limited lung expansion and guarding. Effective, aggressive, and continual pain management should enable avoidance of additional pulmonary compromise because of pain.

References: Radovich, P. (2018). Gastrointestinal system. In T. M. Hartjes (Ed.), *AACN core curriculum for high acuity, progressive, and critical care nursing* (7th ed.). St. Louis: Elsevier.

Tenner, S., & Steinberg, W. (2016). Acute pancreatitis. In M. Feldman, L. Friedman, & L. Brandt (Eds.), *Sleisenger and Fordtran's gastrointestinal and liver disease*, (10th ed.), (pp. 969–993). Philadelphia: Elsevier Saunders.

2-55. **(C)** Cardiac perforation by pacemaker is a rare but potentially fatal complication leading to hemopericardium and tamponade. This would result in symptoms of JVD and hypotension with narrowed pulse pressure. Patients also demonstrate tachycardia; however, this patient would not demonstrate tachycardia due to pacer dependency. Hemothorax or pneumothorax may cause diminished breath sounds on the affected side. Pacer lead infection is not an acute complication of transvenous pacer insertion.

Reference: Efre, A., & Boling, B. (2018). Cardiovascular system. In T. M. Hartjes (Ed.), *AACN core curriculum for high acuity, progressive, and critical care nursing* (7th ed.). St. Louis: Elsevier.

2-56. **(D)** The preceptor needs to use two evidence-based interventions such as observing for signs of respiratory distress, use of capnography if available, measurement of pH of aspirate, and observing the visual characteristics of the aspirate. Radiographic confirmation to assess nasogastric tube placement and prevent potential harm is recommended. Radiographic evaluation is the most definitive way to confirm the position of an NG tube. Option A is refuted by case reports in which bubbling did not occur despite malpositioning of the tube within the airways. AACN practice recommends that practitioners do not use the auscultatory method or the water bubbling method to determine tube location. Option B is incorrect because the literature contains numerous reports of the ineffectiveness of air insufflation and auscultation for verification of tube location. Option C is also not optimal. Although observing for respiratory distress may be useful, there have been reports of failures of this method in that 16- to 18-French NG tubes malpositioned in the respiratory tract did not induce immediate respiratory distress in patients with neurologic debilitation or advanced respiratory disease.

Reference: Metheny, N. (2016). Initial and ongoing verification of feeding tube placement in adults. *Critical Care Nurse, 36*(2), e8–e13. http://dx.doi:10.4037/ccn2016141.

2-57. **(C)** Infection is a major cause of death in patients with acute renal failure and can seriously compromise patients with chronic renal failure. Patients with renal failure have an impaired immune response from uremic toxins and reduced phagocytosis by the reticuloendothelial system. Carbohydrates are encouraged in the renal diet to provide energy for metabolism and healing. Fluid overload may be the precursor of other conditions such as heart failure and respiratory failure, which may lead to risk for infection.

Fluid restriction is a requirement of the renal diet and does not place the patient at risk for infection.

Reference: Boling, B. (2018). Renal system. In T. M. Hartjes (Ed.), *AACN core curriculum for high acuity, progressive, and critical care nursing* (7th ed.). St. Louis: Elsevier.

2-58. **(C)** In patients on diuretic therapy, the vascular system may be depleted and need fluid augmentation despite the presence of rales and heart failure. This patient has an elevated HCT, suggesting hypovolemia; a low serum albumin that would contribute to loss of fluid into the interstitial spaces; and a BUN/creatinine ratio greater than 20 to 1, indicating hypovolemia. Dobutamine infusion would increase the force of ventricular contraction but would not raise BP if the stroke volume remained low because of intravascular volume depletion. Norepinephrine (Levophed) could temporarily increase BP through vasoconstriction, but vasopressors should be used only after volume deficits are corrected. Furosemide (Lasix) would further decrease intravascular volume.

References: Efre, A., & Boling, B. (2018). Cardiovascular system. In T. M. Hartjes (Ed.), *AACN core curriculum for high acuity, progressive, and critical care nursing* (7th ed.). St. Louis: Elsevier.

Carubelli, V., Lombardi, C., Gorga, E., Ravera, A., Metra, M., & Mentz, R. (2016). Cardiorenal interactions. *Heart Failure Clinics, 12*(3), 335–347.

2-59. **(D)** Insofar as it is possible, allowing patients to continue their customary routines and practices when in the hospital is the best approach because it offers COPD patients the greatest amount of control, which can lessen anxiety and maintain a more positive outlook. A mental health consult may be advisable for some COPD patients but is not warranted for others. The health care team should consider continuing antidepressants and other medications during the exacerbation, but benzodiazepines are not indicated for all COPD patients.

References: Dermenchyan, A. (2018). Professional caring and ethical practice. In T. M. Hartjes (Ed.), *AACN core curriculum for high acuity, progressive, and critical care nursing* (7th ed.). St. Louis: Elsevier.

von Leypoldt, A., & Ken, K. (2013). The psychology of chronic obstructive pulmonary disease. *Current Opinion in Psychiatry, 26*(5), 458–463. http://dx.doi.org/10.1097/YCO.0b013e328363c1fc.

2-60. **(C)** Spirituality has potential importance for acute and critically ill patients and families. Spirituality may influence understanding of suffering and illness and how a patient or family copes with the situation. By addressing spiritual issues, critical care nurses can create more holistic and compassionate systems of care. Option A is incorrect because spirituality may promote a patient's clinical stability. Option B is incorrect because spirituality issues can be addressed during all phases of health and illness. Option D is incorrect and demonstrates lack of respect for a patient's beliefs.

References: Dermenchyan, A. (2018). Professional caring and ethical practice. In T. M. Hartjes (Ed.), *AACN core curriculum for high acuity, progressive, and critical care nursing* (7th ed.). St. Louis: Elsevier.

AbdAleati, N., Mohd Zaharim, N., & Mydin, Y. (2016). Religiousness and mental health: Systematic review study. *Journal of Religion & Health, 55*(6), 1929–1937. http://dx.doi.org/10.1007/s10943-014-9896-1.

2-61. **(B)** Intraaortic balloon counterpulsation increases myocardial oxygen supply by increasing coronary artery perfusion when balloon inflation occurs during diastole. Just before ventricular systole, the balloon is deflated, allowing the left ventricle to eject against a low volume in the aorta. This reduction of afterload effectively decreases the left ventricular workload. Balloon augmentation improves contractility by supporting more efficient left ventricular emptying, thus increasing cardiac output. Neither myocardial oxygen supply nor left ventricular filling volume is directly affected. Although the balloon-augmented systolic pressure is higher than the aortic systolic pressure, left ventricular systolic pressure is not increased.

Reference: Efre, A., & Boling, B. (2018). Cardiovascular system. In T. M. Hartjes (Ed.), *AACN core curriculum for high acuity, progressive, and critical care nursing* (7th ed.). St. Louis: Elsevier.

2-62. **(A)** Phenytoin can cause bradycardia, heart block, and hypotension. The patient has a history of "fainting spells" and the etiology of the "spells" from a low heart rate is unknown. The "spells" could be secondary to a hypotensive process or Stokes-Adams syndrome (a periodic fainting spell in which there is a periodic onset and offset of blockage of heart due to disorder of heart rhythm that may last for seconds, hours, days, or even weeks before the conduction returns). In addition, the patient already demonstrates asymptomatic bradycardia. Lorazepam, midazolam, and diazepam would be first-line choices followed by valproic acid or levetiracetam if the patient fails to respond to benzodiazepines.

References: Blissitt, P. A. (2018). Neurologic system. In T. M. Hartjes (Ed.), *AACN core curriculum for high acuity, progressive, and critical care nursing* (7th ed.). St. Louis: Elsevier.

Lawson, T., & Yeager, S. (2016). Status epilepticus in adults: A review of diagnosis and treatment. *Critical Care Nurse, 36*(2), 62–73. http://dx.doi.org/10.4037/ccn2016892.

2-63. **(A)** Option A shows the nurse taking the initiative to find a solution to the patient's problem with compliance in medication administration. Neither Option B nor Option D helps the patient with her vision problem. Option C might be considered as collaboration; however, this patient does not warrant long-term placement until all possible solutions to keep her independent have been exhausted.

Reference: Dermenchyan, A. (2018). Professional caring and ethical practice. In T. M. Hartjes (Ed.), *AACN core curriculum for high acuity, progressive, and critical care nursing* (7th ed.). St. Louis: Elsevier.

2-64. **(C)** Brugada syndrome is a rare but well-defined cause of sudden cardiac death. Diagnosis requires a Brugada-type ECG as well as typical clinical features; such clinical considerations are currently key in guiding risk stratification and, hence, management. Although pharmacologic therapies are under investigation, the only intervention with a robust evidence base remains insertion of an implantable cardioverter defibrillator. Ablation and permanent pacemaker have not been proven to improve outcomes related to Brugada syndrome.

References: Efre, A., & Boling, B. (2018). Cardiovascular system. In T. M. Hartjes (Ed.), *AACN core curriculum for high acuity, progressive, and critical care nursing* (7th ed.). St. Louis: Elsevier.

Mashar, M., Kwok, A., Pinder, R., & Sabir, I. (2014). The Brugada syndrome revisited. *Trends in Cardiovascular Medicine, 24*(5), 191–196. http://dx.doi.org/10.1016/j.tcm.2013.11.001.

2-65. **(C)** Up to 90% of cor pulmonale cases are attributable to chronic obstructive pulmonary disease (COPD). The most common symptom of pulmonary hypertension associated with cor pulmonale is exertional dyspnea. Other clinical manifestations include those characteristics of right heart failure (i.e., fatigue, increased central venous pressures, jugular venous distention, hepatomegaly, splenomegaly, and peripheral edema, especially in dependent areas). Distant heart sounds are heard in pericardial tamponade or effusion. Although patients with COPD may experience cough, that finding reflects their pulmonary rather than cardiac disorder.

References: Efre, A., & Boling, B. (2018). Cardiovascular system. In T. M. Hartjes (Ed.), *AACN core curriculum for high acuity, progressive, and critical care nursing* (7th ed.). St. Louis: Elsevier.

Arshad, R. (2017). Cor pulmonale. In F. Ferri (Ed.), *2017 Ferri's clinical advisor: 5 books in 1* (pp. 320–322). Philadelphia: Elsevier.

2-66. **(A)** Early therapy for aortic dissection is critical and should be initiated when diagnostic tests are being performed. Opioids should be administered in adequate doses to control pain and decrease sympathetic tone. Patients with aortic dissections are typically hypertensive. The two goals of medical management are to reduce blood pressure and decrease the rate of rise of the arterial pulse to diminish shearing forces. A target blood pressure of 100 to 120 mm Hg systolic and a heart rate lower than 60 beats/min are recommended. Beta-adrenergic blockers are the cornerstone of aortic dissection management and are effective when used as the sole agent (in addition to opioid analgesia for pain). Because vasodilators such as sodium nitroprusside reflexively increase the heart rate and may also increase the rise of the arterial pulse; they necessitate concomitant use of a beta-blocker and so are a more complicated form of therapy.

References: Efre, A., & Boling, B. (2018). Cardiovascular system. In T. M. Hartjes (Ed.), *AACN core curriculum for high acuity, progressive, and critical care nursing* (7th ed.). St. Louis: Elsevier.

Marx, J., & Rosen, P. (2014). Aortic dissection. In J. Marx, & P. Rosen (Eds.), *Rosen's emergency medicine: Concepts and clinical practice* (pp. 1124–1128). Philadelphia: Elsevier Saunders.

2-67. **(C)** Normal arterial $PaCO_2$ is 35 to 45 mm Hg. Generally, hyperventilation is avoided in the early hours after head injury in order to prevent ischemia and worsening of related secondary injury. Chronic prophylactic hyperventilation therapy should be avoided during the first 5 days after severe TBI, particularly during the first 24 hours. Mild hyperventilation (arterial $PaCO_2$ 30–35 mm Hg) is considered for management of intracranial hypertension when measures such as osmotic therapy (mannitol), cerebrospinal fluid drainage (in patients with an external ventricular drain), sedation, and chemical paralysis are ineffective. More severe hyperventilation resulting in severe hypocapnia (Options A and B) is generally avoided to prevent ischemia. One study shows that patients who were hyperventilated to a $PaCO_2$ level of 25 mm Hg had worse outcomes than patients who were kept at a nearly normal $PaCO_2$ level. Higher levels of carbon dioxide (Option D) can cause vasodilation, increasing cerebral blood volume and raising ICP. Hyperventilation reduces ICP only temporarily, progressively losing effectiveness after 16 hours of continuous use.

References: Blissitt, P. A. (2018). Neurologic system. In T. M. Hartjes, (Ed.), *AACN core curriculum for high acuity, progressive, and critical care nursing* (7th ed.). St. Louis: Elsevier.

Rangel-Castilla, L., Salinas, P., Hanbali, F., & Gasco, J. (2016). Closed head injury treatment & management. Available from http://www.medscape.com/.

2-68. **(C)** This rhythm strip demonstrates atrial and ventricular lead failure to capture, with concomitant under sensing in both chambers. Undersensing occurs when the pacemaker fails to sense native cardiac activity, which results in asynchronous pacing. Failure to capture is demonstrated by the presence of a pacemaker artifact without a corresponding paced P or QRS. Oversensing occurs when electrical signals are inappropriately recognized as native cardiac activity and pacing is inhibited. These inappropriate signals may be large P or T waves, skeletal muscle activity, or lead contact problems. Runaway pacemaker is a potentially life-threatening malfunction of older-generation pacemakers. It is related to low battery voltage (e.g., overdue pacemaker replacement). The pacemaker delivers paroxysms of pacing spikes at 2000 beats/min, which may provoke ventricular fibrillation. Paradoxically, there may be failure to capture—causing bradycardia—because the pacing spikes are very low in amplitude (due to the depleted battery voltage) and because at very high rates the ventricle may become refractory to stimulation.

References: Efre, A., & Boling, B. (2018). Cardiovascular system. In T. M. Hartjes (Ed.), *AACN core curriculum for high acuity, progressive, and critical care nursing* (7th ed.). St. Louis: Elsevier.

Camm, A., Boyden, P., & Saksena, S. (2012). Electrocardiography of cardiac pacing. In S. Saksena, & A. Camm (Eds.), *Electrophysiological disorders of the heart* (pp. 475–486). Philadelphia: Elsevier Health.

2-69. **(A)** The transient causes of urinary incontinence in the elderly can be listed with the acronym DIAPPERS. The acronym stands for **d**elirium, **i**nfection (urinary), **a**trophic urethritis and vaginitis, **p**harmaceuticals, **p**sychological disorders (depression), **e**ndocrine (hypercalcemia, hypokalemia, glycosuria), **r**estricted mobility, and **s**tool impaction. Renal failure and dehydration cause a decrease in urine output and are not likely to cause urinary incontinence. Pregnancy can cause urinary incontinence but is unlikely in an elderly patient.

References: Bardsley, A. (2016). An overview of urinary incontinence. *British Journal of Nursing, 25*(18), S14–S21.

Alvero, R. (2017). Urinary incontinence. In F. Ferri (Ed.), *2017 Ferri's clinical advisor: 5 books in 1* (pp. 672–673). Philadelphia: Elsevier.

2-70. **(A)** Pulmonary contusion causes impairment of gas exchange at the gas–tissue interface. The most common etiology of pulmonary contusion is trauma related to a motor vehicle crash. The greater the degree of pulmonary contusion, the greater the degree of ventilatory impairment. Administration of pain medication will improve ventilation and decrease splinting, and the administration of oxygen will improve oxygenation and gas exchange. Auscultation of lung sounds is appropriate; however, pulmonary contusions do not require insertion of chest tubes because there is no hemothorax or pneumothorax. Patients can be managed without mechanical ventilation if their PaO_2 is greater than 60 mm Hg on 50% FiO_2, their respiratory rate is less than 24 breaths/min, spontaneous tidal volume is more than 5 mL/kg, and vital capacity exceeds 10 mL/kg. There is no evidence of a pleural effusion. A subsequent intervention would be to obtain a chest x-ray. If a chest x-ray revealed a pleural effusion, then a thoracentesis would be done if the effusion was significantly impairing the patient's ventilatory status.

References: Storzer, D. N. (2018). Pulmonary system. In T. M. Hartjes (Ed.), *AACN core curriculum for high acuity, progressive, and critical care nursing* (7th ed.). St. Louis: Elsevier.

Gallagher, J. (2014). Management of blunt pulmonary injury. *AACN Advanced Critical Care, 25*(4), 375–386. http://dx.doi.org/10.1097/NCI .0000000000000059.

2-71. **(B)** Nosocomial UTIs (composed mostly of asymptomatic bacteriuria), up to 97% of which are associated with instrumentation of the urinary tract, are the most common nosocomial infection worldwide and account for up to 40% of nosocomial infections in U.S. hospitals each year. Before placing a catheter, the nurse must have appropriate indications for the catheter. End-of-life care is an appropriate indication. Daily meatal care helps decrease the incidence of catheter-associated urinary tract infection (CAUTI) but does not prevent it. Option C is incorrect because most catheter-associated urinary tract infections are asymptomatic. Option D is incorrect because the family might not understand the risks associated with a catheter.

References: Dermenchyan, A. (2018). Professional caring and ethical practice. In T. M. Hartjes (Ed.), *AACN core curriculum for high acuity, progressive, and critical care nursing* (7th ed.). St. Louis: Elsevier.

AACN Practice Alert. (2015). Catheter-associated urinary tract infections. Available from http:// www.aacn.org/.

2-72. **(B)** Allowing the group to complete their prayer session supports the patient's cultural

and perhaps religious beliefs and displays cultural sensitivity. Interrupting the prayer (Option A) is inappropriate, unwarranted, and insensitive to the patient's belief system. Option C would not be appropriate because movement into the group could disrupt the prayer session. Observing the session (Option D) appears unwarranted as there is no indication that patient safety has been jeopardized in any way.

References: Dermenchyan, A. (2018). Professional caring and ethical practice. In T. M. Hartjes (Ed.), *AACN core curriculum for high acuity, progressive, and critical care nursing* (7th ed.). St. Louis: Elsevier.

Nelson, R. (2016). Spirituality: Part of nursing practice, but too often neglected. *American Journal of Nursing, 116*(9), 19–20.

2-73. **(D)** Lack of quality sleep is a ubiquitous problem for ICU patients. Increasing the amount of deep sleep is one of the most important treatments for delirium because sleep deprivation affects cognitive functioning and is associated with an increased frequency of delirium. Delirium can be caused by infections, dehydration, and medication changes. Administering additional diuretic could worsen dehydration-related delirium. Unlimited visiting with family and friends could further disrupt sleep patterns. Delirium is a serious and usually sudden disturbance in a patient's thinking ability, involving confusion and disorientation. Dementia, by contrast, is an irreversible, ongoing condition that affects both thinking and physical function, with symptoms such as memory loss, inability to solve simple problems, problems with language and thinking, and personality and behavior changes.

References: Chapa, D., & Akintade, B. (2018). Psychosocial aspects of critical care. In T. M. Hartjes (Ed.), *AACN core curriculum for high acuity, progressive, and critical care nursing* (7th ed.). St. Louis: Elsevier.

McFeely, J. (2016). Patients rarely sleep in the ICU. *Critical Care Alert, 24*(3), 17–19.

2-74. **(B)** The combination of respiratory alkalosis and metabolic acidosis, as evidenced by an elevated anion gap, is the hallmark of salicylate toxicity. Salicylates such as aspirin (acetylsalicylic acid) stimulate the respiratory center and cause hyperventilation, resulting in respiratory alkalosis along with a compensatory renal loss of bicarbonate. Salicylates also cause the uncoupling of oxidative phosphorylation, which leads to deceased ATP production, increased oxygen consumption, increased CO_2 production, and increased heat production. Derangements in the Krebs cycle and in carbohydrate metabolism lead to an accumulation of organic acids, including pyruvate, lactate, and acetoacetate, and result in a metabolic acidosis. Acetaminophen toxicity leads to hepatic necrosis and massive liver damage. Patients will present with GI irritation, lethargy, and diaphoresis or pallor and, in rare cases of massive poisoning, will develop metabolic acidosis (low pH and low HCO_3) within the first 24 hours. Signs and symptoms of NSAID toxicity include metabolic acidosis (low pH and low HCO_3), lethargy, hypotension, bradycardia, apnea, renal failure, and hepatotoxicity. Benzodiazepine overdose manifests as behavior associated with excessive alcohol ingestion, respiratory depression, dilated pupils, and weak and rapid pulse. ABG results would show a respiratory acidosis (low pH and elevated $PaCO_2$) secondary to respiratory depression.

References: Seifter, J. (2016). Acid-base disorders. In L. Goldman (Ed.), *Goldman-Cecil medicine* (25th ed.), (pp. 762–774). Philadelphia: Elsevier Health Sciences.

Kaul, V., Imam, S., Gambhir, H., Sangha, A., & Nandavaram, S. (2013). Negative anion gap metabolic acidosis in salicylate overdose—A zebra! *American Journal of Emergency Medicine, 31*(10), 1536.e3–1536.e4. http://dx.doi.org/10.1016/j.ajem.2013.05.031.

2-75. **(B)** Seizures are defined as a discrete event characterized by an excessive and disorderly discharge of cerebral neurons with associated sensory, motor, and/or behavioral changes. Seizures warrant treatment when they last longer than 3 minutes to avoid the possibility of permanent neurologic injury. Frequent neurologic examinations (Option A) are appropriate in the early postoperative period. High-dose phenobarbital (Option C) may be given if seizures are refractory to other medications. A postoperative imaging study (Option D) may be obtained to evaluate structural changes after surgery and to identify any complications such as a blood clot.

References: Blissitt, P. A. (2018). Neurologic system. In T. M. Hartjes (Ed.), *AACN core curriculum for high acuity, progressive, and critical care nursing* (7th ed.). St. Louis: Elsevier.

Jette, N., Reid, A., & Wiebe, S. (2014). Surgical management of epilepsy. *Canadian Medical Association Journal, 186*(13), 997–1004. http://dx.doi.org/10.1503/cmaj.121291.

2-76. **(D)** Norepinephrine (Levophed) is a potent vasoconstricting agent that rapidly increases blood pressure. Levophed is effective in the setting of cardiogenic shock. Dopamine is indicated in pulmonary edema when blood pressure is at least 70 mm Hg. However, dopamine is proarrhythmic, and cardiomyopathy patients are prone to ventricular arrhythmias. Dobutamine is a positive inotropic agent that is indicated in pulmonary edema when the blood pressure is 70 to 100 mm Hg and signs of shock are *not* present. Nitroglycerin is not a vasopressor and may be indicated in pulmonary edema to reduce systemic vascular resistance and cardiac work when the systolic blood pressure is greater than 90 to 100 mm Hg.

Reference: Hollenberg, S. (2016). Cardiogenic shock. In L. Goldman (Ed.), *Goldman-Cecil medicine* (25th ed.), (pp. 681–685). Philadelphia: Elsevier Health Sciences.

2-77. **(A)** Complementary therapy (e.g., music or touch) has not been shown to be associated with safety concerns and appears to reduce pain and tension during early recovery from open heart surgery. In the synergy model of patient care, the critical care nurse recognizes and appreciates the use of complementary therapies for pain management as a caring practice and response to diversity. Option B is incorrect because it negates the family's interest in providing a therapy that may assist the patient. The first portion of Options C and D are untrue (there are no biomedical or electrical safety concerns) for battery-operated music players, and the latter portion of Option C is not true because there are data to suggest that pain may be reduced in the immediate postoperative period with use of complementary therapies.

References: Dermenchyan, A. (2018). Professional caring and ethical practice. In T. M. Hartjes (Ed.), *AACN core curriculum for high acuity, progressive, and critical care nursing* (7th ed.). St. Louis: Elsevier.

Yang, L., & Petrini, M. A. (2015). Effects of music therapy on pain, anxiety, and vital signs in patients after thoracic surgery. *Complementary Therapies in Medicine, 23*(5), 714–718. http://dx.doi.org/10.1016/jxtim.2015.08.002.

2-78. **(D)** Several tests are available to diagnose PAD. The initial test of choice includes the simple ABI measurement. To calculate the ABI, systolic pressures are determined in both arms and both ankles with the use of a handheld Doppler instrument. The highest readings for the dorsalis pedis (DP) and posterior tibial (PT) arteries are used to calculate the index. The ankle-brachial index is noninvasive, and abnormal findings can be followed up with a more invasive test. Angiography exposes the patient to contrast dye, and a lower extremity x-ray will not show arterial occlusions.

References: Efre, A., & Boling, B. (2018). Cardiovascular system. In T. M. Hartjes (Ed.), *AACN core curriculum for high acuity, progressive, and critical care nursing* (7th ed.). St. Louis: Elsevier.

Kullo, I., & Rooke, T. (2016). Clinical practice. Peripheral artery disease. *New England Journal of Medicine, 374*(9), 861–871. http://dx.doi.org/10.1056/NEJMcp1507631.

2-79. **(A)** Acute MI with papillary muscle rupture requires both revascularization and valve repair or replacement. Immediate treatment may be accomplished with open heart surgery. If immediate cardiac surgery is not available, PCI and IABP may stabilize the patient until transfer to a facility that performs cardiac valve repair can occur. IABP therapy decreases afterload and reduces mitral valve regurgitation. Thrombolytics should not be administered to the patient with papillary muscle rupture because that would delay valve replacement surgery and allow cardiogenic shock to continue without definitive treatment until the half-life of the thrombolytics has transpired. IABP and vasopressor support may be used to stabilize the patient until surgery but will not reperfuse the occluded coronary artery.

References: Efre, A., & Boling, B. (2018). Cardiovascular system. In T. M. Hartjes (Ed.), *AACN core curriculum for high acuity, progressive, and critical care nursing* (7th ed.). St. Louis: Elsevier.

Mitchell, J., Bogar, L., & Burton, N. (2014). Cardiothoracic surgical emergencies in the intensive care unit. *Critical Care Clinics, 30*(3), 499–525. http://dx.doi.org/10.1016/j.ccc.2014.03.004.

2-80. **(C)** Administration of normal saline will help replace fluids, providing volume to improve the blood pressure and urinary output and helping to dilute glucose levels and blood viscosity. Administration of bicarbonate would fail to benefit the patient in that it would result in alkalemia and too rapid a shift of potassium back into the cells and potentially cause cerebral edema, central acidosis, and death. Glargine insulin is a long-acting, basal analog preparation that provides a more physiologic control of glucose; however, it would not provide the rapid correction required for this patient. Correction of serum potassium will be needed as glucose is corrected; however, it would be inappropriate to administer it when the patient is oliguric.

Reference: MacDermott, J. (2018). Endocrine system. In T. M. Hartjes (Ed.), *AACN core curriculum for high acuity, progressive, and critical care nursing* (7th ed.). St. Louis: Elsevier.

2-81. **(C)** Patients with COPD have some degree of nonreversible damage to their lungs, so rather than regaining textbook "normal" function or laboratory or diagnostic study values (Option A), COPD patients—in the best of situations—will regain their former baseline function and laboratory values. Pressure support and spontaneous breathing trials are both used for weaning COPD patients from mechanical ventilation, but other parameters are required to assess readiness for extubation.

References: Storzer, D. N. (2018). Pulmonary system. In T. M. Hartjes (Ed.), *AACN core curriculum for high acuity, progressive, and critical care nursing* (7th ed.). St. Louis: Elsevier.

Dostal, C., Aditi S., & Criner, G. (2014). Care of the challenge-to-wean patient. In P. Lanken, S. Manaker, B. Kohl, & C. Hanson (Eds.), *The intensive care unit manual* (pp. 253–262). Philadelphia, PA: Elsevier Saunders.

2-82. **(D)** Acetaminophen is the most appropriate medication to administer to this elderly patient to reduce pain and permit participation with planned exercise. It will not cloud sensorium and does not affect blood pressure or sodium reabsorption. Nonsteroidal antiinflammatory medications are contraindicated in heart failure because they may cause sodium and water retention, which would exacerbate symptoms of failure.

Corticosteroids will also cause sodium and water retention. Morphine sulfate 5 mg is a large dose for an 80-year-old patient and may cause hypotension and drowsiness, which would impede participation in the exercise program.

References: DeJongh, B., Birkeland, K., & Brenner, M. (2015). Managing comorbidities in patients with chronic heart failure: First, do no harm. *American Journal of Cardiovascular Drugs, 15*(3), 171–184. http://dx.doi.org/10.1007/s40256-015-0115-6.

Jones, M., Ehrhardt, K., Ripoll, J., Sharma, B., Padnos, I., Kaye, R., & Kaye, A. (2016). Pain in the elderly. *Current Pain & Headache Reports, 20*(3), 23. http://dx.doi.org/10.1007/s11916-016-0551-2.

2-83. **(D)** No action is needed for this patient because all the parameters are within acceptable range. Cerebral perfusion pressure (CPP) is defined as the difference between the mean arterial pressure (MAP) and the intracranial pressure (ICP). The target cerebral perfusion pressure is 50 to 70 mm Hg. Normal intracranial pressure is up to 15 mm Hg. Option C is incorrect because, even if ICP were elevated, hyperventilation to achieve a $PaCO_2$ of 30 mm Hg is no longer recommended based on research findings.

References: Blissitt, P. A. (2018). Neurologic system. In T. M. Hartjes (Ed.), *AACN core curriculum for high acuity, progressive, and critical care nursing* (7th ed.). St. Louis: Elsevier.

Bhagat, H., Durga, P., Chawla, R., Prabhakar, H., & Sandhu, K. (2014). Current concepts of optimal cerebral perfusion pressure in traumatic brain injury. *Journal of Anaesthesiology Clinical Pharmacology, 30*(3), 318. http://dx.doi.org/10.4103/0970-9185.137260.

2-84. **(B)** Leukemia patients are at high risk for infection. Because 80% of infections are due to the patient's endogenous flora, frequent bathing (with 2% chlorhexidine gluconate solution) and mouth care can help prevent infection. Visits from friends and family members also carry risks, including the introduction and sharing of dangerous bacteria. Fabrics, such as clothing, drapes, pillowcases, and bedsheets, are potential sources of pathogenic bacteria and viruses. Pillows and cosmetics are a source of bacteria and fungi.

References: Dressler, D. (2018). Hematological and immunological systems. In T. M. Hartjes (Ed.), *AACN core curriculum for high acuity, progressive, and critical care nursing* (7th ed.). St. Louis: Elsevier.

Berliner, N. (2016). Leukocytosis and leukopenia. In L. Goldman (Ed.), *Goldman-Cecil medicine* (25th ed.) (pp. 1129–1138). Philadelphia: Elsevier Health Sciences.

2-85. **(D)** Nicardipine, a second-generation dihydropyridine derivative calcium-channel blocker with high vascular selectivity and strong cerebral and coronary vasodilatory activity, is used in hypertensive crises, particularly in patients with cardiac or neurologic comorbidities. Sodium nitroprusside, an arterial and venous vasodilator, is used for the treatment of hypertensive emergency or hypertensive urgency only when other intravenous antihypertensive agents are not available and then only in specific clinical circumstances in patients with normal renal and hepatic function. IV hydralazine is administered in single doses and not available in a titratable infusion. A titratable infusion is preferred as the patient's oral medications are restarted. Labetalol is contraindicated in heart failure and could cause bradycardia in a patient with a heart rate of 65 beats/min.

References: Efre, A., & Boling, B. (2018). Cardiovascular system. In T. M. Hartjes (Ed.), *AACN core curriculum for high acuity, progressive, and critical care nursing* (7th ed.). St. Louis: Elsevier.

Loftus, T. (2015). Responding to a hypertensive crisis. *American Nurse Today, 10*(1), 36.

2-86. **(B)** The patient's presenting symptoms and history describe restrictive cardiomyopathy, the least common form of cardiomyopathy. Restrictive cardiomyopathy is usually caused by an infiltrative process, most often amyloidosis. Lifestyle choices do not cause the underlying disease process. Option A describes hypertrophic cardiomyopathy caused by hypertension. Option C describes ischemic cardiomyopathy (dilated cardiomyopathy) caused by coronary artery disease. Option D describes alcohol-induced cardiomyopathy (dilated cardiomyopathy).

References: Efre, A., & Boling, B. (2018). Cardiovascular system. In T. M. Hartjes (Ed.), *AACN core curriculum for high acuity, progressive, and critical care nursing* (7th ed.). St. Louis: Elsevier.

Modesto, K., & Sengupta, P. (2013). Myocardial mechanics in cardiomyopathies. *Progress in Cardiovascular Diseases, 57*(1), 111–124. http://dx.doi.org/10.1016/j.pcad.2014.03.00.

2-87. **(A)** Hypomagnesemia can be caused by diuretics, pancreatitis, and alcoholism. Magnesium needs to be administered because this patient is exhibiting ECG evidence that suggests hypomagnesemia. Hypertonic saline would be administered for hypoosmolar disorders such as syndrome of inappropriate ADH (SIADH). Sodium polystyrene sulfonate (kayexalate) is indicated in hyperkalemia, which would be unlikely in the setting of high dose diuretics. Hyperkalemia would manifest on the EKG as peaked T waves. Acetazolamide is used to treat hyperphosphatemia.

    Reference: Boling, B. (2018). Renal system. In T. M. Hartjes (Ed.), *AACN core curriculum for high acuity, progressive, and critical care nursing* (7th ed.). St. Louis: Elsevier.

2-88. **(D)** This patient's ABG shows hypoxemia that may respond to judicious increases in FiO_2. The elevated $PaCO_2$ is not accompanied by a commensurately acidotic pH, so the patient likely retains high levels of CO_2 on a chronic basis, negating any need for intubation. Because the patient is tachypneic, the CO_2 level does not reflect a diminished respiratory drive. There are no data provided that suggest a need for diuresis.

    Reference: Storzer, D. N. (2018). Pulmonary system. In T. M. Hartjes (Ed.), *AACN core curriculum for high acuity, progressive, and critical care nursing* (7th ed.). St. Louis: Elsevier.

2-89. **(A)** Numerous medical and psychiatric conditions can cause agitation; some of these causes are life threatening. It is important to be able to differentiate between medical and nonmedical causes of agitation so that patients can receive appropriate and timely treatment. If symptoms, such as loss of memory, disorientation, muscle stiffness, weight loss, psychosis or difficulty breathing, are found or suspected at initial intake triage, immediate evaluation by a clinician is indicated. Oxygenation level and blood sugar level should also be obtained if possible. The initial examination should be directed at identifying factors that could indicate serious, possibly life-threatening, conditions such as head trauma, meningitis, encephalopathy, hypoxia, thyroid disease, seizure, hypoglycemia, and medication overdose.

    Reference: Chapa, D., & Akintade, B. (2018). Psychosocial aspects of critical care. In T. M. Hartjes (Ed.), *AACN core curriculum for high acuity, progressive, and critical care nursing* (7th ed.). St. Louis: Elsevier.

2-90. **(A)** The hallmark symptom of compartment syndrome is pain not controlled by narcotic administration. Other symptoms in compartment syndrome are subtle and include a wood-like muscle mass. Pulse pressure decrease and loss of motor function are usually late signs. Graft occlusion would cause loss or decrease of distal pulses and signs of poor perfusion in the extremity such as increased capillary refill time, pallor, paresthesia, and weakness. False aneurysm would cause a pulsatile mass at the suture site, hematoma, and a tense thigh or calf. Signs of heparin-induced thrombocytopenia include oozing at the suture sites, petechiae, and decreased platelet count.

    References: Efre, A., & Boling, B. (2018). Cardiovascular system. In T. M. Hartjes (Ed.), *AACN core curriculum for high acuity, progressive, and critical care nursing* (7th ed.). St. Louis: Elsevier.

    Stracciolini, A., & Hammerberg, E. (2016). Acute compartment syndrome of the extremities. Available from http://www.uptodate.com/home.

2-91. **(C)** Although the usefulness of antibiotics for treatment of acute exacerbations of asthma continues to be debated, there is no consensus advocating their use. This patient's exacerbation is most likely secondary to the cat allergy. Treatment aims primarily toward relieving the bronchoconstriction experienced by patients with status asthmaticus. All of the other interventions (bronchodilators, magnesium, and oral corticosteroids) can be used effectively to relax the airways and reduce inflammation (Options A, B, D).

    Reference: Storzer, D. N. (2018). Pulmonary system. In T. M. Hartjes (Ed.), *AACN core curriculum for high acuity, progressive, and critical care nursing* (7th ed.). St. Louis: Elsevier.

2-92. **(C)** The social commitment of the physician is to sustain life and relieve suffering. A major source of common ethical conflict occurs when the physician and patient or patient surrogate disagree. With beneficence, the person is trying to do good for the other person as the physician is attempting to do in this situation. Option A is incorrect because the nurse is acting as a surrogate. Option B is incorrect because the nurse is displaying justice in her comments but is not advocating according to the family's expressed wishes. Option D is incorrect in that the nurse is advocating for the physician rather than the patient.

Reference: Dermenchyan, A. (2018). Professional caring and ethical practice. In T. M. Hartjes (Ed.), *AACN core curriculum for high acuity, progressive, and critical care nursing* (7th ed.). St. Louis: Elsevier.

2-93. **(A)** The combination of heparin, eptifibatide, and aspirin increases the risk of bleeding. Cardiac catheterization and PCI use the groin for access, and the groin site may exhibit signs of bleeding such as oozing and hematoma formation. Risk of coronary artery spasm is reduced with infusion of nitroglycerin. Abrupt closure may be seen in the immediate post-PCI period but is rare. Restenosis may occur days to years after PCI. Heparin-induced thrombocytopenia may occur in a patient who has received prior heparin therapy or after receiving heparin therapy for greater than 24 hours.

Reference: Efre, A., & Boling, B. (2018). Cardiovascular system. In T. M. Hartjes (Ed.), *AACN core curriculum for high acuity, progressive, and critical care nursing* (7th ed.). St. Louis: Elsevier.

2-94. **(D)** Thrombocytopenia is a common problem in cancer patients. Thrombocytopenia occurs 10 to 14 days after chemotherapy. Each chemotherapy agent differs in how it causes thrombocytopenia: alkylating agents affect stem cells; cyclophosphamide affects later megakaryocyte progenitors; bortezomib prevents platelet release from megakaryocytes; and some treatments promote platelet apoptosis. Thrombopoietin is the main regulator of platelet production. In numerous studies, recombinant thrombopoietin raised the platelet count nadir, reduced the need for platelet transfusions, reduced the duration of thrombocytopenia, and allowed maintenance of chemotherapy dose intensity. A bone marrow biopsy is invasive and would not accurately demonstrate the marrow function in the setting of chemotherapy. A spleen ultrasound would determine whether platelets are being sequestered in the spleen. In this case the cause of the thrombocytopenia would be thought to be primarily chemotherapy induced. An endoscopy would

determine whether blood and thrombocyte loss is related to bleeding. However, it is also invasive, and the thrombocytopenia could be explained by the presence of chemotherapy.

References: Dressler, D. (2018). Hematological and immunological systems. In T. M. Hartjes (Ed.), *AACN core curriculum for high acuity, progressive, and critical care nursing* (7th ed.). St. Louis: Elsevier.

Kuter, D. (2015). Managing thrombocytopenia associated with cancer chemotherapy. *Oncology (08909091), 29*(4), 282–294. http://dx.doi.org/dx.doi.org/204748.

2-95. **(A)** Atrial fibrillation commonly occurs within 3 days after open heart surgery. Multiple trials have compared the effects of various pharmacologic agents to treat or prevent the occurrence of atrial fibrillation, including digoxin, beta blockers, amiodarone, and magnesium, but none has been shown to be clearly superior. Supraventricular dysrhythmias such as AVNRT and SVT may occur after coronary artery bypass surgery but more commonly occur with surgery involving the cardiac septum. Atrial flutter may occur with digoxin toxicity.

References: Efre, A., & Boling, B. (2018). Cardiovascular system. In T. M. Hartjes (Ed.), *AACN core curriculum for high acuity, progressive, and critical care nursing* (7th ed.). St. Louis: Elsevier.

Ozben, B., Akaslan, D., Sunbul, M., et al.(2016). Postoperative atrial fibrillation after coronary artery bypass grafting surgery: A two-dimensional speckle tracking echocardiography study. *Heart, Lung & Circulation, 25*(10), 993–999. http://dx.doi.org/10.1016/j.hlc.2016.02.003.

2-96. **(D)** In SIADH, an excess of antidiuretic hormone causes resorption of water at the kidney tubule, leading to a dilutional hyponatremia. Fluid restriction is a required part of the treatment of SIADH. The total amount of fluid intake should be less than the patient's total output (urine and insensible losses). Fluid restriction of 800 to 1200 mL/d is effective in both acute and chronic SIADH. However, patients with SIADH have normal thirst, so fluid restriction can discomfort the patient and may be difficult to maintain. Fluid restriction may be especially difficult to maintain in the ICU because of continuous infusions, IV antibiotics, and other medications that are a part of the intake for the patient. Mary and her family should be educated on the rationale for the fluid restriction. The nurse can provide wet mouth swabs, frequent mouth care, and mouth moisturizer to relieve Mary's oral discomfort.

Reference: MacDermott, J. (2018). Endocrine system. In T. M. Hartjes (Ed.), *AACN core curriculum for high acuity, progressive, and critical care nursing* (7th ed.). St. Louis: Elsevier.

2-97. **(B)** Any form of abdominal surgery can lead to a bowel perforation. Free air in the abdomen, elevated WBC, abdominal pain, and fever can be indicative of a bowel perforation with peritonitis. Bowel perforation is a surgical emergency due to the bowel contents spilling into the abdomen and leading to peritonitis. Enema administration can be dangerous in the setting of bowel perforation. An abdominal CT scan will show vascular problems, infection, masses, or pancreatic pseudocyst. Nasogastric tube placement does not treat a bowel perforation.

References: Radovich, P. (2018). Gastrointestinal system. In T. M. Hartjes (Ed.), *AACN core curriculum for high acuity, progressive, and critical care nursing* (7th ed.). St. Louis: Elsevier.

Collins, D. (2014). Bowel perforation following Cesarean leads to death. *Contemporary OB/GYN, 59*(10), 12.

2-98. **(A)** Packed red blood cells do not contain clotting factors, so replacement of clotting factors with transfusion of fresh-frozen plasma and platelets should occur after administration of each unit of packed red blood cells. In addition, one quarter of severely injured patients present in the emergency room with acute coagulopathy of trauma (ACOT). The drivers of ACOT are tissue hypoperfusion, inflammation, and activation of the neurohumoral system. Acetaminophen and diphenhydramine (Benadryl) are generally administered after transfusion to treat transfusion reaction. Furosemide (Lasix) is indicated if pulmonary congestion is apparent after transfusion. Normal saline is administered concurrently with transfusion to prevent hemolysis and increased blood viscosity. Salt-poor albumin is indicated to increase blood volume in hypovolemic patients with excess interstitial fluid volume and is not

indicated if blood replacement has been adequate. Calcium chloride is sometimes administered to patients who receive large volumes of banked blood containing citrate as a preservative.

References: Holleran, R. (2018). Multisystem: Multisystem trauma. In T. M. Hartjes (Ed.), *AACN core curriculum for high acuity, progressive, and critical care nursing* (7th ed.). St. Louis: Elsevier.

Katrancha, E., & Gonzalez, L., III. (2014). Trauma-induced coagulopathy. *Critical Care Nurse, 34*(4), 54–63.

2-99. **(C)** The critical care nurse needs to allow family members to be present for death, only if they choose. While the nurse may be comfortable with death, it would be more harmful to try to convince a loved one of the beauty of the experience. Any attempt to convince them may be leading them to believe that the nurse not accepting of their choice and/or that the nurse is judging them. Options A, B, and D are coercive, as grief is an individual experience, and the husband should be supported in his choice.

Reference: Wyckoff, M., & Hartjes, T. M. (2018). Critical care patients with special needs: Palliative and end-of life care in the ICU. In T. M. Hartjes (Ed.), *AACN core curriculum for high acuity, progressive, and critical care nursing* (7th ed.). St. Louis: Elsevier.

2-100. **(B)** The normal C-reactive protein level is 0.03 to 1.1 mg/dL. C-reactive protein elevation indicates the presence of inflammation in the coronary arteries due to plaque, which may be ready to embolize. The normal brain natriuretic peptide (BNP) is less than 100 pg/mL. BNP elevation indicates LV dysfunction because of strain on the ventricle from volume or pressure overload and indicates risk of heart failure. The desired cholesterol level to reduce risk of CAD is less than 200 mg/dL. The desired value of HDL to reduce risk of coronary artery disease is greater than 40 mg/dL. Total cholesterol value of 180 mg/dL and HDL of 60 mg/dL indicate low risk of coronary artery disease.

References: Efre, A., & Boling, B. (2018). Cardiovascular system. In T. M. Hartjes (Ed.), *AACN core curriculum for high acuity, progressive, and critical care nursing* (7th ed.). St. Louis: Elsevier.

Ridker, P. (2016). A test in context: High-sensitivity C-reactive protein. *Journal of the American College of Cardiology (JACC), 67*(6), 712–723. http://dx.doi.org/10.1016/j.jacc.2015.11.037.

2-101. **(D)** Rotation therapy is thought to improve oxygenation through better matching of ventilation to perfusion and to prevent pulmonary complications associated with bed rest and mechanical ventilation. Hemodynamic instability that persists for 10 minutes, as demonstrated by tachycardia and hypotension, indicates that the patient is not tolerating rotational therapy and should be returned to a supine position. Hemodynamic values obtained when the patient is in the lateral or prone position is reliable if the zero level is maintained at the phlebostatic axis. Neither side-lying nor prone positioning increases the risk of aspiration. SpO_2 is not a good indicator of positioning tolerance and, for this reason, arterial blood gases are used to gauge the effectiveness of rotational therapy.

References: Stacy, K. (2018). Pulmonary therapeutic management. In L. Urden, K. Stacy, & M. Lough (Eds.), *Critical care nursing: Diagnosis and management* St. Louis, MO: Mosby/Elsevier. Elsevier.

Lamba, T., Sharara, R., Leap, J., & Singh, A. (2016). Management of respiratory failure. *Critical Care Nursing Quarterly, 39*(2), 94–109. http://dx.doi.org/10.1097/CNQ.000000000000103.

2-102. **(A)** Patients who have undergone bariatric surgery may develop deficiencies in calcium, iron, vitamin B_{12}, and folate because of the bypassing of the gastric fundus, body, and antrum, as well as the duodenum and variable lengths of the proximal jejunum. Bypassing these structures results in malabsorption. Option B identifies symptoms characteristic of hyperglycemia. Option C lists symptoms associated with pancreatic cancer. Option D includes findings associated with hepatic encephalopathy.

Reference: Benefield, A. (2018). Critical care patients with special needs: Bariatric patients. In T. M. Hartjes (Ed.), *AACN core curriculum for high acuity, progressive, and critical care nursing* (7th ed.). St. Louis: Elsevier.

2-103. **(B)** Because the patient has an elevated FT_4 and low TSH, the nurse needs to search the literature to identify drugs associated with thyroid dysfunction. Nurses should be vigilant in seeking information on drug–drug and drug–food interactions. Clinical inquiry seeks to validate whether available literature can answer the clinical question. Holding medications one at a time (Option A) could be both time consuming and dangerous and suggests a lack of direction in searching for relevant evidence. Option C would not afford sufficient information to identify the problem. Option D is inappropriate because Wolf- Chaikoff is a protective mechanism against the development of hyperthyroidism.

References: Dermenchyan, A. (2018). Professional caring and ethical practice. In T. M. Hartjes (Ed.), *AACN core curriculum for high acuity, progressive, and critical care nursing* (7th ed.). St. Louis: Elsevier.

Javier, M., Jae Youn, K., Toone, E., & Granger, B. (2016). Overcoming barriers to using patient-reported outcomes for clinical inquiry. *AACN Advanced Critical Care*, 230–235. http://dx.doi.org/10.4037/aacnacc2016265.

2-104. **(A)** Right ventricular failure may occur after mitral valve replacement in patients with pulmonary hypertension. When the right ventricle fails, it requires larger volumes to ensure adequate output. This is easily accomplished with crystalloid fluid boluses to maintain the pulmonary artery diastolic pressure at 15 to 18 mm Hg. Nitroglycerin may be ordered with fluid bolus to reduce right ventricular afterload. Furosemide would decrease preload and worsen right ventricular failure. Norepinephrine or vasopressin would increase vasoconstriction and worsen right ventricular failure.

References: Efre, A., & Boling, B. (2018). Cardiovascular system. In T. M. Hartjes (Ed.), *AACN core curriculum for high acuity, progressive, and critical care nursing* (7th ed.). St. Louis: Elsevier.

Hyllén, S., Nozohoor, S., Ingvarsson, A., Meurling, C., Wierup, P., & Sjögren, J. (2014). Right ventricular performance after valve repair for chronic degenerative mitral regurgitation. *The Annals of Thoracic Surgery, 98*(6), 2023–2030. http://dx.doi.org/10.1016/j.athoracsur.2014.07.075.

2-105. **(A)** Because complications from HHNK result from an increase in blood viscosity, IV normal saline will help to replace fluids lost to polyuria, diminish blood viscosity, and improve perfusion. Severe dehydration is often associated with HHNK, and deficits of 10 L or more can exist in patients presenting with this condition. Regular insulin, rather than glargine, would be used in insulin drips because regular insulin does not promote antigen development and is short acting. Unless the patient has other concurrent health problems, oxygen administration and seizure precautions are usually not needed for hyperosmolar patients.

References: MacDermott, J. (2018). Endocrine system. In T. M. Hartjes (Ed.), *AACN core curriculum for high acuity, progressive, and critical care nursing* (7th ed.). St. Louis: Elsevier.

Scott, A. (2015). Management of hyperosmolar hyperglycaemic state in adults with diabetes. *Diabetic Medicine, 32*(6), 714–724. http://dx.doi.org/10.1111/dme.12757.

2-106. **(D)** Torsades de pointes is a polymorphic ventricular rhythm characterized by varying QRS morphology and is associated with prolonged QT intervals. Magnesium sulfate is the medication utilized to treat dysrhythmias associated with long QT syndromes. Common drugs that can cause a prolonged QT include class Ia, Ic, or III antiarrhythmic agents, tricyclic antidepressants, phenothiazines, and certain antivirals and antifungals. Amiodarone and sotalol are antiarrhythmics associated with known or possible risks of torsades de pointes. Adenosine is used to manage supraventricular tachycardias.

Reference: Efre, A., & Boling, B. (2018). Cardiovascular system. In T. M. Hartjes (Ed.), *AACN core curriculum for high acuity, progressive, and critical care nursing* (7th ed.). St. Louis: Elsevier.

2-107. **(B)** The patient is presenting with the hallmarks of cryptogenic organizing pneumonia (COP), previously termed bronchiolitis obliterating organizing pneumonia (BOOP). Her laboratory results suggest an inflammatory rather than an infectious process (Option A), and there is no evidence suggesting cardiac failure (Options C and D). Because certain infections may be contributive factors to COP, Option B is the best answer.

References: Storzer, D. N. (2018). Pulmonary system. In T. M. Hartjes (Ed.), *AACN core curriculum for high acuity, progressive, and critical care nursing* (7th ed.). St. Louis: Elsevier.

Ellis, J., & Ridman, M. (2016). Cryptogenic organizing pneumonia. *Clinical Advisor, 19*(3), 64–73.

2-108. **(A)** The guideline state that patients with malignancy in the past 2 years except squamous cell and basal tumors are not eligible for transplant. The other options (B, C, and D) are all contraindications for lung transplant.

Reference: Storzer, D. N. (2018). Pulmonary system. In T. M. Hartjes (Ed.), *AACN core curriculum for high acuity, progressive, and critical care nursing* (7th ed.). St. Louis: Elsevier.

2-109. **(C)** The catheterization laboratory picture shows an occlusion of the proximal left anterior descending artery. This artery perfuses the anterior wall of the left ventricle. Occlusion of the right coronary artery would cause an inferior wall MI. The left circumflex perfuses the high lateral wall, posterior wall, and occasionally the inferior wall. The left anterior descending artery also perfuses the low lateral wall and septal wall.

References: Efre, A., & Boling, B. (2018). Cardiovascular System. In T. M. Hartjes (Ed.), *AACN core curriculum for high acuity, progressive, and critical care nursing* (7th ed.). St. Louis: Elsevier.

Werns, S. (2014). Acute coronary syndromes and acute myocardial infarction. In J. Parillo, & R. Delllinger (Eds.), *Critical care medicine: Principles of diagnosis and management in the adult* (pp. 470–514). Philadelphia: Elsevier Saunders.

2-110. **(D)** Patients with symptomatic PAD frequently have concomitant cerebrovascular or coronary artery disease (CAD) that places them at high risk for adverse cardiovascular outcomes after surgery. Theses events include MI, congestive heart failure, and CVA. Rehabilitation should begin as soon as possible for the postoperative patient. Prolonged bedrest is not indicated after surgery. Pneumothorax is not a complication from of femoropopliteal bypass. In patients with known renal insufficiency, elective surgery should not immediately follow diagnostic angiography; if possible, it should be delayed to allow recovery from the nephrotoxic effects of the contrast load.

References: Menard, M., & Belkin, M. (2014). Aortoiliac disease. In R. Rutherford, J. Cronenwett, & K. Wayne (Eds.), *Rutherford's vascular surgery* (pp. 1701–1720). Philadelphia: Elsevier Saunders.

Efre, A., Boling, B. (2018). Cardiovascular System. In Hartjes, T.M. (ed.), *AACN Core Curriculum for High Acuity, Progressive, and Critical Care Nursing* (7th ed.). St. Louis: Elsevier.

2-111. **(B)** The syndrome of inappropriate antidiuretic hormone (ADH) secretion (SIADH) is defined by the hyponatremia and hypoosmolality resulting from inappropriate, continued secretion or action of the hormone despite normal or increased plasma volume, which results in impaired water excretion. After the identification of hyponatremia, the approach to the patient depends on the clinically assessed volume status. If the duration of hyponatremia is unknown and the patient is asymptomatic, it is reasonable to presume chronic SIADH. Diagnosis and treatment of the underlying cause of SIADH are important to reverse the condition. Prominent physical findings may be seen only in severe or rapid-onset hyponatremia. In an emergency setting, rapid serum sodium correction (Option A) should always be weighed against the risk of inducing central pontine myelinolysis (a complication of treatment of patients with profound, life-threatening hyponatremia that occurs as a consequence of a rapid rise in serum tonicity from intracellular adaptations to the prevailing hypotonicity). This patient is not demonstrating any signs of severe hyponatremia such as confusion, delirium, seizures, coma, muscle weakness, ataxia, tremor, or Cheyne-Stokes respirations. A CT scan of the head (Option C) would be warranted to find an underlying cause of SIADH and rule out cerebral edema as a complication. However, this patient does not have any neurologic deficits; she is demonstrating signs of pneumonia as an underlying cause of SIADH, so the chest x-ray is a first priority. Administration of an IV steroid (Option D) is not indicated for treatment of SIADH.

References: MacDermott, J. (2018). Endocrine system. In T. M. Hartjes (Ed.), *AACN core curriculum for high acuity, progressive, and critical care nursing* (7th ed.). St. Louis: Elsevier.

Verbalis, J., Greenberg, A., Burst, V., et al. (2016). Diagnosing and treating the syndrome of inappropriate antidiuretic hormone secretion. *American Journal of Medicine, 129*(5), 537.e9–537.e23. http://dx.doi.org/10.1016/j.amjmed.2015.11.005.

2-112. **(D)** Mental status and renal perfusion are the best indicators of cardiac output because the brain and kidneys receive one-fourth of the cardiac output. Patients with pulmonary edema due to diastolic dysfunction may have normal ejection fractions. Peripheral edema may be absent in left ventricular failure if it is not accompanied by right ventricular failure. Although a respiratory rate of 20 breaths/min or less and an SpO_2 of 94% may be therapeutic target goals for this patient, they do not indicate cardiac output adequacy in the mechanically ventilated patient.

Reference: Efre, A., & Boling, B. (2018). Cardiovascular system. In T. M. Hartjes (Ed.), *AACN core curriculum for high acuity, progressive, and critical care nursing* (7th ed.). St. Louis: Elsevier.

2-113. **(A)** Recent data suggest that target temperature management to 32° to 36°C can improve neurologic outcomes and survival after hospital discharge for cardiac arrest patients. These patients are at risk for a decrease in white blood cell and platelet counts because of immune response suppression secondary to hypothermia therapy. Insulin resistance and decreased insulin release will contribute to hyperglycemia. Blood sugar levels are ideally maintained at 80 to 110 mg/dL. Option B is incorrect because based on the data provided, the patient is not at risk for development of hyperkalemia; hypothermia patients are at risk for hypokalemia. The risk for hyperkalemia occurs during rewarming.

References: Schenone, A., Cohen, A., Patarroyo, G., et al. (2016). Therapeutic hypothermia after cardiac arrest: A systematic review/meta-analysis exploring the impact of expanded criteria and targeted temperature. *Resuscitation,* 108102–108110. http://dx.doi.org/10.1016/j.resuscitation.2016.07.238.

Radigan, K. (2016). Postcardiac arrest targeted temperature management. *Critical Care Alert, 24*(6), 1–5.

2-114. **(C)** Defibrillator pads or paddles must be placed 1 to 2 inches (2.5 to 5 cm) from the pacemaker site on the chest. Option A is untrue. Option B is incorrect. The pacemaker magnet is used to program the pacemaker to an asynchronous mode. Option D is incorrect because only an implantable cardioverter defibrillator has defibrillation and pacemaker functions combined.

Reference: Efre, A., & Boling, B. (2018). Cardiovascular system. In T. M. Hartjes (Ed.), *AACN core curriculum for high acuity, progressive, and critical care nursing* (7th ed.). St. Louis: Elsevier.

2-115. **(C)** Although the decision to draft an advanced directive should have been made before this admission, that point is not the issue at this time. The patient has a need to confer with his family, physician, and significant others so that they understand his wishes. Attempting to placate the patient by saying he will probably change his mind later belittles the decision-making process that led to this conclusion. Although he is experiencing an alteration in oxygenation, he may not be legally responsible to make such a decision; however, he may have been thinking about and discussing this issue over a period. Ascertaining the patient's true wishes and supporting that decision will enable the nurse to serve more effectively as an advocate for the needs of patients and their families.

Reference: Dermenchyan, A. (2018). Professional caring and ethical practice. In T. M. Hartjes (Ed.), *AACN core curriculum for high acuity, progressive, and critical care nursing* (7th ed.). St. Louis: Elsevier.

2-116. **(C)** Glucagon works by stimulating the liver to produce glucose, so the patient may not respond to it for 10 to 20 minutes. Glucagon can cause vomiting, so after injection, position patients on their side to prevent aspiration. Each of the other choices can be appropriate measures at a later time. Ongoing assessment of neurologic status would represent the next appropriate intervention, with a recheck of capillary glucose to evaluate the effectiveness of the glucagon dose in 30 minutes and then preparation to feed the patient after he or she regains consciousness.

Reference: MacDermott, J. (2018). Endocrine system. In T. M. Hartjes (Ed.), *AACN core curriculum for high acuity, progressive, and critical care nursing* (7th ed.). St. Louis: Elsevier.

2-117. **(B)** Each of the options will be part of the process, but it is important for all of the units that will be using the new equipment to be part of the evaluation process from the beginning. Central to any successful change process are communication and input. Because multiple units may be involved in the change, it is essential that the decision be based on input from each of the involved areas.

Reference: Dermenchyan, A. (2018). Professional caring and ethical practice. In T. M. Hartjes (Ed.), *AACN core curriculum for high acuity, progressive, and critical care nursing* (7th ed.). St. Louis: Elsevier.

2-118. **(D)** Neuromuscular blocking agents may cause prolonged myopathy (critical illness myopathy) in any patient, so their relative benefit must always be weighed against their potential for harm. As a result, NMBs should be used with caution and only after other options have proven ineffective. The myopathy associated with NMBs is particularly problematic for patients concomitantly receiving steroids (Option A), so NMB use would only be as a last resort. Because of the risks associated with NMBs, they are not used routinely (Option B). NMBs act on skeletal, rather than smooth, muscle (Option C).

References: Naguib, M., Luig, C. A., & Meistelman, C. (2015). Pharmacology of neuromuscular blocking drugs. In R. D. Miller (Author), *Miller's anesthesia* (pp. 958–994). Philadelphia: Elsevier Saunders.

Annane, D. (2016). What is the evidence for harm of neuromuscular blockade and corticosteroid use in the intensive care unit? *Seminars in Respiratory & Critical Care Medicine, 37*(1), 51–56. http://dx.doi.org/10.1055/s-0035-1570355.

2-119. **(A)** Pulmonary artery hypertension causes enlargement of the pulmonary artery, which makes obtaining pulmonary artery diastolic pressures unreliable or unobtainable. The pulmonary artery diastolic pressure approximates mean left atrial pressure; therefore a left atrial line is used to obtain left ventricular end diastolic pressures to reflect preload status. Left atrial lines predispose the patient to development of air embolus but are not used to evacuate left atrial air emboli. A left atrial line is not superior to a pulmonary artery catheter in diagnosing pericardial tamponade. During cardiac surgery, there is no need for continuous monitoring of cardiac chambers because the patient is on cardiopulmonary bypass.

Reference: Lough, M., & Thompson, C. (2018). Cardiovascular diagnostic procedures. In L. Urden, K. Stacy, & M. Lough (Eds.), *Critical care nursing: Diagnosis and management* St. Louis: Mosby/Elsevier.

2-120. **(C)** The hemodynamic values indicate that the patient is experiencing a decrease in cardiac output (in relation to the SVR) as a result of decreased preload (CVP: 4 mm Hg). Administering a fluid bolus of normal saline is the most appropriate intervention that would improve the patient's hemodynamic status. If the patient were anemic, then the fluid of choice would be PRBCs. Based on the 2016 surviving sepsis guidelines, resuscitation targets are a MAP ≥65 mm Hg and a normalized lactate. Other hemodynamic values that reflect the patient's inadequate fluid resuscitation are HR, BP, and PAP. Norepinephrine would increase the patient's BP and SVR but would likely increase rather than reduce the patient's tachycardia. Administering fluid would lessen the need for vasopressor therapy. Metoprolol is a negative chronotropic and inotropic agent (beta blocker) that is not indicated for this patient. The patient is hypotensive and would not tolerate the administration of a beta blocker. Dobutamine results in a positive inotropic and chronotropic effect with afterload reduction. The patient is tachycardic and has a low SVR secondary to the septic shock. Administering dobutamine would result in an increased HR and lower SVR, which would further compromise the patient's clinical status.

References: Johnson, A. (2018). Multisystem: Systemic inflammatory response syndrome and septic shock. In T. M. Hartjes (Ed.), *AACN core curriculum for high acuity, progressive, and critical care nursing* (7th ed.). St. Louis: Elsevier.

Surviving Sepsis Campaign: International Guidelines for Management of Severe Sepsis and Septic Shock: 2016. (February 2016). Retrieved March 19, 2017, from http://survivingsepsis.org/guidelines/Pages/default.aspx.

2-121. **(B)** The tidal volume settings for a patient with ARDS should be 5 to 7 mL/kg. An optimal tidal volume for this patient then is 350 to 490 mL. Excessive tidal volumes and high PEEP levels increase the risk of volutrauma and barotrauma, so the PEEP should not be increased until the tidal volume is adjusted and PaO_2 levels do not improve. Studies show that early and limited duration use of neuromuscular blockade may improve outcomes in ARDS. Vecuronium is an appropriate neuromuscular blockade agent.

References: Storzer, D. N. (2018). Pulmonary system. In T. M. Hartjes (Ed.), *AACN core curriculum for high acuity, progressive, and critical care nursing* (7th ed.). St. Louis: Elsevier.

Aoun, N. (2017). Acute respiratory distress syndrome. In F. Ferri (Ed.), *2017 Ferri's clinical advisor: 5 books in 1* (pp. 38–41). Philadelphia: Elsevier.

2-122. **(A)** Prevention of stroke is the primary concern when a patient presents with hypertensive crisis with hypertensive encephalopathy. Neurologic symptoms are frequent and of poor prognosis. Prevention centers on rapid lowering of systolic blood pressure (25% over 8 hours). End-organ failure is generally preventable when blood pressure and vasoconstriction are reduced in a timely manner. Renal failure from chronic hypertension may precipitate the hypertensive event. Seizures are not common with hypertensive crisis but may occur if there is intracerebral bleeding or encephalopathy. Left ventricular hypertrophy is common in patients with chronic hypertension and may result in heart failure.

References: Efre, A., & Boling, B. (2018). Cardiovascular system. In T. M. Hartjes (Ed.), *AACN core curriculum for high acuity, progressive, and critical care nursing* (7th ed.). St. Louis: Elsevier.

Loftus, T. (2015). Responding to a hypertensive crisis. *American Nurse Today, 10*(1), 36.

2-123. **(B)** The purpose of informed consent in health care is to ensure that patient autonomy is respected in decisions about their health care. Because effective informed consent depends on a patient's ability to make decisions about treatment free of pressure and based on logical reasoning, patients should receive adequate information about the nature, alternatives, risks, and benefits of the proposed treatment. The nurse recognizes that explanation of significant risks should be discussed with the patient and family to ensure informed consent. Allowing the physician to leave without discussing the risks of the procedure does not advocate for the patient. Option C provides collaboration with another discipline but does not provide informed consent. Option D facilitates knowledge of the family but does not ensure that the risks of the procedure are reviewed by the physician before signing consent.

Reference: Dermenchyan, A. (2018). Professional caring and ethical practice. In T. M. Hartjes (Ed.), *AACN core curriculum for high acuity, progressive, and critical care nursing* (7th ed.). St. Louis: Elsevier.

2-124. **(C)** The prevalence of diverticulosis, or colonic outpouching, increases with age; in Western society, approximately two-thirds of the population has diverticulosis by age 85 years. Risk factors for bleeding diverticulosis include advanced age, the use of nonsteroidal antiinflammatory drugs (NSAIDs) or anticoagulation therapy, diabetes mellitus, and ischemic heart disease. Diverticula bleeding is the most common cause of acute massive colonic blood loss. Intestinal polyps cause intermittent or occult bleeding. Crohn disease is a less common cause of lower GI bleeding. Angiodysplasia (arteriovenous malformation of the mucosa) is a common cause of chronic or intermittent low-grade bleeding in aged patients.

References: Radovich, P. (2018). Gastrointestinal system. In T. M. Hartjes (Ed.), *AACN core curriculum for high acuity, progressive, and critical care nursing* (7th ed.). St. Louis: Elsevier.

Wilson, A. M., & Lynch, K. (2017). The management of lower gastrointestinal bleeding. In A. M. Cameron, & J. L. Cameron (Authors), *Current surgical therapy* (pp. 322–325). Philadelphia: Elsevier Saunders.

2-125. **(B)** Ischemic colitis may occur after aortic surgery because of embolization, occlusion, or ligation of mesenteric vessels or because of hypoperfusion from long aortic cross-clamp times or hypovolemia. Initial symptoms of ischemic colitis may include edema, elevated white blood cell (WBC) count, tachycardia, pain, acidosis, hypotension, and diarrhea. Graft infection is not usually evident within 2 days, but symptoms would include tachycardia, hypotension, and elevated WBC count without GI symptoms. Fistula formation is also a late-onset finding and may cause signs of peritonitis, GI bleeding, or visible fistula formation. Abdominal compartment syndrome may present as abdominal pain, rigidity, and myoglobinuria.

References: Radovich, P. (2018). Gastrointestinal system. In T. M. Hartjes (Ed.), *AACN core curriculum for high acuity, progressive, and critical care nursing* (7th ed.). St. Louis: Elsevier.

Moghadamyeghaneh, Z., Sgroi, M., Chen, S., Kabutey, N., Stamos, M., & Fujitani, R. (2016). Risk factors and outcomes of postoperative ischemic colitis in contemporary open and endovascular abdominal aortic aneurysm repair. *Journal of Vascular Surgery, 63*(4), 866–872. http://dx.doi.org/10.1016/j.jvs.2015.10.064.

2-126. **(D)** MODS occurs in patients with multiple trauma. Infection is the leading cause of MODS after trauma. All the other nursing interventions are important, but infection prevention has the most effect on MODS prevention for this patient. Multiple trauma leads to a body-wide systemic immune response. Secondary infection increases the mortality risk for these patients.

Reference: Johnson, A. (2018). Multisystem: Multiple organ dysfunction syndrome. In T. M. Hartjes (Ed.), *AACN core curriculum for high acuity, progressive, and critical care nursing (7th ed.).* St. Louis: Elsevier.

2-127. **(A)** ACE inhibitors should be discontinued if the serum creatinine level increases higher than 3.0 mg/dL because they prevent conversion of angiotensin I to angiotensin II, which decreases glomerular filtration and may potentiate renal insufficiency. Serum creatinine is an indicator of renal function. Serum potassium levels less than 3.5 mEq/L indicate a need for potassium replacement. An SpO_2 of 95% is still adequate to maintain oxygenation. An increased number of atrial premature contractions could herald the onset of atrial fibrillation and warrants continued monitoring, but a reduced heart rate indicates that therapy is appropriate.

Reference: Efre, A., & Boling, B. (2018). Cardiovascular system. In T. M. Hartjes (Ed.), *AACN core curriculum for high acuity, progressive, and critical care nursing* (7th ed.). St. Louis: Elsevier.

2-128. **(A)** Patients with cardiogenic shock or hemodynamic instability are generally excluded from hybrid procedures. One of the most common off pump, minimally invasive surgical procedures involves the anastomosis of the left internal mammary artery to the left anterior descending (LAD) artery (Option B). The transcatheter aortic valve replacement (TAVR) is an option for patients who require an aortic valve replacement but could not tolerate traditional open heart surgery (Option C). Mitral valve repair procedures (Option D) can also be treated by a minimally invasive approach.

References: Lough, M. (2018). Cardiovascular therapeutic management. In L. Urden, K. Stacy, & M. Lough (Eds.), *Critical care nursing: Diagnosis and management.* St. Louis, MO: Mosby/Elsevier.

Wong, K. (2015). Minimally invasive cardiac surgery: Where we are and future direction. *Operating Theatre Journal,* (293), 14.

2-129. **(A)** HELLP syndrome derives its name from severe preeclampsia characterized by **h**emolytic anemia, **e**levated **l**iver enzymes, and a **l**ow **p**latelet count. Decreased hemoglobin and hematocrit are related to blood loss and hemodilution because of crystalloid and colloidal infusions to replace depleted circulating volume. Magnesium levels rise if a magnesium drip is used to slow electrical impulses and prevent seizure activity; however, this laboratory value increases secondary to magnesium administration, not from pathophysiology. Albuminuria and increased serum creatinine levels occur related to the renal response to hypertension. Generally, BUN is elevated rather than decreased with renal impairment.

References: Houston, J. F. (2018). Critical care patients with special needs: High-risk obstetric patients. In T. M. Hartjes (Ed.), *AACN core curriculum for high acuity, progressive, and critical care nursing* (7th ed.). St. Louis: Elsevier.

Snyder, S., Kivlehan, S., & Collopy, K. (2015). HELLP syndrome. *EMS World, 44*(6), 39–45.

2-130. **(A)** The patient is alkalotic with a pH of 7.60. Acetazolamide (Diamox) is a diuretic used in alkalosis to decrease hydrogen ion loss that may occur with diuresis. Alkalosis hinders release of oxygen to tissues, so it should be avoided in patients with pulmonary edema who may be hypoxemic. Additional furosemide (Lasix) will continue diuresis without correcting alkalosis. Endotracheal intubation will improve oxygenation but is not indicated when PaO_2 is 78 mm Hg and $PaCO_2$ is normal. Hydrochlorothiazide is a thiazide diuretic that will induce diuresis but not preserve hydrogen ions and thus would increase alkalosis.

References: Efre, A., & Boling, B. (2018). Cardiovascular system. In T. M. Hartjes (Ed.), *AACN core curriculum for high acuity, progressive, and critical care nursing* (7th ed.). St. Louis: Elsevier.

Peixoto, A., & Alpern, R. (2013). Treatment of severe metabolic alkalosis in a patient with congestive heart failure. *American Journal of Kidney Diseases, 61*(5), 822–827. http://dx.doi.org/10.1053/j.ajkd.2012.10.028.

2-131. **(A)** Regardless of the cause or type of diabetes insipidus, the patient's electrolyte values will govern appropriate treatment for this disorder. In nephrogenic diabetes insipidus, the kidney has been damaged and no longer responds to vasopressin, so aggressive replacement of fluids is required to sustain life. Neurogenic diabetes insipidus is a problem caused when too little vasopressin is released by the pituitary gland, possibly due to increased

intracranial pressure; therefore, supplemental vasopressin administration sustains life. Whether because of a lack of vasopressin or a lack of response, urinary output exceeds 500 mL/hr, resulting in dehydration and altered electrolytes. The goal of therapy is to reestablish and maintain a normal fluid and electrolyte balance.

References: MacDermott, J. (2018). Endocrine system. In T. M. Hartjes (Ed.), *AACN core curriculum for high acuity, progressive, and critical care nursing* (7th ed.). St. Louis: Elsevier.

Lough, M. E. (2018). Endocrine disorders and therapeutic management. In L. D. Urden, K. M. Stacy, & M. E. Lough (Authors), *Critical care nursing: diagnosis and management*. St. Louis, MO: Elsevier.

2-132. **(C)** Hemodialysis is the "gold standard" for management of chronic renal failure because it is the most effective of all renal replacement therapies. Although the patient managed her renal failure using CAPD at home, peritoneal dialysis is not currently an option due to the patient's abdominal surgery. SCUF is used in patients with volume overload and some degree of renal function, but it has minimal effect on urea and creatinine levels. CVVH is used for patients who require fluid removal and are hemodynamically unstable.

Reference: Lough, M. E. (2018). Kidney disorders and therapeutic management. In L. D. Urden, K. M. Stacy, & M. E. Lough (Authors), *Critical care nursing: diagnosis and management*. St. Louis, MO: Elsevier.

2-133. **(B)** The goal of ventilator management with persistent air leaks is to minimize airway pressures in order to prevent further injury to the affected area (Option B). Maximizing PEEP or using large tidal volumes may worsen the clinical situation by increasing the volume lost through the air leak (Options A and D). Using the minimal effective FiO_2 is always a good idea, but it will not aid management of an air leak (Option C).

Reference: Storzer, D. N. (2018). Pulmonary system. In T. M. Hartjes (Ed.), *AACN core curriculum for high acuity, progressive, and critical care nursing* (7th ed.). St. Louis: Elsevier.

2-134. **(D)** The GI tract harbors organisms that may trigger an inflammatory focus if they are translocated from the gut into the portal circulation from which they may not be adequately cleared by the liver. This process is microbial translocation. Common enteric organisms with this potential include *Enterococcus spp., Escherichia coli, Clostridium perfringens,* and *Enterobacter cloacae.* Bacterial translocation has been associated with drugs commonly used in critically ill patients such as antibiotics and antacids. Antibiotics alter the function of normal protective bacteria located in the gut. Antacids increase the intragastric pH, allowing ingested bacteria to survive in the GI tract and potentially become pathologic. Conditions thought to increase gut permeability and microbial translocation include mucosal ischemia, mucosal hypoperfusion, immunoglobulin A deficit (associated with TPN), thermal injury, glucocorticoid administration, endotoxin release, glutamine, and fiber deficiencies. TPN (option C) could cause microbial translocation. In addition, sepsis guidelines recommend the administration of early full enteral nutrition rather than parenteral nutrition in patients that can be fed enterally. Therefore, nutrition initiation should not be held or delayed (option A and B).

References: Johnson, A. (2018). Multisystem: Systemic inflammatory response syndrome and septic shock. In T. M. Hartjes (Ed.), *AACN core curriculum for high acuity, progressive, and critical care nursing* (7th ed.). St. Louis: Elsevier.

Klingensmith, N., & Coopersmith, C. (2016). The gut as the motor of multiple organ dysfunction in critical illness. *Critical Care Clinics, 32*(2), 203–212. http://dx.doi.org/10.1016/j.ccc.2015.11.004.

2-135. **(C)** In Haiti, education is limited, and 85% of the population is illiterate; however, Haitians place a high value on education to improve social status. Education is much more difficult to obtain in rural communities, and often families must pay to send their children to school, which they will even sacrifice food to do so. A Haitian immigrant and her family may be illiterate and written information could be construed as insulting because of their lack of education. In Haiti, women usually make health care decisions for themselves and their children; however, when there is a husband, he usually will want to make major health decisions such as those regarding surgery for his wife (Option A). Haitian patients welcome and often expect eye contact during caregiving interactions and view touch as conveying warmth and friendliness (Option B). Obtaining an accurate personal or family health history may be difficult—if not impossible—because many people have parents or other close family members who died in Haiti without medical care or a formal diagnosis (Option D).

References: Dermenchyan, A. (2018). Professional caring and ethical practice. In T. M. Hartjes (Ed.), *AACN core curriculum for high acuity, progressive, and critical care nursing* (7th ed.). St. Louis: Elsevier.

Mendes, A. (2015). Culture and religion in nursing: providing culturally sensitive care. *British Journal of Nursing, 24*(8), 459. http://dx.doi.org/10.12968/bjon.2015.24.8.459.

2-136. **(D)** Rapid culture and antibiotic administration (Option A) are important interventions in treating any pneumonia; however, preventing hypoxia and hypoperfusion are the priorities (Option D) for this patient. Completing confirmatory diagnostic tests such as a chest x-ray and treating the patient's fever are secondary priorities (Options B and C).

Reference: Storzer, D. N. (2018). Pulmonary system. In T. M. Hartjes (Ed.), *AACN core curriculum for high acuity, progressive, and critical care nursing* (7th ed.). St. Louis: Elsevier.

2-137. **(A)** The nurse knows that sensitivity to family needs is required when brain death is declared. Family members have the option to obtain a second opinion about brain death. Documentation of the discussion (Option B) is an important aspect but is superseded by the need to advocate on behalf of the family during a time of crisis. Options C and D may come later in the course of this patient's care. Organ donation should not be discussed immediately after the family has just learned of a flat EEG. Option D is inappropriate because there is no apparent conflict in this situation that needs to be resolved.

References: Dermenchyan, A. (2018). Professional caring and ethical practice. In T. M. Hartjes (Ed.), *AACN core curriculum for high acuity, progressive, and critical care nursing* (7th ed.). St. Louis: Elsevier.

Lewis, A., Varelas, P., & Greer, D. (2016). Prolonging support after brain death: When families ask for more. *Neurocritical Care, 24*(3), 481–487. http://dx.doi.org/10.1007/s12028-015-0209-7.

2-138. **(C)** Ideally, corrective surgery for aortic dissection should not be delayed. One exception is when a patient with aortic dissection develops profound hypotension or pulseless electrical activity (PEA). In this instance, emergency pericardiocentesis may be performed before surgery. Pericardial tamponade is an anticipated complication of aortic dissection, so clinical evidence of this disorder as increased right atrial pressure or widened mediastinum on chest x-ray would not represent reasons for delay. Stable patients should proceed directly to surgery.

Reference: Efre, A., & Boling, B. (2018). Cardiovascular system. In T. M. Hartjes (Ed.), *AACN core curriculum for high acuity, progressive, and critical care nursing* (7th ed.). St. Louis: Elsevier.

2-139. **(C)** In this example of failure to sense, atrial and ventricular pacing spikes are seen around the intrinsic QRS complexes. Pacemaker activity does not sense the inherent rhythm. A failure to capture complication occurs when a pacemaker fires as expected but fails to depolarize the myocardium. A failure to pace complication is noted when a pacemaker spike is not seen after the lower rate-limiting interval has been exceeded.

Reference: Mulpuru, S. K., Madhavan, M., McLeod, C. J., Cha, Y., & Friedman, P. A. (2017). Cardiac pacemakers: Function, troubleshooting, and management: Part 1 of a 2-part series. *Journal of the American College of Cardiology (JACC), 69*(2), 189–210. http://dx.doi.org/10.1016/j.jacc.2016.10.061.

2-140. **(A)** Administration of normal saline fluid bolus is used to treat prerenal acute renal failure (ARF). The fluid bolus will increase the patient's blood pressure and renal perfusion. Urine in prerenal ARF is concentrated with low sodium. Restricting the patient's fluid or administering a diuretic such as furosemide will further exacerbate the patient's prerenal condition. Both fluid restriction and administration of diuretics are used for patients who are in ARF and are fluid overloaded. Discontinuing the administration of cefazolin, which is nephrotoxic, would be appropriate if the patient was in intrarenal ARF.

Reference: Boling, B. (2018). Renal system. In T. M. Hartjes (Ed.), *AACN core curriculum for high acuity, progressive, and critical care nursing* (7th ed.). St. Louis: Elsevier.

2-141. **(A)** The location of the AVM suggests which deficit the nurse needs to anticipate. A lesion in the right frontal area would be expected to affect voluntary motor control on the left side of the body. Comprehension of spoken language (Option B) is controlled in the dominant temporal lobe; in most patients, this would be in the left hemisphere. A visual field deficit such as a homonymous hemianopsia (Option C) would result from a temporal lobe or optic tract disorder. The sensory deficits described in Option D would most likely result from a lesion in the parietal lobe. AVMs are abnormal vascular networks connecting arteries directly to veins. The lack of a capillary network bridging the high-pressure arterial system to the low-pressure venous system creates a risk of bleeding at that junction, where aneurysms are found in these malformations. Small AVMs commonly present with intracranial hemorrhage, whereas large AVMs present most often with seizures.

References: Blissitt, P.A. (2018). Neurologic system. In T. M. Hartjes (Ed.), *AACN core curriculum for high acuity, progressive, and critical care nursing* (7th ed.). St. Louis: Elsevier.

Stacy, K. (2018). Neurologic disorders and therapeutic management. In L. Urden, K. Stacy, & M. Lough (Eds.), *Critical care nursing: Diagnosis and management*. St. Louis, MO: Mosby/Elsevier.

2-142. **(C)** Acute intraabdominal blood loss results in decreased venous return to the heart and reduces preload and thus cardiac output. This reduction in cardiac output results in the clinical signs of hypovolemia, hypotension, and diminished cerebral blood flow and triggers compensatory changes such as tachycardia and narrow pulse pressure. The compensatory vasoconstriction that increases blood flow to vital organs also reduces blood flow to peripheral tissues, causing cold, clammy, pale skin. Increased intracranial pressure is often associated with a widened pulse pressure and the development of bradycardia. In this scenario, the patient's pulse pressure narrows and the heart rate increases, reflective of a hypovolemic shock state. In acute MI, the patient typically exhibits chest pain, diaphoresis, nausea, vomiting, and shortness of breath. A patient with pulmonary embolism will exhibit symptoms of tachypnea, anxiety, light-headedness, sharp chest pain, hemoptysis, and rales.

References: Efre, A., & Boling, B. (2018). Cardiovascular system. In T. M. Hartjes (Ed.), *AACN core curriculum for high acuity, progressive, and critical care nursing* (7th ed.). St. Louis: Elsevier.

McGrath, A., & Whiting, D. (2015). Recognizing and assessing blunt abdominal trauma. *Emergency Nurse, 22*(10), 18–24. http://dx.doi.org/10.7748/en.22.10.18.e1377.

2-143. **(D)** Administration of sedation/analgesia will treat operative pain and allow the patient to tolerate mechanical ventilation; a bronchodilator can help to open constricted airways to improve ventilation and oxygenation, and postoperative antibiotics are a standard treatment after contaminated bowel surgery. IV steroids (Option A) have not demonstrated definitive benefits in patients with ARDS and are not a priority intervention for this patient. Diuretics (Option B) are not indicated in a fresh postoperative patient who has no evidence of fluid overload. Volume status needs to be assessed before administration of additional fluids (Option C) to minimize volume overload in ARDS.

References: Storzer, D. N. (2018). Pulmonary system. In T. M. Hartjes (Ed.), *AACN core curriculum for high acuity, progressive, and critical care nursing* (7th ed.). St. Louis: Elsevier.

Radovich, P. (2018). Gastrointestinal system. In T. M. Hartjes (Ed.), *AACN core curriculum for high acuity, progressive, and critical care nursing* (7th ed.). St. Louis: Elsevier.

2-144. **(D)** The clinical manifestations described are a vasoocclusive crisis. A hematologic crisis (Option A) is manifested by sudden exacerbation of anemia with a corresponding drop in hemoglobin level. Infectious crisis (Option B) is due to a compromised immune system that is susceptible to common infectious agent such as *Haemophilus influenza, Streptococcus pneumoniae, Salmonella typhimurium, Staphylococcus aureus,* and *Escherichia coli.* Aplastic anemia is part of sickle cell disease, but it is not called aplastic crisis (Option C).

References: Dressler, D. (2018). Hematological and immunological systems. In T. M. Hartjes (Ed.), *AACN core curriculum for high acuity, progressive, and critical care nursing* (7th ed.). St. Louis: Elsevier.

Yawn, B., & John-Sowah, J. (2015). Management of sickle cell disease: Recommendations from the 2014 expert panel report. *American Family Physician, 92*(12), 1069–1076.

2-145. **(D)** The nurse competency of clinical inquiry relates to the nurse applying a change in practice when evidence exists to support the change. Especially because the preceptor is not familiar with the practice change, the best course is for the nurse to conduct a literature review to identify studies that support or refute the use of the lower arm for noninvasive blood pressure monitoring. Option A is likely not necessary because there is no evidence that the orientee does not know how to perform standard BP measurement. Option B would be of limited value because it affords a single set of measurements, although current literature indicates that upper and lower arm readings are not interchangeable in either the supine position or with the head of bed elevated 45 degrees. Rather, a difference in measurements of up to 33 mm Hg can exist between the upper arm and lower arm locations. Designing a research study would be a time-consuming activity that may not be justified if literature addressing the issue is already available.

Reference: Dermenchyan, A. (2018). Professional caring and ethical practice. In T. M. Hartjes (Ed.), *AACN core curriculum for high acuity, progressive, and critical care nursing* (7th ed.). St. Louis: Elsevier.

2-146. **(D)** Febrile nonhemolytic reactions occur in about 1% of transfusions and manifest with a temperature increase of more than 1°C (2° F) during or shortly after a transfusion. The reaction is thought to represent the action of antibodies against white cells or the actions of cytokines either present in the transfused component or generated by the recipient to the transfused component. The initial nursing intervention for this patient would be to immediately stop the transfusion to prevent additional exposure to the offending antigen or infectious agent. After the termination of the transfusion, the physician would be contacted for additional orders to administer antipyretics and/or antihistamines. Individual institutions have policies and procedures regarding the disposition of the remaining unit contents and post reaction testing.

Reference: Miller, R. (2015). Patient blood management. In R. Miller, & N. Cohen (Eds.), *Miller's anesthesia* (8th ed.), (pp. 1830–1867). Philadelphia: Elsevier Saunders.

2-147. **(A)** Hepatitis A virus infection has a fecal–oral transmission route. It can also be transmitted by ingestion of raw or undercooked shellfish contaminated by sewage dumped in the ocean. Parenteral transmission of hepatitis A is rare. Hepatitis B, C, and D are associated with parenteral transmission.

References: Radovich, P. (2018). Gastrointestinal system. In T. M. Hartjes (Ed.), *AACN core curriculum for high acuity, progressive, and critical care nursing* (7th ed.). St. Louis: Elsevier.

Fort, G. (2017). Hepatitis A. In F. Ferri (Ed.), *2017 Ferri's clinical advisor: 5 books in 1* (pp. 568–569). Philadelphia: Elsevier.

2-148. **(D)** Pressure = regulated volume = controlled ventilation is an appropriate choice for a patient with chronic obstructive bronchitis because it prevents hyperventilation and barotrauma by adjusting flow rates to provide consistent tidal volumes. A rate of 10 breaths/min permits the patient to have a physiologically regulated exhalation time. Patients with obstructive disorders may develop lung injury with volume cycle modes of ventilation. Chronic obstructive disease generally results in elevated $PaCO_2$, which is compensated by elevated bicarbonate. When the CO_2 is corrected, this results in a metabolic alkalosis, which is to be expected in this patient. Increasing the FiO_2 in this patient may decrease the patient's respiratory drive and prevent weaning. Short-term ventilation as the obstruction causing respiratory failure is relieved is the goal for the patient. Increasing FiO_2 would delay the patient's spontaneous respiratory drive and prolong mechanical ventilation.

References: Storzer, D. N. (2018). Pulmonary system. In T. M. Hartjes (Ed.), *AACN core curriculum for high acuity, progressive, and critical care nursing* (7th ed.). St. Louis: Elsevier.

Hill, N. (2016). Acute ventilatory failure. In R. Masor, V. Broaddus, T. Martin, T. King, D. Schraufnagel, J. Murray, & J. Nadel (Eds.), *Murray and Nadel's textbook of respiratory medicine* (pp. 1723–1729). Philadelphia: Elsevier Saunders.

2-149. **(C)** The ICU nurse is an important mentor and role model. The ICU nurse explains that fluid repletion decreases blood sugar levels independently of insulin administration (Option A), prevents or treats intravascular collapse (Option D), and improves organ perfusion (Option B). Option C is the incorrect reply because fluid resuscitation does not affect fat breakdown.

References: MacDermott, J. (2018). Endocrine system. In T. M. Hartjes (Ed.), *AACN core curriculum for high acuity, progressive, and critical care nursing* (7th ed.). St. Louis: Elsevier.

Sanuth, B., Bidlencik, A., & Volk, A. (2014). Management of acute hyperglycemic emergencies. *AACN Advanced Critical Care, 25*(3), 197–202. http://dx.doi.org/10.1097/nci.0000000000000045.

2-150. **(A)** Risk factors for heparin-induced thrombocytopenia (HIT) include longer duration of exposure to heparin, type of heparin (unfractionated heparin has a greater risk), and type of patient (surgical patients, especially cardiac and orthopedic surgery, are at higher risk than medical patients). A patient who has received heparin in the past has an increased risk of developing HIT because prior exposure causes development of antibodies that are already present when the patient is next exposed to heparin. Patients undergoing coronary artery bypass grafting receive heparin during the surgery. Chronic conditions such as asthma, diabetes, hypertension, and renal failure do not influence the development of heparin-induced thrombocytopenia.

References: Dressler, D. (2018). Hematological and immunological systems. In T. M. Hartjes (Ed.), *AACN core curriculum for high acuity, progressive, and critical care nursing* (7th ed.). St. Louis: Elsevier.

Rehfeldt, K., & Barbara, D. (2016). Cardiopulmonary bypass without heparin. *Seminars in Cardiothoracic & Vascular Anesthesia, 20*(1), 40–51. http://dx.doi.org/10.1177/1089253215573326.

3 Core Review Test 3

3-1. The critical care nurse in the emergency room is anticipating the admission of a violent patient with an anxiety disorder. Which of these nursing interventions is not effective for deescalation of violence?
   A. Permit patient to wear own clothing instead of hospital gown
   B. Remove all dangerous items from the examination room
   C. Offer food and blankets
   D. Set limits and ramifications for inappropriate behavior

3-2. A patient is admitted to the ICU after an attempted drug overdose. He develops generalized muscle rigidity followed by a rhythmic muscle jerking. The nurse observes this activity for 1 minute and pages the physician managing the patient's care. The activity continues for 10 minutes despite administration of lorazepam 4 mg IV. The next course of action the nurse should anticipate is
   A. STAT EEG to confirm that the patient is having a seizure and to localize foci
   B. STAT serum and urine labs, including myoglobin
   C. Infusion of midazolam with phenytoin 15 mg/kg IV
   D. Infusion of pentobarbital 20 mg/kg IV

3-3. A patient is admitted after exhibiting several neuropsychiatric symptoms, including motor coordination difficulties, delayed reaction times, headache, and impaired cognitive skills. During the nurse's conversations with the family to secure a patient history, the patient's spouse mentioned that they are in the process of renovating a home that has been in the family for over 75 years. This information suggests that the most likely etiology for this patient's symptoms is
   A. Cyanide poisoning
   B. Carbon monoxide exposure
   C. Exposure to pesticides
   D. Lead poisoning

3-4. A patient in the ICU is receiving IV antibiotics. His history includes current IV drug abuse, and obtaining IV access is difficult. He has a peripheral IV in the antecubital area that was placed yesterday with ultrasound guidance. The patient is currently complaining of slight pain near the IV site. The nurse checks the site, and it flushes easily and has good blood return. The site has slight erythema proximal to the catheter. Which of these interventions is most appropriate?
   A. Notify the doctor to assess the site
   B. Inform the patient that bending his arm will cause pain and redness and place an arm board
   C. Continue to monitor the site
   D. Remove the cannula and place a new IV site

3-5. A diabetic patient is admitted for treatment of diabetic ketoacidosis. Which of these

findings does the critical care nurse anticipate for the patient?
A. Anion gap 14, pH 7.41, blood glucose
410 mg/dL
B. Anion gap 8, pH 7.29, blood glucose
320 mg/dL
C. Anion gap18, pH 7.29, blood glucose
280 mg/dL
D. Anion gap 18, pH 7.35, blood glucose
380 mg/dL

3-6. A 56-year-old patient is admitted to the ICU
after an open surgical repair of an abdominal
aortic aneurysm. Two hours after arrival, the
patient is hemodynamically stable. Nursing
care of the patient at this time should focus on
A. Preventing peripheral vascular damage
with a bed cradle and toe padding
B. Ensuring return of bowel function by
instituting a bowel protocol
C. Frequent suctioning to prevent pneumonia
D. Pain control

3-7. A COPD patient has been admitted for an
acute exacerbation. She is minimally responsive, tachypneic, and tachycardic. The critical care nurse obtains a stat ABG. Arterial
blood gas results include pH 7.20; PaO$_2$
55 mm Hg; and PaCO$_2$ 68 mm Hg. The nurse
anticipates the next intervention to be
A. Instituting BiPAP
B. Endotracheal intubation
C. Application of low-flow oxygen by nasal
cannula
D. Administration of 50 mEq of sodium
bicarbonate injection to correct acidosis

3-8. A 35-year-old Asian man is admitted with
jaundice, elevated liver enzyme levels, malaise, and lack of appetite. His total bilirubin is
34 mg/dL, aspartate aminotransferase (AST)
is 874 U/L, alanine aminotransferase (ALT)
is 789 IU/L, prothrombin time (PT) is 23 sec,
international ratio (INR) is 3.2. His HAV IgM
is negative, HAV IgG is positive, HCV Ab is
negative, HBsAg is positive, HBsAb is negative. The probable cause of these findings is
A. Hepatitis A
B. Hepatitis B
C. Hepatitis C
D. Hepatitis D

3-9. A patient in the ICU is admitted with a diagnosis of hypertensive crisis. He is known
to be noncompliant with his blood pressure

medications and has multiple hospital admis-
sions. Which of these findings indicate that
he is now experiencing end-organ damage?
A. Blurred vision
B. BUN 20 mg/dL
C. Patient complaints of lethargy
D. R wave in V$_5$ plus S wave in V$_1$ are
greater than 35 mm

3-10. A patient is admitted from the operating
room after aneurysmal subarachnoid hemorrhage and has been stable after her craniotomy for left middle cerebral artery aneurysm
clipping. On the nurse's most recent assessment, he notices that the patient has developed new right lower extremity weakness,
perseveration, and a rather flat affect. Which
of these interpretations of these new findings
will best aid the nurse in planning appropriate care?
A. Hyponatremia related to cerebral salt
wasting
B. Rebleeding of the left middle cerebral
artery aneurysm
C. New onset of hydrocephalus
D. Vasospasm of the left anterior cerebral
artery

3-11. Mr. Jones is a patient with known chronic
liver failure who has been admitted for
treatment of hepatic encephalopathy. The
patient has a decreased level of consciousness, but he opens his eyes spontaneously.
Mr. Jones is disoriented to time and place.
He demonstrates amnesia for past events
and has impaired performance on subtrac-
tion tasks. The patient also demonstrates
decreased inhibitions and subtle personality changes. He is paranoid and apathetic
and has hypoactive reflexes and ataxia.
Which of the following describes the
grade of his clinical assessment of hepatic
encephalopathy?
A. Grade I
B. Grade II
C. Grade III
D. Grade IV

3-12. Which of these hemodynamic profiles would
the nurse anticipate for a patient with a pulmonary history of COPD?
A. PAP 40/20 mm Hg, PAOP 20 mm Hg,
CVP 18 mm Hg, CI 1.8 L/min/m^2
B. PAP 20/7 mm Hg, PAOP 4 mm Hg, CVP
1 mm Hg, CI 1.8 L/min/m^2

C. PAP 40/25 mm Hg, PAOP 7 mm Hg, CVP 4 mm Hg, CI 1.8 L/min/m^2

D. PAP 30/15 mm Hg, PAOP 14 mm Hg, CVP 4 mm Hg, CI 1.8 L/min/m^2

3-13. The ICU nurse is caring for a 77-year-old patient who has been intubated on mechanical ventilation for the past 6 days. The nurse is planning interventions to prevent delirium. Which of the following is not part of the delirium prevention bundle?

A. Delirium screening assessment tool every 12 hours

B. Sedation awakening trial every 24 hours

C. Early mobilization of all intubated patients with stable vital signs

D. Pain assessment every 4 hours

3-14. A patient was in the ICU with newly diagnosed diabetes and diabetic ketoacidosis and is now ready for discharge. The patient lives alone and is unable to see the numbers on the syringes to self-administer insulin. Which of the following is indicated at this time to decrease the chance of hospital readmission?

A. Determine whether the patient may be placed in a skilled nursing facility

B. Provide the patient with a video on insulin administration to reinforce the information

C. Consult with the case manager for a visiting nurse to see this patient

D. Request that the patient's daughter live with the patient until she can self-administer her insulin

3-15. An elderly patient was admitted to the ICU 3 days ago after a bowel resection for perforated bowel. During the past 4 hours, the patient has developed progressive hypotension that is not responding to fluid boluses. The patient has become oliguric and is demonstrating signs of MODS, The nurse's priority for care now centers on which of the following as the most important intervention in reducing mortality of patients with SIRS and/or MODS?

A. Pain management

B. Maintenance of tissue oxygenation

C. Nutritional and metabolic support

D. Identification and treatment of underlying source

3-16. An elderly patient is admitted to the ICU after an emergency hemicolectomy. The patient has a history of current tobacco abuse, diabetes, myocardial infarction, coronary artery disease, severe arthritis, and obesity. The ICU nurse is planning care for this postoperative patient. The nurse anticipates monitoring the surgical patient for which of the most common postoperative complications for this patient?

A. Perioperative MI

B. Pneumonia

C. Infection

D. Severe hyperglycemia

3-17. A challenge in nursing care of patients undergoing bariatric surgery is adequately meeting the patient's psychosocial needs. In caring for this patient population, the nurse can anticipate needs related to

A. Low self-esteem

B. Dependence

C. Personal autonomy

D. Trusting others

3-18. The nurse is conducting discharge teaching for a patient newly diagnosed with COPD. Among the recommendations are smoking cessation, pulmonary rehabilitation therapy, and counseling. At the end of the session, the patient asks if giving up cigarettes will make the COPD "go away." What is the nurse's best response?

A. "Yes, if you stop smoking, your lungs will slowly but eventually return to normal."

B. "Most of the damage is permanent, so stopping smoking won't affect your COPD."

C. "If you stop smoking, the rate of damage slows, but your lungs will not be normal again."

D. "As long as you don't have alpha-1 antitrypsin deficiency, cessation of smoking can restore nearly normal lung tissues after about 2 years."

3-19. After partial gastrectomy, a surgical patient develops a paralytic ileus. Current vital signs include temperature 36.6°C; HR 122/min, sinus tachycardia; BP 82/64 mm Hg; RR 30/min and shallow because of abdominal distention. SpO$_2$ is 94% on 4 L oxygen by nasal prongs. Lungs are clear with decreased sounds in the bases. Urine output is 30 mL and 26 mL for the past 2 hours. The patient is restless and complains of abdominal pain. The most likely cause of these findings is

A. Sepsis

B. Hypovolemia

C. GI hemorrhage

D. Acute respiratory failure

3-20. A 78-year-old ICU patient with type 2 diabetes, recent coronary stents, and ischemic cardiomyopathy is scheduled for a CT angiogram of the abdomen and pelvis. The critical care nurse is concerned about the patient's medication regimen. Which of these orders should be held until the nurse has conferred with the physician?

A. Clopidogrel (Plavix) 75 mg daily

B. Enoxaparin (Lovenox) 40 mg subcutaneous daily

C. Metformin (Glucophage) 500 mg daily

D. IV Pantoprazole (Protonix) 40 mg IV daily

3-21. An unresponsive patient in the ICU is at the end of life. The family has requested that no heroic measures be initiated, that no unnecessary monitoring be used, and that withdrawal of support be initiated. One family member asks why the bispectral index (BIS) monitor is still in use. The nurse's best response is that

A. "It will tell us when your loved one is brain dead."

B. "It is used to ensure that the patient is not experiencing any pain."

C. "We used it to measure pressures inside the skull."

D. "It's used routinely on all comatose patients."

3-22. The critical care nurse is assisting with a bedside thoracentesis for a patient with a large pleural effusion. The patient is sitting on the edge of the bed with her hands and arms supported on a padded overbed table. The physician has obtained 1000 mL of pleural fluid when the patient begins to experience coughing and shortness of breath. Her vital signs remain unchanged, and the oxygen saturation is 97% on 2-L nasal cannula. The nurse anticipates which of these interventions?

A. Reposition the patient before continuing the thoracentesis

B. Administer IV midazolam 0.5 mg before continuing the thoracentesis

C. Discontinue the thoracentesis

D. Administer IV morphine 2 mg before continuing the thoracentesis

3-23. A patient admitted with necrotizing pancreatitis has just returned from the operating room after an aggressive debridement of peripancreatic tissue was performed. The patient's postoperative care includes antibiotics, IV fluids, and mechanical ventilation. In managing care for this patient over the next few days, which of these findings should the nurse recognize as the most reliable indicator of a poor prognosis for this patient?

A. Elevated serum amylase

B. Elevated APACHE-II score

C. Decreased PaO_2 level

D. Decreased serum C-reactive protein (CRP) level

3-24. A patient comes to ICU after left pneumonectomy for a hilar mass. The patient has stable vital signs and is awake, oriented, intubated, and ventilated on assist-control mode at a rate of 18, tidal volume 6 mL/kg, PEEP +5, and FiO_2 0.40. The patient's heart rate and respiratory rate suddenly increase, and his oxygen saturation decreases. The nurse notes that a new central line was placed to the right subclavian site. While she is increasing the oxygen and preparing for chest tube insertion, the nurse formulates an ongoing plan of care. Which of these interventions is least likely to be helpful in preventing further pulmonary complications in this patient?

A. Prompt ventilator weaning

B. Aggressive pulmonary toilet

C. Increase PEEP

D. Pain management

3-25. A patient in the ICU has been diagnosed with idiopathic pulmonary fibrosis. The nurse caring for the patient collaborates with the physician to plan care that would most benefit the patient. Which of the following would be most beneficial?

A. Provide incentive spirometry and demonstrate use

B. Assist with palliative care consult

C. Administer anxiolytics

D. Administer prophylactic antibiotics

3-26. A patient is admitted in critical condition after a severe construction site accident with multiple crush injuries. The nurse notes oozing of blood from trauma sites, an IV catheter, and surgical drains. The patient is diagnosed with a hypercoagulable state that is a hematologic finding for this type of injury. Which of these sets of laboratory findings suggests that this patient has developed one of these coagulation disorders?

A. ↑aPTT, ↑PT, ↓platelets, ↑FDPs (fibrindegradation products)

B. ↓aPTT, ↓PT, ↑platelets, ↓FDPs

C. ↑aPTT, ↑PT, ↑platelets, ↑FDPs

D. ↓aPTT, ↓PT, ↓platelets, ↓FDPs

3-27. A recent patient satisfaction survey report shows that the patients are not satisfied with their overall experience in the progressive care unit. The unit clinical practice committee meets to identify strategies to improve the patients' satisfaction. Which of the following strategies would be most effective to develop a core plan to improve patient satisfaction?

A. Assist patients with completing a unit specific survey prior to transfer from the unit

B. Invite unit RN staff from all shifts to a planning meeting

C. Invite members from different departments, including dietary, phlebotomy, environmental services, patient relations, and physicians to a planning meeting

D. Implement new practices identified by the committee to improve satisfaction

3-28. A patient is admitted to the ICU for respiratory distress. Upon assessment, the critical care nurse notes an agonal respiratory pattern. A stat arterial blood gas is obtained. The critical care nurse anticipates which of these findings?

A. pH 7.5, $PaCO_2$ 30 mm/Hg, PaO_2 60 mm/Hg, HCO_3 24 mEq/

B. pH 7.3, $PaCO_2$ 20 mm/Hg, PaO_2 80 mm/Hg, HCO_3 16 mEq/L

C. pH 7.3, $PaCO_2$ 60 mm/Hg, PaO_2 50 mm/Hg, HCO_3 26 mEq/L

D. pH 7.4, $PaCO_2$ 58 mm/Hg, PaO_2 70 mm/Hg, HCO_3 29 mEq/L

3-29. The ICU nurse has received a patient post pneumonectomy. Which of these interventions would most likely be held until the nurse contacts the surgeon?

A. Position patient on the operative side and do not turn the patient

B. Administer IV normal saline at 150 mL/hr

C. IV hydromorphone 0.5 mg every hour PRN

D. Place chest tube to -20 cm H_2O suction

3-30. An ICU patient admitted for a GI bleed is diagnosed with idiopathic thrombocytopenic purpura (ITP). Nursing interventions primarily focus on

A. Maintaining a patent airway

B. Controlling the respiratory rate

C. Replenishing circulating blood volume

D. Coping with alterations in body image

3-31. A patient with severe traumatic brain injury has persistent hyperthermia. Extensive medical workup has revealed no source of infection. The critical care nurse anticipates which of these damaged brain structures is responsible for thermoregulation?

A. Thalamus

B. Hypothalamus

C. Subthalamus

D. Epithalamus

3-32. A patient is admitted to the ICU after surgery to remove a bullet from a gunshot wound to the chest. The patient remains intubated on mechanical ventilation with chest tube drainage of 75 mL/hr. Two hours later, the nurse notes that the patient's tidal volumes are decreasing, chest tube output has increased to 300 mL/hr, and BP has decreased from 123/78 to 70/50 mm Hg. After notification of the trauma surgeon, the nurse immediately prepares for

A. Insertion of a second chest tube

B. Returning the patient to the operating room

C. Initiation of a dopamine drip

D. Assisting with a bronchoscopy

3-33. An ICU patient has become confused and lethargic 5 days after aneurysmal subarachnoid hemorrhage and aneurysm coil embolization. Which of these approaches should the nurse anticipate discussing with the acute care nurse practitioner managing this patient's care?

A. Discontinue nimodipine therapy

B. Reduce the volume of IV fluids to prevent hyperemia and risk of rebleed

C. Perform CT angiography to evaluate for evidence of vasospasm

D. Prepare for lumbar puncture to evaluate for evidence of meningitis

3-34. An 83-year-old patient with a history of chronic heart failure, longstanding COPD, and osteoarthritis is admitted to the ICU with pneumonia. The patient has undergone tracheostomy and has since failed three attempts to wean from the ventilator.

Although the patient is alert and oriented, he seems too fatigued to assist with the weaning process. Nursing staff are feeling increasingly frustrated in their attempts to help this patient progress. Which of the following would likely help the ICU nursing staff improve outcomes for this patient?

A. Contact the social worker to help prepare the patient for discharge to a long-term acute care facility

B. Suggest that the intensivist request a consult from the multidisciplinary ventilator team

C. Speak with the family to determine feasibility of taking the patient home on a ventilator

D. Suggest a nutrition team consult to build the patient's strength for successful weaning

3-35. The nurses in an ICU have expressed concerns about delays in ventilator weaning for mechanically ventilated patients. Staff members express frustrations about delays in obtaining ventilator weaning orders from the physicians. A committee of nurses is established to investigate these delays. The committee determines that nurse-driven protocols for ventilator weaning would improve patient outcomes. The next best intervention would be

A. Arrange a meeting with the ICU physicians to discuss the concerns

B. Discuss the committee's concerns with nursing management

C. Invite respiratory therapists to join the committee

D. Perform an extensive search for evidence-based practice related to nurse-driven ventilator weaning

3-36. A patient with type 1 diabetes is frequently hospitalized for diabetic ketoacidosis. The patient refuses to administer insulin, perform capillary glucose measurement, or follow the diabetic diet after initial diagnosis of the disease. This admission's initial laboratory results are as follows: glucose 200 mg/dL, pH 7.1, $PaCO_2$ 25.7 mm Hg, PaO_2 94 mm Hg, and bicarbonate 15.0 mEq/L. Which of these orders should the nurse perform first?

A. Administer 8 units of NPH insulin subcutaneously using a sliding scale

B. Encourage oral clear liquids in order to maintain nutritional status

C. Obtain specimen for blood gas interpretation and chemistry in 1 hour

D. Administer IV fluids

3-37. An elderly Orthodox Jewish patient in the ICU has died. One family member has remained in the room after the others have left. The family member refuses to leave the patient. What is the most appropriate way to address this family member?

A. "I am sorry but you must leave because we have to transfer your loved one to the morgue within a certain time frame."

B. "You may visit with your loved one for another hour."

C. "I will arrange for you to remain with the body if you would like."

D. "If you are concerned about the circumstances of your family member's death, we can perform an autopsy."

3-38. A patient with end-stage cardiomyopathy has an ejection fraction of 10%. She has refused LVAD (left ventricular assist device) placement and does not want further interventions. She is in the ICU intubated on mechanical ventilation and remains awake and alert, and she writes clear messages on a clipboard. The patient and the family request comfort measures, and the patient has asked to be extubated. Her family is supportive of her decision because this has been her fifth intubation in the last month. The patient is placed on morphine and extubated. After extubating and high-dose morphine titration, the patient continues to gasp and demonstrate severe suffering and distress. Her family asks if there is anything more that can be done to ease her suffering. Your best response is

A. "She is on maximum dose analgesia now."

B. "It would be illegal to provide lethal dose analgesia."

C. "We will consult palliative care."

D. "I will contact the physician to order sedation now."

3-39. Patients who experience cardiac arrest related to trauma before arriving at the hospital rarely survive despite rapid and effective emergency management. Among the interventions designed to improve survival for these patients, which of the following is most important?

A. Performing the primary and secondary survey

B. Determining the extent of injury by removing the patient's clothing

C. Providing aggressive IV fluid resuscitation

D. Transporting the patient to the ER or tertiary care facility

3-40. A patient is admitted to the ICU after major vascular surgery. The patient has multiple risk factors for coronary artery disease. Which of these elevated serum values would suggest a diagnosis of perioperative myocardial infarction?

A. Troponin

B. Total CK

C. C-reactive protein

D. Myoglobin

3-41. A patient is in the ICU with septic shock from toxoplasmosis. The patient has a history of AIDS and is intubated and on mechanical ventilation. The patient communicates concern about missing doses of his antiretroviral treatment after being intubated. The nurse's best response is

A. "I am sure we can give you your medications enterally."

B. "We will hold your antiretroviral medications, so we can prevent any potential drug interactions with your current therapy."

C. "Most antiretroviral medications are available in intravenous form."

D. "Because you are critically ill right now, you are at increased risk for pancreatitis if we continue your antiretroviral treatment."

3-42. The nursing staff in a cardiac surgical ICU have been refusing to follow new orders for postoperative patients regarding mobility to the chair immediately after extubation. The staff reports that the early mobilization causes undue stress and pain for the patients and can lead to hemodynamic compromise. Which of the following would be the best intervention to support positive patient outcomes?

A. Discuss the concerns with the surgeon

B. Document negative outcomes and patient experiences of pain associated with the new orders and present them to the surgeon

C. Perform an evidence-based literature review related to early mobilization after cardiac surgery and present the findings to the staff

D. Encourage the staff to use their best judgment in each patient situation

3-43. A trauma surgeon states that nurses do not know how to care for patients with chest tubes and requests that only two specific nurses be assigned to care for his patients when they are in the ICU. The unit's nursing staff can best manage this situation by

A. Suggesting that the surgeon meet with the nurse manager

B. Convening a task force to review unit standards of care for these patients

C. Discussing the surgeon's specific concerns with him

D. Scheduling a mandatory in-service for all unit nurses about the care of these patients

3-44. A patient is recovering from an acute exacerbation of COPD. The physician requests that the patient begin ambulating around his room. The nurse knows that this activity

A. Often triggers a relapse of bronchitis

B. Represents a key component of pulmonary rehabilitation

C. Requires support with supplemental oxygen

D. Should be preceded by premedication with bronchodilators

3-45. Cardiac resynchronization therapy is indicated for heart failure associated with all these conditions except

A. Left bundle branch block

B. Systolic dysfunction

C. QRS duration greater than 150 ms

D. QRS duration less than 120 ms; left ventricular hypertrophy and documented ventricular tachycardia

3-46. A patient in the ICU is experiencing insomnia and associated agitation. The patient prefers not to take a controlled substance as a sleep aid. In addition to reducing noise and interruptions, which of these interventions has been shown to be both valuable and feasible in this situation?

A. Massage

B. Aromatherapy

C. Alternative sedatives

D. Progressive muscle relaxation

3-47. An intensive care unit (ICU) visit is a stressful time for patients and families. Added to the depersonalization of a hospital gown, unpredictability through changing of routines, and uncertainty of self-preservation, a patient is tossed into a state of disempowerment. Medications that had been independently taken at home are administered by a nurse; privacy can become compromised with changing from a home-like setting to a group environment, and often the stay invokes a sense of decreased resilience and powerlessness. The risk of delirium and dementia can occur secondary to a patient's time spent in the ICU. Which of these nursing interventions is not effective to prevent ICU delirium or dementia?

A. Perform all ADLs for the patient to prevent fatigue
B. Play reminiscent or ambient music in the room
C. Provide puzzles, simple board games, and cards
D. Provide uninterrupted rest at night

3-48. An older patient is admitted after a fall that resulted in a momentary loss of consciousness. The patient's medications include atenolol, furosemide, digoxin, Motrin, and paroxetine. Vital signs are BP 110/72 mm Hg, HR 56 beats/min, RR 18 breaths/min. During the nursing history, the patient describes yesterday's bowel movement as sticky and black in color. Based on these findings, the nurse would initiate interventions aimed at monitoring this patient's

A. Intracranial pressure and level of consciousness.
B. 12-lead ECG to evaluate the bradycardia
C. Diet and nutritional support systems in the home
D. Hemoglobin and hematocrit to evaluate blood loss

3-49. The echocardiogram of a patient with acute infectious endocarditis demonstrates tricuspid and pulmonary insufficiency. The patient is intubated and placed on mechanical ventilation and receives propofol and lorazepam for sedation as well as antibiotic therapy. Which of the following is potentially an immediate, life-threatening problem for this patient?

A. Acute drug withdrawal and seizures
B. Abscess formation and septicemia
C. Pulmonary infarction
D. Stroke

3-50. A 42-year-old patient admitted with hypertensive crisis admits to noncompliance with his medical regimen. Which of these statements is most helpful to prevent future noncompliance?

A. "If you don't take your medications, you will develop kidney failure and heart disease."
B. "If you can't afford your medications, we can find less expensive alternatives."
C. "Let's talk about the barriers to adherence with your medical regimen."
D. "Young people often have difficulty coping with a chronic disease."

3-51. During an initial neurologic assessment, the nurse finds that the patient has a positive Brudzinski sign and a positive Kernig sign. Otherwise, the patient's examination is nonfocal. Because the lumbar puncture performed earlier showed high protein and low glucose in the CSF, the nurse's most appropriate action at this time is to

A. Prepare for brain MRI to rule out mass lesion
B. Arrange for initiation of plasmapheresis
C. Prepare to administer intravenous antibiotics
D. Prepare the patient for a repeat LP to withdraw accumulating CSF

3-52. Which of these findings best indicates that fluid resuscitation for hypovolemic shock has been appropriate?

A. SVO_2 45%, CO 3.0 L/min, SVR 800 dynes/sec/cm^{-5}
B. SVO_2 45%, CO 5.0 L/min, SVR 1900 dynes/sec/cm^{-5}
C. SVO_2 68%, CO 5.0 L/min, SVR 2100 dynes/sec/cm^{-5}
D. SVO_2 68%, CO 4.4 L/min, SVR 1100 dynes/sec/cm^{-5}

3-53. A shock patient on an IV infusion of norepinephrine at 4 mcg/min has been stable for the past 24 hours. The nurse observes a trend of decreasing blood pressure over the past 2 hours and suspects tachyphylaxis. After conferring with the intensivist, which of these interventions would the nurse anticipate?

A. Immediate discontinuation of the drip and change to a different vasopressor
B. Increase the norepinephrine and titrate to the MAP goals previously ordered

C. Administer IV Benadryl 50 mg and continue the norepinephrine at the current rate

D. Continue the current norepinephrine rate and monitor the patient

3-54. A patient in the ICU has been receiving non-invasive ventilation (NIV). Which of these sets of arterial blood gas results indicate acute respiratory failure that requires immediate endotracheal intubation?

A. pH 7.30, PaO_2 69 mm Hg, $PaCO_2$ 48 mm Hg

B. pH 7.50, PaO_2 64 mm Hg, $PaCO_2$ 52 mm Hg

C. pH 7.20, PaO_2 60 mm Hg, $PaCO_2$ 53 mm Hg

D. pH 7.50, PaO_2 65 mm Hg, $PaCO_2$ 20 mm Hg

3-55. The patient with fulminating liver disease secondary to hepatitis B infection mentions to the nurse that he has been sharing needles with friends. Which of the following will help protect the friends from developing an active hepatitis B infection?

A. Acetaminophen administration to prevent inflammation

B. IV penicillin infusion

C. Immunoglobulins to increase available antibodies

D. Exchange transfusions to replace infected blood with noninfected blood

3-56. A patient admitted to the emergency room after a traumatic brain injury has been successfully resuscitated. Which of these studies would be most helpful at this point?

A. Magnetic resonance imaging (MRI) of the brain

B. Computed tomography (CT) scan of the head

C. Lumbar puncture (LP)

D. Cerebral angiography

3-57. A family has donated monies to support the redesign of an ICU. The intensivist has been working with the contractor on the unit design. The nurse on the design team reviews the plans and has concerns that they are not conducive to the comfort needs of visitors to the unit. Which of the following would be the best approach for the nurse to communicate these concerns to the design team?

A. Speak with the nurse manager regarding these concerns

B. Assemble a team of nurses to revise the plan

C. Mention these concerns at the next scheduled team design meeting

D. Gather data on the needs of family members who visit ICU

3-58. A patient is admitted for hypertensive crisis secondary to newly diagnosed hypertension. The young patient and his wife have asked the critical care nurse to answer some concerns. They confide that they heard that beta blockers cause sexual dysfunction. The critical care nurse performs a literature search to accurately answer the patient and wife's concern. What would be the best response?

A. "Unfortunately, beta blockers cause sexual dysfunction."

B. "Beta blockers cause sexual dysfunction in less than 0.5% of patients."

C. "If you experience sexual dysfunction, you can stop taking the beta blocker."

D. "Beta blockers cause sexual dysfunction, but Viagra can help in that situation."

3-59. An end-stage renal disease (ESRD) patient receiving hemodialysis three times per week is admitted to the CCU with an acute anterior wall myocardial infarction. The patient's BP is 108/46 mm Hg, HR is 62/min, and RR is 24/min. The critical care nurse should anticipate that this patient's dialysis will be managed by

A. Slow continuous ultrafiltration

B. Continuous venovenous hemodialysis

C. Hemodialysis

D. Peritoneal dialysis

3-60. Which of these intrinsic or extrinsic factors does not affect wound healing in the ICU patient?

A. Sickle cell disease

B. Chronic venous insufficiency

C. Smoking

D. Low carbohydrate diet

3-61. A 71-year-old female is admitted to the progressive care unit with complaints of epigastric pressure. An ECG is performed, and the nurse notes changes from the patient's baseline ECG. ST and T-wave abnormalities are of greatest concern for the nurse in patients with

A. Dilated cardiomyopathy

B. Arrhythmogenic right ventricular cardiomyopathy

C. Left bundle branch block

D. Pericarditis

3-62. A 56-year-old male with a history of diverticulitis is admitted to the ICU with a diagnosis of acute abdomen and dehydration. On assessment, the nurse notes that he is complaining of sudden onset of severe (9/10) left lower quadrant pain with abdominal wall tenderness, diaphoresis, nausea, and pallor. He is becoming increasingly more agitated. His blood pressure has dropped from 135/86 mm Hg to 90/54 mm Hg, and his HR has risen from 92 beats/min to 135 beats/min; his temperature is 38.3°C. Which of these interventions should the nurse focus on at this point?

A. Restoring circulating volume

B. Completing an abdominal assessment

C. Instituting cooling measures

D. Obtaining the patient's medication list

3-63. A patient admitted with fever, dyspnea, and a cough productive of large amounts of rust-colored sputum now complains of severe pleuritic chest pain. After 1 L of normal saline, his temperature is 39.5°C, HR is 120/min, RR is 40/min, SpO_2 is 95% on 50% FiO_2, and BP is 100/40 mm Hg. His breath sounds are diminished bilaterally with fine, inspiratory crackles in both bases, and a chest x-ray is obtained. Which of these interventions should the critical care nurse anticipate next?

A. Thoracentesis for a likely pulmonary effusion

B. Chest tube insertion for a pneumothorax

C. Administration of an analgesic agent

D. Administration of a diuretic

3-64. An ICU patient with pulmonary hypertension is placed on inhaled nitric oxide. The critical care nurse is concerned that the patient could develop which of the following?

A. Rebound pulmonary hypertension when nitric oxide is discontinued

B. Hypotension caused by nitric oxide administration

C. Decreased oxygen saturation related to nitric oxide uptake

D. Pulmonary embolus related to nitric oxide effects on platelet aggregation

3-65. The critical care nurse assists the physician with the placement of a feeding tube in an unresponsive patient. The nurse verifies the placement of the tube with an air bolus and auscultation. Once verified, the nurse initiates enteral feeding at 30 cc/hr. The patient develops a sudden onset of severe respiratory distress and is emergently intubated. Enteral feed is suctioned from the patient's lungs. The physician asks the nurse if the radiograph that was ordered for the confirmation of the tube placement was completed before feeding. The nurse admits that the patient was fed before radiograph confirmation. The patient develops aspiration pneumonia and eventually dies. This scenario is an example of which of these areas of professional liability?

A. Malpractice

B. Breach of duty

C. Duty

D. Injury

3-66. A pregnant woman (28 weeks' gestation) is admitted to the ICU after sustaining a head injury. The patient is receiving intracranial monitoring, is intubated, and receives mechanical ventilation. Intracranial pressure readings this hour range from 12 to 14 mm Hg. The nurse assigned to this patient is the most experienced ICU nurse on duty that evening but has not provided care to a critically ill obstetric patient before. Which of these responses by this nurse will serve the patient best?

A. Contact the perinatal clinical nurse specialist for collaboration in providing care

B. Speak to the intensivist regarding setup and use of fetal monitoring equipment

C. Collaborate with the emergency department nursing staff regarding patient care needs

D. Contact the neurosurgical nurse practitioner for collaboration in patient monitoring

3-67. A critically ill stroke patient in the ICU is surrounded by her family and friends. She remains unresponsive, and her family has opted for comfort measures. The critical care nurse focuses on providing end-of-life care. Which of the following will have the most effect on the patient and family's perceptions of end-of-life care?

A. Follow up meetings after the patient dies

B. Privacy for the patient and family during end of life

C. Family presence during all procedures and care

D. Communication between staff and family

3-68. The ICU nurse is responsible for the delegation of appropriate tasks to trained support staff. Which of the following is not an appropriately delegated task?

A. Delegating suctioning of a stable head injury patient with a tracheostomy to a licensed practical nurse

B. Delegating a bedside blood glucose test to a nursing student

C. Delegating the documentation of a patient assessment for a patient with a right- and left-sided ventricular support device to an unlicensed patient care technician

D. Delegating feeding assistance for a patient with bilateral arm fractures to an unlicensed patient care technician

3-69. A gay teenager involved in a motor vehicle crash is admitted to the ICU for observation. His partner visits frequently, and the couple hold hands during those visits. Visitors of other patients complain about this behavior and demand that the nurse "do something" about it. The ICU nurse can best resolve this situation by

A. Convening a multidisciplinary staff meeting to determine an approach to this issue

B. Explaining to the patient and his visitor that their behavior is upsetting to others and must cease

C. Listening to the visitors' concerns and clarifying that the behavior they describe is a comfort gesture

D. Moving the patient to another ICU cubicle where the occupants are less visible to others

3-70. A patient is admitted to the ICU for evaluation of suspected acute liver rejection. The patient had a liver transplant 3 years ago and reports he has been healthy since then. The patient complains of fever and lethargy, and admission laboratory results reveal elevated liver function tests. Which of the following should the nurse do next?

A. Prepare the patient for transport for magnetic resonance imaging

B. Ensure the patient's bladder is empty in preparation for percutaneous liver biopsy

C. Gather supplies and equipment for placement of a central line and a pulmonary artery catheter

D. Obtain baseline measurements of abdominal girth and intraabdominal pressure

3-71. An end-stage lung cancer patient on home hospice has arrived in the emergency room. His wife called 911 when he began experiencing respiratory distress and severe anxiety that he rated as 10/10. Escalating doses of opioids and benzodiazepines at home failed to relieve his suffering. He confirms that he wishes to remain a DNR and DNI, but he can't bear the fear and suffering. Which of these interventions could the nurse suggest to alleviate his suffering and provide comfort?

A. Short-term intubation

B. High-dose IV propofol

C. Short-term noninvasive positive pressure ventilation

D. Encourage patient to withdraw DNR and accept full treatment

3-72. A 100-kg patient on mechanical ventilation has been weaning from continuous ventilation. Which of these findings demonstrate that the patient is not ready for extubation?

A. Maximum inspiratory pressure of -12 cm H_2O

B. 5 cm H_2O PEEP

C. Spontaneous V_T 6 liters

D. FiO_2 0.4

3-73. During episodes of shock because of acute blood loss, compensatory mechanisms attempt to increase oxygen delivery to vital organs. When the nurse provides care to a patient in hemorrhagic shock, which of the following is an anticipated finding attributable to such compensation?

A. Widened pulse pressure

B. Vasodilatation of arteries

C. Decreased heart rate

D. Decreased urine sodium

3-74. An 86-year-old man with a history of esophageal cancer is admitted to the surgical ICU post esophagogastrectomy. His vital signs are temperature 37.2°C; BP 146/76 mm Hg; pulse 122 beats/min. His incisional pain is 8/10. Which of these interventions would be a key to reducing this patient's risk of mortality and morbidity?

A. Pulmonary care

B. Pain management

C. Administration of large amounts of IV fluids

D. Immediate institution of tube feedings

3-75. A patient admitted to the ICU is suspected to have an ischemic stroke. A CT scan has ruled out intracranial hemorrhage. Which of these assessment findings would alert the nurse to a contraindication for rt-PA?

A. NIH stroke scale score of 1

B. History of seizure disorder

C. A mild traumatic brain injury from a motor vehicle collision 6 months ago

D. INR greater than 1.3

3-76. A patient is admitted to the intensive care unit for severe respiratory distress secondary to COPD exacerbation. It is her third admission in the past 2 months for the same. The patient is on noninvasive positive-pressure ventilation, and arterial blood gas results demonstrate that the patient will require intubation and mechanical ventilation. The nurse is planning care for this patient. Which of the following will have the greatest effect on hospital acquired complication prevention?

A. The choice of endotracheal tube used

B. Initiation of enteral feeding within 4 hours

C. Mobilization to the chair within 8 hours

D. IV heparin for DVT prophylaxis

3-77. An ICU patient's low arterial blood pressure alarm is indicating a significant decrease in blood pressure. You notice that the nurse assigned to the care of the patient is ignoring the alarm. After checking on the patient and obtaining a manual cuff pressure, you discover that the arterial line is intermittently positional leading to false readings. You notify the nurse responsible for that patient. The nurse replies, "That arterial line is positional, just ignore the alarm." You express your concern about the patient to the colleague. The alarm sounds again and your colleague ignores it. After checking on the patient, your next best action should be

A. Monitor the alarm and check on the colleague's patient frequently

B. Immediately notify the nurse manager

C. Contact the intensivist and ask them to change the arterial line

D. Consider the arterial line to be positional and do not react to the alarms

3-78. A critical care nurse is working a double shift with two assigned patients, and the time is 1800 hours. One is a 15-year-old patient newly diagnosed diabetic with diabetic ketoacidosis, requiring hourly blood glucose monitoring; the other is a 20-year-old patient who needs hourly neurologic checks for a closed head injury and whose mother needs constant reassurance. A recently graduated nurse has asked this nurse to help her change a colostomy bag on a fresh postoperative patient; in addition, the nurse manager stops by the unit to ask the nurse to look over the staffing schedule for the next 6 weeks. As the nurse considers this work-load, she realizes that some of the work will need to be delegated to ensure that the priority patient needs are met. Which of the following best reflects an appropriate and safe delegation strategy?

A. Hourly glucose checks delegated to another RN

B. Hourly neurologic check delegated to the UAP

C. Helping new nurse delegated to another RN

D. Staffing schedule review delegated to the new nurse

3-79. A young man was admitted 3 days ago after a motorcycle accident in which he sustained a closed head injury and a fracture of his right femur. The patient develops tachycardia with increased oxygen demands. On assessment, the nurse notes a petechial skin rash over his chest and neck. The patient is now disoriented to both person and place, which is a change from the previous shift. His platelet count had dropped from 290,000/mm^3 to 49,580/mm^3. Which of the following is the most likely explanation for this patient's development of hypoxia?

A. Thrombus resulting from venous stasis obstructed pulmonary blood flow

B. Injury to the endothelial lining of pulmonary capillaries caused alveolar flooding

C. Bronchociliary clearance mechanisms are overwhelmed

D. Blood is being shunted through poorly ventilated areas of pulmonary consolidation

3-80. A patient with a history of multiple intubations with extubation failure has been readmitted to the ICU for COPD exacerbation. He is intubated on mechanical ventilation.

The patient met the criteria for ventilator liberation and has been extubated. Which of these therapies does the critical care nurse anticipate for this patient?

A. Reintubation
B. Noninvasive positive pressure ventilation
C. High-flow nasal cannula
D. Partial rebreather mask

3-81. Assessment parameters for a patient in septic shock reveal these hemodynamic values: HR 90/min, BP 80/50 mm Hg, PAP 36/15 mm Hg, CVP 13 mm Hg, CO 2.5 L/min, CI 1.9 L/min/m^2, SVR 1000 dynes/sec/cm^{-5}, SVO$_2$ 60% Which of these treatments should the nurse expect to administer to this patient?

A. Norepinephrine and dobutamine
B. Dopamine and 500-mL fluid bolus
C. Dobutamine and 500-mL fluid bolus
D. Norepinephrine and sodium bicarbonate

3-82. You are orienting a new nurse on the unit. The patient you are caring for has a pulmonary artery catheter in place. When educating the new nurse about pulmonary artery catheters, which of these interventions do you explain should be performed to ensure accurate readings?

A. Perform a square wave test before obtaining each reading
B. Level the transducer to the left atrium
C. Maintain the patient in a flat supine position whenever measurements are taken
D. Obtain readings at the end of inhalation

3-83. A patient is admitted to the ICU after rupture of a cerebral aneurysm with a subarachnoid hemorrhage (SAH). The critical care nurse knows that the most common site of aneurysm rupture is the

A. Middle cerebral artery
B. Anterior communicating artery
C. Posterior communicating artery
D. Anterior cerebral artery

3-84. A patient remains in ICU 1 week after undergoing thoracotomy for repair of a traumatic aortic tear. She has been extubated for 2 days and remains on an aerosol mask with FiO$_2$ 0.50. Her vitals are HR 88 beats/min, BP 130/82 mm Hg, O$_2$ sat 97%, temperature 37.9°C. Pain control has been an issue, but she is currently comfortable with a morphine PCA and long-acting narcotics. Over the past 3 hours, she has become increasingly agitated and now complains of difficulty breathing. Her vitals now are HR 140 beats/min, BP 95/50 mm Hg, and O$_2$ sat 88%. The nurse telephones the physician and anticipates which of these orders?

A. Increase the FiO$_2$, call anesthesia to intubate STAT, and alert the operating room
B. Administer an anxiolytic, change to a short-acting narcotic, and call for a STAT anesthesia consult
C. Increase the FiO$_2$, PA and lateral chest x-ray, and prepare the patient for CT angiogram of the chest
D. PA and lateral chest x-ray, discontinue the PCA, and prepare the patient for emergency surgery

3-85. A 36-year-old patient with a past medical history of schizophrenia with psychosis (last episode, 3 years ago), occasional IV drug abuse, smoking, and ETOH abuse is admitted to the ICU complaining of fever, malaise, chills, and night sweats. His absolute neutrophil count is 400 cells/mm3. He lives with his sister, who affirms that he is compliant with his home medication regimen, including clozapine, olanzapine, and quetiapine. Which of these interventions does the critical care nurse anticipate first for this patient?

A. HIV testing
B. Cessation of the current schizophrenia medications
C. Blood cultures
D. Bone marrow biopsy

3-86. A 28-year-old patient presents to the ICU confused, combative, and unable to report any personal information or medical history. Results of toxicology screen and blood alcohol levels are negative, and no focal deficits are apparent. If this patient is demonstrating an encephalopathy, which of these investigations should the nurse now anticipate for this patient?

A. Intracranial pressure monitoring
B. Serum osmolality and ammonia testing
C. Lumbar puncture for immunoassay
D. Cerebral angiographic evaluation

3-87. The critical care nurse is planning care for a patient with acute renal failure after cardiac surgery. Which of these findings demonstrate that the nurse has achieved the outcome criteria to improve the patient's condition?

A. CVP is 1 mm Hg
B. CI is 2.8 L/min/m^2

C. MAP is 60 mm Hg

D. PAOP is 6 mm Hg

3-88. A 38-year-old male is in the ICU for treatment of an NSTEMI. His ex-wife has left their 8-year-old child at the hospital in the patient's room on a school day. She states, "It's his turn to watch her." The child is extremely thin, wearing dirty and torn clothing, and does not have a coat despite the winter weather. The patient's lunch tray arrives, and the child eats the entire tray and asks the nurse for more food. She states, "I am not allowed to ask my mom for food. I am so hungry." The nurse notices bruising and perfectly round, uniform scabs on the child's arms in the shape and size of a cigarette tip. The nurse discusses her suspicion of abuse with the supervisor, who advises her not to upset the patient by reporting these alleged concerns. The nurse's next appropriate action should be

A. Collect used clothing and coats from other nurses on the unit to give to the child

B. Discuss the suspicion of abuse or neglect with the patient

C. Discuss the suspicion of abuse or neglect with the patient's physician and ask him to report the neglect

D. Call the child abuse report hotline and make a report of the abuse and neglect concerns

3-89. A patient in the ICU receiving treatment for heart failure has a pulmonary artery catheter. A critical care nurse walking by a patient's room observes a pulmonary artery occlusion pressure waveform on the monitor. After verifying that the catheter balloon is deflated, which of the following would be the next intervention?

A. Immediately call the cardiologist for catheter repositioning by advancing the catheter

B. Immediately call the cardiologist for catheter repositioning by withdrawal of the catheter

C. Immediately call the cardiologist for treatment of the PAOP result

D. Immediately call the cardiologist for discontinuation of the PA catheter

3-90. A patient's family requests the patient's withdrawal from mechanical ventilation. To prepare them for what to expect, the nurse should include

A. The name of the person who will be performing the procedure

B. The anticipated time frame to death

C. Manifestations the patient will likely exhibit

D. The need to insert an airway to remove secretions that cause a "death rattle"

3-91. An ICU patient with end-stage heart failure was admitted 3 days ago for medical management of an acute exacerbation of CHF. The patient is currently stable and receiving IV milrinone therapy. The cardiologist has placed an order for transfer to the telemetry unit and home milrinone therapy. The nurse enters the room to assess the patient and notices a respiratory pattern of increasing ventilation followed by progressively shallow breaths until a short period of apnea occurs. This pattern repeats itself. The patient's pulse oximetry is 97% on room air. The nurse anticipates which of these interventions?

A. Stat arterial blood gas

B. Stat chest x-ray

C. Continue with patient transfer and home milrinone therapy

D. Delay transfer for 24 hours to monitor patient

3-92. Mr. Patel is an Indian heart failure patient who has been in the hospital for 4 months after experiencing complications from surgical placement of a left ventricular assist device. Mr. Patel complains of fatigue, exhaustion, aches, pains, and anorexia. He has been refusing his physical therapy, stating he is too tired. The nurse suspects that Mr. Patel is depressed. Which of these interventions could have the most effect on his current depression?

A. Discuss initiating an antidepressant with the physician

B. Discuss depression with the patient's family and encourage them to try to help "cheer him up"

C. Collaborate with the medical team to plan a trip outside and have the family bring the beloved dog for a visit

D. Encourage the family to bring in Mr. Patel's favorite meal

3-93. Tumor necrosis factor-α (TNF-α) is a polypeptide secretory product of the monocyte-macrophage system that is released during SIRS. Nurses who work with critically ill patients need to be especially vigilant regarding clinical situations that may precipitate release of TNF because one of the most serious cellular responses to this mediator is
   A. Microvascular vasodilation
   B. Metabolic alkalosis
   C. Decreased oxygen consumption
   D. Increased capillary permeability

3-94. A patient in the ICU was admitted 10 days ago after a motor vehicle accident. The patient experienced severe thoracic trauma and is still recovering in the ICU. The patient's recovery is complicated by a persistent air leak in the chest tube. The patient and the family are very discouraged and ask the nurse to explain the alternatives available to treat a persistent air leak. Which of the following would be the least likely treatment for this disorder?
   A. Bronchoscopy
   B. Instillation of antibiotics into the chest tube
   C. Progressive advancement of the chest tube
   D. Surgery

3-95. A 68-year-old end-stage renal disease (ESRD) patient who receives hemodialysis for 3 hours, three times per week, presents to the ED with a complaint of sharp, stabbing chest pain that increases on inspiration and dyspnea on exertion. The patient's vital signs are BP 110/68 mm Hg, HR 122/min, RR 28/min and labored, temperature 37.9°C. The patient has a pericardial friction rub. Management of this patient will now include
   A. Four hours of hemodialysis three times per week
   B. Four hours of hemodialysis done daily
   C. Peritoneal dialysis, four exchanges per day
   D. Peritoneal dialysis, five exchanges per day

3-96. The critical care nurse is orienting a new nurse on the unit. He is teaching the new nurse how to meet the psychosocial needs of the family members of critically ill patients. Which of the following is not part of the new nurse's education?
   A. The family needs to obtain information
   B. The family needs clergy support
   C. The family needs to receive support and reassurance
   D. The family needs to be with the patient

3-97. A 46-year-old Desert Storm veteran has been admitted to the ICU after a severe motor vehicle accident. He was drinking and speeding when he hit a tree in his vehicle. He is currently recovering from multiple fractures. The night shift nurse reports that she has observed nightmares and fitful rest the past 3 nights. Which of these interventions would be most helpful for this patient?
   A. Referral to Alcoholics Anonymous
   B. Obtain an order for a benzodiazepine
   C. Referral to veterans support foundation
   D. Psychiatry consult

3-98. A patient with heart failure has been admitted to the ICU. You are the preceptor assigned with a new nurse to care for this patient. The patient develops flash pulmonary edema, and the intensivist orders furosemide 80-mg IV push. You notice that the new nurse has already given the drug. She tells you that she was very concerned that the patient would require intubation so she pushed the drug quickly over less than 1 minute. You are immediately concerned that the patient may develop
   A. Hypotension
   B. Hearing loss
   C. Renal failure
   D. Severe hypokalemia and arrhythmia

3-99. A patient in the ICU is admitted for acute hemorrhagic stroke. He presents with dizziness, vertigo, ataxia, occipital headache, nystagmus, and dysarthria. The critical care nurse anticipates the stroke is located in which cortical structure?
   A. Cerebellum
   B. Pons
   C. Thalamus
   D. Putamen

3-100. The critical care nurse is caring for a patient with a diagnosis of meningococcal meningitis. The nurse is diligently monitoring for the development of a serious complication of meningitis that can lead to sepsis and shock. Which of the following is a potential complication of meningitis that can lead to shock and increased mortality?

A. Korsakoff syndrome
B. Brudzinski sign
C. Waterhouse-Friderichsen syndrome
D. Brown-Séquard syndrome

3-101. A 28-year-old woman is admitted to the ICU after a motorcycle accident in which she sustained a severe pelvic fracture and blunt trauma to her lower extremities. She is on bed rest and has been started on a clear liquid diet. Her hemoglobin continues to drift down over the past 36 hours from a high after transfusion of 11 g/dL to 9.3 g/dL. The physician has ordered continued monitoring of her hemoglobin and administration of 2 units of packed cells. Her BP is 110/72 mm Hg, pulse is 98 beats/min, and RR is 18 breaths/min. Her risks for development of pulmonary emboli are increased because of

A. Venous stasis, vein injury, and a hypercoagulable state
B. Intravascular cannulation, dehydration, and age
C. Hypoxia, interstitial edema, and right ventricular dysfunction
D. Pulmonary artery hypertension, atelectasis, and immobility

3-102. The ICU nurse knows through evidence-based practice that one critical nursing intervention prevents multiple patient complications and improves patient outcomes, especially in intubated patients. This intervention reduces the incidence and severity of ICU acquired weakness, decreases length of stay in the hospital, reduces mechanical ventilation duration, improves long-term functional independence, prevents ICU-acquired pneumonia, improves glycemic control, and can reduce mortality as it improves the quality of life post discharge. Which of the following describes that intervention?

A. DVT prophylaxis
B. Fall prevention
C. VAE prevention
D. Early mobilization

3-103. A patient is admitted after exploratory laparotomy and debridement for severe necrosing pancreatitis. Intraoperative blood loss was 4000 mL. Upon return to ICU, the patient's BP is 76/45 mm Hg, pulse is 145 beats/min, respirations are 32 breaths/min, and urine output is 20 mL/hr for the past 2 hours. She receives 4 units of packed cells, 1 unit of fresh-frozen plasma, and 2000 mL of crystalloid volume replacement. The patient's urine output remains 20 mL/hr, and vital signs are BP 100/67 mm Hg, pulse 128 beats/min, and respirations 28 breaths/min. Based on recent laboratory results, the physician decides to initiate continuous veno-venous hemofiltration (CVVH). The rationale for choosing CVVH is that this therapy

A. Provides ultrafiltration and solute removal by convection without significant hemodynamic consequences
B. Avoids complications such as clotting and infection associated with other forms of renal replacement
C. Is the optimal treatment for chronic renal failure
D. Will more effectively maintain the BUN level at less than 100 mg/dL

3-104. A 58-year-old man is admitted with shortness of breath, oxygen saturation of 82%, respirations 32/min, and moderate confusion. A chest x-ray shows the patient has a large pleural effusion. A thoracentesis is planned to remove the fluid. The patient is a newlywed of 4 months, and his wife, after signing the consent form, requests to be present during the procedure. Which of the following is the best response that the patient's nurse could make to the wife's request?

A. "Our unit policy states that during procedures, family wait in the waiting room."
B. "Have you ever seen a thoracentesis before? The procedure uses needles."
C. "Because the procedure requires a sterile field, family must stay in the waiting room."
D. "Family members usually are not present during these procedures, but let me talk to the physician about your staying."

3-105. The critical care nurse knows that patients in the ICU are at risk for complications such as deep vein thrombosis. Which of the following is an important enzyme in the blood responsible for degrading fibrin blood clots?

A. Plasmin
B. Thrombin
C. Antithrombin III
D. Phospholipid

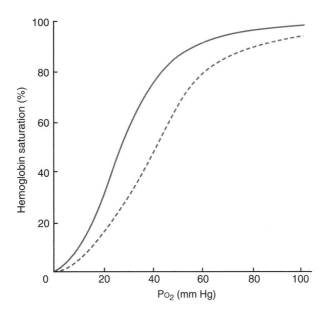

3-106. A 70-kg patient with acute respiratory distress syndrome is mechanically ventilated on these settings: FiO_2 70%; tidal volume 450 mL, rate 10/min; PEEP 20 cm H_2O. On these settings, the patient's PaO_2 is 76 mm Hg. The patient currently has a core temperature of 37°C, heart rate of 116/min, and blood pressure of 78/58 mm Hg. Which of these interventions should the nurse now anticipate?
   A. Decrease PEEP to decrease intrathoracic pressure
   B. Administer 500-mL fluid bolus of normal saline
   C. Initiate a norepinephrine infusion to maintain systolic BP at least 80 mm Hg
   D. Increase tidal volume to 700 mL

3-107. In the oxyhemoglobin dissociation curve below, the dotted blue line represents a shift caused by which of these conditions?
   A. Hyperventilation
   B. Alkalosis
   C. Hyperthermia
   D. Carbon monoxide poisoning

3-108. A patient in the ICU has a history of stroke with expressive aphasia and bilateral extremity weakness. She has been admitted with fever, elevated WBC, cough, shortness of breath, and acute renal failure. You are the ICU nurse assigned to her care today. The intensivist has ordered two sets of blood cultures. After explaining the procedure to the patient, she extends her arm for blood draw as requested. You prepare to obtain the second set of cultures, but the patient does not comply by extending her arm. Which of the following would be your most appropriate intervention?
   A. Gently coax her arm into an extended position to obtain the sample
   B. Notify the intensivist that the patient has refused the second set of cultures
   C. Ask another colleague to obtain the second set of cultures
   D. Obtain the second set of blood cultures from the central line

3-109. An older patient with longstanding obstructive pulmonary disease is admitted to the hospital with an exacerbation of COPD. His initial ABGs are pH 7.28, PaO_2 75 mm Hg, $PaCO_2$ 70 mm Hg, HCO_3 30 mEq/L. Which of the following represents the primary goal for nursing management of patients with an acute exacerbation of COPD?

A. Optimize arterial blood gases based on patient baseline values

B. Identify triggers of the exacerbation so these can be avoided

C. Administer broad-spectrum antibiotics early based on WBC count

D. Administer bronchodilators only if necessary to avoid cardiovascular effects

3-110. A patient with suspected meningitis had a lumbar puncture performed 2 hours ago. The patient is complaining of a headache, and the nurse is concerned about a cerebrospinal fluid leak. The progressive care nurse understands that the functions of cerebrospinal fluid are all of the following except

A. Enables the diffusion of water-soluble metabolites

B. Serves as a channel for neurochemical communication

C. Provide ATP for impulse formation

D. Provides cushioning from injury

3-111. A patient is admitted to the ICU after an anaphylactic reaction to a bee sting. Which of these components of the immunologic system stimulate the inflammatory response that leads to anaphylaxis?

A. Neutrophils

B. T cells

C. Macrophages

D. Basophils

3-112. Mr. Jones is an 85-year-old patient admitted to the ICU for septic shock. He is a full-time nursing home resident because of a history of severe dementia, stroke, bilateral AKA, renal failure with hemodialysis, failure to thrive with peg tube placement, end-stage heart failure, and multiple decubitus ulcers. He is intubated and placed on multiple vasopressors. Goals of care meetings are held with the patient's family, and they continue to want a full code status and "everything done." The family continued to receive full information from the medical team. The family reports that the patient's wishes were always to be kept alive by every means possible because the patient believed that "a cure for everything

would be found eventually." According to the ethical principal of beneficence, which of the following would be most appropriate for this patient?

A. Hospital ethics committee consult

B. Hospice consult

C. Continue full life support interventions

D. Begin to withdraw treatments without the family's knowledge

3-113. A patient is admitted to the progressive care unit after an ablation procedure for atrial fibrillation. The progressive care nurse is monitoring for post-procedural complications. Which of the following is the most life-threatening complication of radiofrequency ablation of cardiac accessory pathways?

A. Development of second-degree heart block type II

B. Pericardial tamponade

C. Cardiac valve damage

D. Dislodgement of micro emboli

3-114. An Asian immigrant been admitted to the ICU for acute ST elevation MI. He has a cardiac catheterization that reveals three-vessel coronary artery disease. The cardiac surgeon arrives to obtain consent for coronary artery bypass graft surgery. An Asian translator from language services has arrived to translate. After providing a clear description of the facts, implications, and consequences of the surgery, the patient nods and smiles. The surgeon leaves the room and arrives later with the consent. He placed the consent in front of the patient and hands him a pen. The patient signs the consent and the surgeon asks you to witness the consent. Which of the following would be most appropriate at this time?

A. Sign the consent as a witness to the patient's informed consent

B. Ask language services to send a translator to verify the patient's informed consent

C. Refuse to sign the consent

D. Ask an Asian colleague to witness the consent

3-115. A patient with an elevated ICP is admitted to the ICU. The critical care nurse understands that ICP elevations cause displacement of brain structures. The patient has this

herniation description: bilateral cerebral lesions that displace both hemispheres, the diencephalon, and the midbrain downward through the tentorial notch, which causes midbrain compression. Which herniation syndrome was described?
A. Cingulate or subfalcine herniation
B. Uncal or lateral transtentorial herniation
C. Central transtentorial herniation
D. Tonsillar herniation

3-116. The respiratory therapist is at a patient's bedside to check the endotracheal tube cuff pressure. The manometer reading is 20 cm H_2O. The nurse anticipates which of these interventions?
A. 1cc of air added to the ET tube cuff
B. 1cc of air removed from the ET tube cuff
C. Recheck cuff pressure in 8 hours
D. No further intervention

3-117. A 70-year-old patient with end-stage renal disease (ESRD), diabetes, and heart failure presents to the ED with complaints of nausea, vomiting, and abdominal cramps. He is lethargic and mildly confused. When waiting to be seen by the ED physician, the patient becomes unresponsive, with no detectable blood pressure, and the cardiac monitor shows sinus bradycardia with a heart rate of 32 beats/min. Which of the following will the nurse now need to administer for initial management of this patient?
A. Insulin and glucose
B. Lidocaine
C. Polystyrene sulfonate (Kayexalate)
D. Amiodarone

3-118. A patient with a traumatic brain injury is admitted to the ICU. An ICP monitor is placed, and the critical care nurse is at the bedside. Which of these findings must be reported to the physician?
A. A rise to 15 mm Hg while the patient is suctioned that returns to 8 mm Hg after suctioning is completed
B. A rise to 18 mm Hg that is sustained for greater than 15 minutes
C. A rise to 20 mm Hg that immediately decreases to 10 mm Hg
D. A rise to 25 mm Hg that is sustained for 10 minutes

3-119. A patient in the ICU is intubated and mechanically ventilated for treatment of community-acquired pneumonia and COPD. Which of these sedation agents would be most appropriate for the patient?
A. Midazolam infusion
B. Dexmedetomidine infusion
C. Vecuronium infusion
D. Lorazepam infusion

3-120. You are a critical care nurse working in an ICU that has seen an increase in morbidly obese patients and bariatric surgical patients. When a bariatric patient is admitted to the ICU, specialty equipment (bariatric beds, commodes, bedpans, gowns, lifts, walkers, chairs, wheelchairs) must be ordered from a rental company, but they can only be ordered after a patient is admitted. The nursing staff has been unable to provide sensitive, compassionate, and safe care because of frequent delays in the delivery of the equipment. Which of the following would be most helpful to obtain the equipment needed to provide the appropriate care for this patient population?
A. Contact the ethics committee about the inadequate care of bariatric patients and yse their assistance to convey the need to purchase the necessary bariatric equipment
B. Complete a literature search for evidence-based practice for the care of bariatric patients and convene a multidisciplinary team to create a protocol for a cost-effective method to provide the supplies needed in a timely manner
C. Contact the physician director of the ICU and explain the ongoing situation
D. Complete an incident report every time a patient's care is compromised by the situation to document the frequency and urgency of this situation

3-121. A postoperative patient has experienced nerve damage secondary to endotracheal intubation. In the cranial nervous system, which of the following nerves is most likely damaged?
A. Abducens nerve
B. Trochlear nerve

C. Hypoglossal nerve

D. Oculomotor nerve

3-122. A 78-year-old resident of a skilled nursing facility receives enteral feedings via a gastrostomy tube. This morning his regular caregivers noticed a decrease in his level of consciousness that may have begun the day before, with shallow, rapid respirations; a blood pressure of 98/38 mm Hg; and continual incontinence of urine. The nurse's assessment finds no visible signs of head or other trauma from a possible unreported fall, so the nurse suspects this patient is experiencing

A. Diabetic ketoacidosis

B. Syndrome of inappropriate antidiuretic hormone

C. Hyperglycemic, hyperosmolar nonketotic coma

D. Diabetes insipidus

3-123. When considering Erikson's eight stages of the life cycle, which of these approaches is not appropriate for an 80-year-old patient?

A. Encourage expression of life experiences

B. Address as Mr./Mrs./Ms.

C. Encourage significant others to participate in the decision-making process

D. Recognize the importance of personal grooming

3-124. You are caring for a patient with an intraaortic balloon pump. A new nurse on the unit has asked you to explain the pump function. Which of the following explains the timing of the balloon inflation?

A. After aortic valve closure

B. At the end of systole

C. At the end of diastole

D. Before the opening of the aortic valve

3-125. A patient with leukemia was admitted to the ICU 1 week after the last chemotherapy treatment. On admission 90 minutes ago, the patient complained of fatigue and was pale with a blood pressure of 110/72 mm Hg and a pulse of 88 beats/min. The BP is now 100/58mm Hg; the pulse is 110 beats/min; and the patient is passing dark, tarry stools. The nurse's plan of care will center on this patient's most immediate needs related to

A. Malnutrition

B. Gastrointestinal bleeding

C. Anemia

D. Immunosuppression

3-126. In a patient with acute hypercapnic respiratory failure, oxygen administration at an FiO_2 of 100% may increase $PaCO_2$ levels because

A. FiO_2 of 100% is needed to replace CO_2 with O_2

B. Alveolar hypoventilation is not corrected by oxygen administration

C. Increased ventilation in anemia does not lower $PaCO_2$

D. In patients with a decreased A-a gradient, carbon dioxide does not diffuse

3-127. Geriatric syndromes are broad categories of signs and symptoms that may have a variety of contributing factors, including normal aging changes, multiple diagnoses, and adverse effects of therapeutic interventions. Syndromes are a major focus of nursing research and best practice guidelines. SPICES is an evidence-based tool for assessing major geriatric syndromes. Which of these syndromes is not part of the SPICES tool?

A. S: Sleep disorders

B. I: Intelligence issues

C. C: Confusion

D. E: Evidence of falls

3-128. When providing nursing care for a patient with suspected stroke, the most important factor related to the use of fibrinolytic therapy is to

A. Begin the therapy within 90 minutes of the patient's arrival

B. Obtain a detailed history of the patient's allergies

C. Establish the nature and time of symptom commencement

D. Start a large-bore central IV line

3-129. You are the nurse caring for a patient scheduled for an aortic valve replacement secondary to aortic stenosis. Which of the following describes the location to best appreciate the heart murmur?

A. Fourth intercostal space, left sternal border

B. Second intercostal space, right sternal border

C. Second intercostal space, left sternal border

D. Apex radiating to left axilla

3-130. A patient in the ICU was treated for a pneumothorax after a motor vehicle accident 5 days prior. He is scheduled to have his chest tube removed. Which of the following would be the most appropriate intervention for the patient?
   A. Clamp the chest tube for 2 hours and obtain chest x-ray before removal
   B. Ensure that the physician obtains consent before removal
   C. Call blood bank to verify that two units of packed red blood cells is available for emergency transfusion
   D. Administer analgesia 1 hour before chest tube removal

3-131. An older patient in the ICU has had an extended stay related to difficulty weaning from mechanical ventilation. Once extubated, which of the following is the most essential initial consult that will be required?
   A. Nutritionist to evaluate nutritional status
   B. Physical therapist to assist with progressive activity tolerance
   C. Speech and swallow to evaluate the patient's ability to swallow
   D. Respiratory therapy to evaluate for laryngeal edema

3-132. After a patient undergoes aortic valve replacement for aortic regurgitation, these hemodynamic values are obtained: HR 70 beats/min 100% paced, BP 90/40 mm Hg, MAP 56 mm Hg; PCWP 18 mm Hg. Urine output is 100 mL/hr. Which of these interventions is most appropriate to increase the patient's blood pressure?
   A. Administering 250 mL normal saline bolus
   B. Initiating a dobutamine infusion
   C. Initiating an infusion of norepinephrine
   D. Increasing the pacing rate to 80/min

3-133. Approximately 48 hours after admission to the ICU after a surgical procedure, a patient with a known history of ETOH abuse begins to exhibit signs and symptoms of alcohol withdrawal syndrome: anxiety, disorientation, tremors, and irritability. Knowing that delirium tremens (DTs) is a life-threatening emergency, the initial intervention that the critical care nurse should provide to prevent DTs is to
   A. Administer haloperidol
   B. Apply restraints for patient safety

   C. Turn on the television to distract the patient
   D. Administer benzodiazepines

3-134. A 58-year-old morbidly obese patient with a BMI greater than 40 is admitted to the ICU for atrial fibrillation. She has a past medical history of congestive heart failure, hypertension, diabetes, COPD, sleep apnea, and chronic renal insufficiency. The cardiologist has decided to perform synchronized cardioversion at the bedside. Informed consent is signed; a large-bore IV site is present, the necessary equipment for conscious sedation and cardioversion are at the bedside, and sedation medication with reversals has arrived from the pharmacy. The cardiologist asks you to administer midazolam 2 mg IV. Which of the following would be most appropriate at this time?
   A. Administer midazolam as ordered
   B. Suggest diazepam instead of midazolam
   C. Refuse to administer the sedation
   D. Suggest a combination of midazolam and fentanyl

3-135. A patient in the ICU with sepsis and respiratory failure secondary to acute respiratory distress syndrome has been unstable for several days despite receiving maximal mechanical ventilator support. The family, who seems to understand the patient's condition, refuses to sign a do-not-resuscitate order at a family meeting with the multidisciplinary team. The patient's SpO_2 acutely drops to 84%, and the physician orders the FiO_2 to be decreased to 21%. Which of the following should the nurse do at this time?
   A. Call respiratory therapy to reduce the FiO_2
   B. Request that the family speak with the physician
   C. Ask the physician to provide a rationale for the change
   D. Administer doses of sedation and pain medication to avoid discomfort

3-136. A 22-year-old patient has been admitted to the ICU after a motorcycle accident. He has a severe closed head injury and multiple organ system trauma, and his family remains at the bedside at all times. The local organ procurement organization has been consulted and is following the case. A stat

CT scan of the head at 3 AM reveals impending herniation. The nurse informs the intensivist that she is calling the organ procurement organization to speak to the family about donation. The intensivist instructs the nurse not to call because it will further upset a family dealing with the imminent death of their loved one. He instructs the nurse to wait until after he has an end-of-life conversation with the family. Which of the following actions is most appropriate?

A. Call the organ procurement organization
B. Discuss organ donation with the family
C. Delay the call to organ procurement as requested by the intensivist
D. Address the issue with the nurse manager when she arrives at 8 AM

3-137. A patient in the ICU is noted to have a cool, blue great toe on his right foot. Dorsalis pedis and posterior tibial pulses are not palpable. Which of these interventions is contraindicated for this patient?

A. Elevation of the right foot on pillows to decrease edema
B. Placing the bed in reverse Trendelenburg position
C. Administration of heparin
D. Administration of vasodilators

3-138. A critical care nurse can delegate tasks to assistive personnel. A critical care nurse must supervise the performance of the task delegated. Which of the following is not a characteristic of task supervision?

A. Provide directions and clear expectations of how the task is to be performed
B. Intervene if necessary
C. Monitor performance of the task to assure compliance with established standard of practice, policies, and procedures.
D. Monitor the delegatee as he or she documents the task

3-139. A new trauma patient is being turned during a bath when the nurse notices a small wound approximately 2 cm on the left posterolateral chest wall with bubbles around the site. Upon closer examination of the wound, the nurse can hear a faint sucking sound. The patient's BP is 100/70 mm Hg, pulse is 120 beats/min, RR is 24 breaths/min. The nurse's next intervention should be to

A. Continue with the bath
B. Apply an occlusive dressing to the wound

C. Notify the physician and prepare for a chest tube insertion
D. Notify the physician and prepare for intubation

3-140. The picture below represents the cardiac conduction system. Which components of the cardiac conduction system are identified by the black arrows?

A. SA and AV nodes
B. His bundles
C. Bundle branches
D. Purkinje fibers

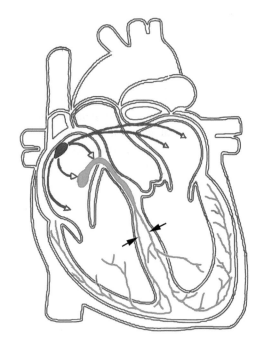

3-141. You work in a busy ICU that has been placing LVADs (left ventricular assist devices) for end-stage heart failure patients. The transplant candidates with these devices are transferred to another facility that specializes in heart transplant surgery. The transfer process is very involved and difficult to coordinate. You would like to develop an LVAD patient transport tool with guidelines for providing the appropriate level of care for an LVAD patient being transferred to another facility. Which of the following should be completed first?

A. Convene a multidisciplinary team to identify the level of care involved for this patient population
B. Create a survey for all personnel that participate in the transport to

identify the level of care involved for this patient population

C. Consult the LVAD specialist to identify the level of care involved for this patient population

D. Perform an extensive literature search to identify the level of care involved for this patient population

3-142. Which of these interventions would the nurse anticipate for effective management of a patient who exhibited the rhythm strip below?

A. Initiate transcutaneous pacing at a rate of 70/min

B. Administer atropine 0.5 mg IV

C. Prepare for insertion of transvenous pacemaker

D. Continue to monitor the patient

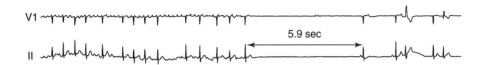

3-143. A 76-year-old patient in the ICU is admitted for cardiogenic shock, multiple organ system failure, and ARDS. The patient is decompensating and facing imminent death. The patient's son is a physician, and he is demanding that the medical staff place ECMO (extracorporeal membranous oxygenation) life support. The intensivist and the ICU team caring for the patient have determined ECMO would be futile care for the patient. Multiple goals of care discussions have been held with the family member, and a joint decision cannot be reached with the patient's son. The critical care nurse anticipates any of the following EXCEPT

A. Consulting the ethics committee to assist with mutual resolution

B. Supporting transfer of care to a different physician

C. Initiating ECMO and evaluate the patient's response in 24 hours

D. Supporting the transfer of care to an alternative institution

3-144. A CVA patient with COPD has a tracheostomy and a gastrostomy tube. She has been in the hospital for 3 months with multiple complications, including PE, pneumonia, and recurrent *Clostridium difficile* infection. Which of the following is not a primary indication for fecal microbiota transplant (FMT)?

A. Multiple recurrent *C. difficile* infections

B. Moderate *C. difficile* infection with no response to standard therapy (vancomycin or fidaxomicin) for at least 1 week

C. Severe or fulminant *C. difficile* infection with no response to standard therapy in 48 hours

D. Moderate *C. difficile* infection in patient allergic to vancomycin

3-145. A patient is admitted to the ICU after a stab wound to the left chest at the level of the fifth rib. Treatment received in the ED included a bolus of 500-mL normal saline and chest tube placement. The patient has 75 mL of bloody drainage in the chest tube collection chamber and a minimal air leak. The anterior chest wound dressing is dry and intact. Upon arrival in the ICU, the patient's vital signs are HR 120 beats/min, BP 98/76 mm Hg, and RR 24 breaths/min on a 100% nonrebreather mask. SpO_2 is 100%. A follow-up chest x-ray obtained on arrival in the ICU shows an enlarged cardiac silhouette and 10% pneumothorax despite chest tube placement. The most likely cause of the patient's low blood pressure is which of the following?

A. Pericardial tamponade

B. Tension pneumothorax

C. Hemothorax

D. Hypovolemia

3-146. Joan was in the ICU for six weeks after a cardiac arrest secondary to an ST elevation MI with subsequent cardiogenic shock. Her recovery was complicated by failure to wean from the ventilator, and she spent 2 months in a rehabilitation facility prior to her discharge home. Joan continues to experience cognitive and psychological impairment indicative of post–intensive care syndrome. Which of the following is true about post intensive care syndrome?

A. Post–intensive care syndrome is usually experienced by patients during the first 24 to 48 hours after transfer out of the ICU

B. Intubated patients on continuous sedation experience less post intensive care syndrome symptoms than patients not on sedation

C. Music therapy can help prevent post intensive care syndrome

D. Nursing care does not prevent the development of post–intensive care syndrome

3-147. The respiratory status of a patient with chronic obstructive pulmonary disease has improved, and she is using 2 L/min of oxygen via cannula. She has been receiving steroid therapy to decrease inflammation. This morning the patient's previously normal laboratory results reveal serum glucose of 280 mg/dL and these arterial blood gas results: pH 7.22, $PaCO_2$ 46 mm Hg, PaO_2 91 mm Hg, and HCO_3 21 mEq/L. Which of these first interventions is warranted to manage these findings?

A. IV fluid and electrolyte replacement

B. Administration of 6 units of regular insulin IV bolus

C. Low-dose insulin in normal saline drip

D. 50-mL bicarbonate solution bolus

3-148. After thoracic aortic repair, a motor vehicle crash victim is on continuous cardiac and hemodynamic pressure monitoring, as well as CSF pressure monitoring. Which of these interventions is contraindicated in the care of this patient?

A. Administration of 200 mL/hr of normal saline

B. Administration of nitroglycerin to maintain SBP less than 170 mm Hg

C. Drainage of 100 mL of CSF to maintain CSF pressure less than 10 mm Hg

D. Administration of fresh-frozen plasma (FFP) and platelets at 75 mL/hr

3-149. A COPD patient arrives to the ICU with respiratory distress. The intensivist orders noninvasive positive-pressure ventilation (NPPV). The therapeutic effect of NIPPV augments treatment by

A. Decreasing air trapping by dropping resistance to exhalation

B. Maximizing ventilation and perfusion matching

C. Increasing alveolar recruitment

D. Resolving mucous plugging in the distal airways

3-150. A 46-year-old prisoner on death row for a triple homicide is admitted to the hospital with severe chest pain. He is diagnosed with an acute ST elevation myocardial infarction and rushed to the catheterization laboratory. A cardiac catheterization reveals diffuse three-vessel disease, including critical left main disease requiring urgent surgical intervention. The cardiologist discusses surgical options with the patient. The patient refuses surgery and states that he would like to return to the prison. He tells the physician that he is not afraid of dying. The physician leaves the room and places an order for a consult to the cardiothoracic surgeon. This demonstrates which ethical principal?

A. Beneficence

B. Paternalism

C. Nonmaleficence

D. Patient autonomy

3 Answers to Core Review Test 3

3-1. **(A)** For patients, a policy of routine undressing and gowning will minimize the likelihood of using hidden weapons when performed in an unbiased manner, regardless of the chief complaint. Preparation of the examination room can facilitate safety. As many objects as possible should be removed from examination rooms that routinely hold violent or agitated patients. Essential violence prevention techniques include interpersonal skills that convey respect and unconditional positive regard. Offer food or drink both as an expression of caring and to minimize irritability. Even as the person receives genuine, unconditional care, boundaries of acceptable behavior should be set, and consequences must be consistent. Inappropriate behavior is unacceptable and patients should be told the ramifications. Some patients do not have the ability to cope with the stressful environment and become verbally or physically uncontrolled. Other patients respond to limit setting and rules.

References: Chapa, D., & Akintade, B. (2018). Psychosocial aspects of critical care. In T. M. Hartjes (Ed.), *AACN core curriculum for high acuity, progressive, and critical care nursing* (7th ed.). St. Louis: Elsevier.

Isaacs, E. (2014). The violent patient. In J. Adams (Ed.), *Emergency medicine* (2nd ed.). (pp. 1630–1638). Philadelphia: Elsevier Saunders.

3-2. **(C)** The patient appears to be in status epilepticus. Status epilepticus is defined as seizure activity lasting longer than 5 to 10 minutes or repetitive seizures occurring without full recovery between ictal episodes. These may be generalized convulsive, nonconvulsive (without visible movement), or focal motor seizures. Benzodiazepines are commonly given to stop acute seizures (usually concurrently with an anticonvulsant drug such as phenytoin) and may be repeated after 10 minutes if seizure activity persists. Although an EEG (Option A) is helpful in diagnosis and treatment planning for patients with seizure disorders, a STAT EEG would not provide any additional information during the acute period. Although some electrolyte disturbances can cause seizures, the description of patient activity is characteristic for status epilepticus, so STAT labs (Option B) are not as high a priority as terminating the seizure activity. The longer a seizure lasts, the more difficult it is to control. Most commonly, seizures refractory to these treatments are stopped with barbiturate infusion. However, the previously mentioned measures are attempted before treatment with barbiturates (Option D). Additionally, the barbiturate dose is twice the recommended dosing (10 mg/kg over 30 minutes followed by a continuous infusion at a lower rate).

References: Blissitt, P. A. (2018). Neurologic system. In T. M. Hartjes (Ed.), *AACN core curriculum for high acuity, progressive, and critical care nursing* (7th ed.). St. Louis: Elsevier.

3-3. **(D)** Up to 70% of houses built before 1960 have surfaces covered in lead-based paint. Chipping paint or simple renovations result in the formation of lead dust, which adults can inhale or consume. Lead poisoning does not produce a classic toxidrome that facilitates easy diagnosis. Lead is compartmentalized into three main areas: bones, soft tissue (including the brain), and blood. Organic lead is assimilated rapidly by the CNS and can produce a host of neuropsychiatric manifestations as described. Cyanide poisoning presents with signs and symptoms that are primarily cardiopulmonary in nature: dysrhythmias, asystole, hypotension, and cardiovascular collapse. Carbon monoxide (CO) exposure results in tissue hypoxia and cellular toxicity. CO binds with hemoglobin in place of oxygen. The organs with the greatest sensitivity to hypoxia—the CNS and cardiovascular system—are affected the most. In addition to neuropsychiatric manifestations, patients with CO poisoning present with dyspnea, tachycardia, and cardiac ischemia. Pesticide exposure produces a cholinergic crisis. Signs and symptoms would include sweating, pupillary constriction, excessive salivation, bradycardia, and blurred vision.

References: Berryman, L. (2018). Multisystem: toxin exposure. In T. M. Hartjes (Ed.), *AACN core curriculum for high acuity, progressive, and critical care nursing* (7th ed.). St. Louis: Elsevier.

O'Brien, S. (2016). Lead poisoning: current practice guidelines. *Clinical Advisor, 19*(10), 16–28.

3-4. **(D)** Staphylococcal infection associated with cannula sepsis and thrombophlebitis is an important and, unfortunately, extremely common reason for morbidity after hospital admission. Staphylococci have a predilection for plastic, rapidly forming a biofilm that remains as a source of bacteremia as long as the plastic is in situ. The visual infusion phlebitis scale recommends changing the site of the catheter if two signs of phlebitis (pain and erythema) are evident. The site should be removed as soon as possible. The notification of a doctor to assess the site prior to site removal is not necessary because it is a nursing intervention to prevent IV site infection. Arm bending may cause pain and or redness at the site. However, these are signs of potential infection and thus cannot be ignored.

References: Mattox, E. A. (2017). Complications of peripheral venous access devices: prevention, detection, and recovery strategies. *Critical Care Nurse, 37*(2), e1–e14. http://dx.doi.org/10.4037/ccn2017657.

3-5. **(C)** Diabetic ketoacidosis (DKA) is the most serious metabolic complication of type 1 diabetes mellitus. Diagnostic study findings include an anion gap greater than 10, an arterial pH less than 7.3, and a plasma glucose level greater than 250 mg/dL. Treatment goals include normalizing the blood glucose level, restoring the acid-base balance, and restoring the fluid balance. The anion gap helps to determine the cause of metabolic acidosis.

References: MacDermott, J. (2018). Endocrine system. In T. M. Hartjes (Ed.), *AACN core curriculum for high acuity, progressive, and critical care nursing* (7th ed.). St. Louis: Elsevier.

3-6. **(D)** The incision in abdominal aortic aneurysm extends from the thorax to the umbilicus. Pain control is a priority for a hemodynamically stable patient in the immediate postoperative period. Return of circulation to the extremities after aneurysm repair is dependent on the preoperative circulatory status. Coughing and deep breathing and use of incentive spirometry are required after extubation and may require premedication with analgesics to prevent incisional pain. The patient is usually extubated within 24 hours unless preexisting pulmonary disease is present. Because the patient is NPO a bowel protocol is usually instituted 2 or more days after surgery.

References: Efre, A., & Boling, B. (2018). Cardiovascular system. In T. M. Hartjes (Ed.), *AACN core curriculum for high acuity, progressive, and critical care nursing* (7th ed.). St. Louis: Elsevier.

3-7. **(B)** Because this patient is minimally responsive, endotracheal intubation is indicated for acute respiratory failure. The diagnosis of acute respiratory failure is supported by the ABG findings of respiratory acidosis and hypoxemia. BiPAP may be used in respiratory failure patients who are responsive. An inability to protect the airway, impaired cough or swallowing, poor clearance of secretions, depressed sensorium, and lethargy are contraindications for noninvasive ventilation. Although low-flow oxygen is frequently used in COPD, this patient is in acute respiratory failure, and the low-flow delivery would not be beneficial in correcting the $PaCO_2$. Correction of pH is best accomplished by decreasing the $PaCO_2$. If the pH was lower than 7.20, sodium bicarbonate might also be indicated.

References: Storzer, D. N. (2018). Pulmonary system. In T. M. Hartjes (Ed.), *AACN core curriculum for high acuity, progressive, and critical care nursing* (7th ed.). St. Louis: Elsevier.

Thompson, W. (2016). Noninvasive positive pressure ventilation in acute respiratory failure. *Critical Care Alert, 24*(7), 1–5.

3-8. **(B)** Hepatitis B infections are prevalent in persons of Asian descent. Many individuals are infected at birth and remain unaware of the infection until they develop symptoms. Acute presentation includes jaundice, elevated transaminases, positive HBVsAg, and positive HBV DNA quantitative level of virus. Hepatitis A (Option A) would be the diagnosis if the HAV IgM was positive, and the HAV IgG was negative. This would indicate an acute infection with hepatitis A virus. The positive HAV IgG in this case indicates a past infection with hepatitis A. Hepatitis C infection (Option C) is usually asymptomatic and noted in a laboratory result of HCV Ab (antibody) that is positive. In this case, the antibody result is negative. Hepatitis D (Option D) is associated with hepatitis B but is not reflected in the laboratory results.

References: Radovich, P. (2018). Gastrointestinal System. In T. M. Hartjes (Ed.), *AACN core curriculum for high acuity, progressive, and critical care nursing* (7th ed.). St. Louis: Elsevier.

Jorgensen, C., Chen, S., Carnes, C., & Block, J. (2016). Know hepatitis B: a multilingual communications campaign promoting testing for Hepatitis B among Asian Americans and Pacific islanders. *Public Health Reports,* 13135–13140.

3-9. **(D)** The most reliable evidence of end-organ damage at this time appears to be the presence of LV hypertrophy. Left ventricular hypertrophy pattern on the ECG indicates that myocardial end-organ dysfunction has occurred. Blurred vision may be caused by vitreal hemorrhages or cotton-wool patches common in hypertensive crisis. These are usually reversible when hypertension is controlled. The BUN is normal and does not indicate renal end organ dysfunction. It is anticipated that patients will feel lethargic after blood pressure reduction for hypertensive crisis.

References: Efre, A., & Boling, B. (2018). Cardiovascular system. In T. M. Hartjes (Ed.), *AACN core curriculum for high acuity, progressive, and critical care nursing* (7th ed.). St. Louis: Elsevier.

3-10. **(D)** Contralateral symptoms in the lower extremity usually relate to anterior cerebral artery circulation problems. These findings can occur after aneurysmal subarachnoid hemorrhage, but the clinical signs described are most commonly associated with vasospasm of the right anterior cerebral artery. Hyponatremia (Option A) does occur in this patient population but is not a likely cause of a focal deficit or acute change. Rebleed (Option B) as well as hydrocephalus (Option C) would likely cause deficits of a more global nature.

References: Blissitt, P. A. (2018). Neurologic system. In T. M. Hartjes (Ed.), *AACN core curriculum for high acuity, progressive, and critical care nursing* (7th ed.). St. Louis: Elsevier.

Lin, C., Dumont, A., Zhang, J., Zuccarello, M., & Muroi, C. (2014). Cerebral vasospasm after aneurysmal subarachnoid hemorrhage: mechanism and therapies. *Biomed Research International,* ***Article ID 679014. http://dx.doi.org/2014/679014.

3-11. **(B)** The clinical assessment in the scenario is grade II. Grade I describes an awake and oriented patient with slight lack of awareness. A grade I patient has some mental clouding, subtle changes in intellectual function, restlessness and irritability, euphoria, anxiety, and muscular incoordination. A grade III clinical assessment demonstrates somnolence to semi-stupor. The grade III patient is completely disoriented when aroused, unable to perform computations, lethargic with bizarre behavior, and unable to coordinate neuromuscular function. A grade IV patient is comatose and may demonstrate decerebrate or decorticate response to pain.

> **References:** Radovich, P. (2018). Gastrointestinal system. In T. M. Hartjes (Ed.), *AACN core curriculum for high acuity, progressive, and critical care nursing* (7th ed.). St. Louis: Elsevier.
> Ferri, F. (2017). Hepatic encephalopathy. In F. Ferri (Ed.), *2017 Ferri's clinical advisor: 5 books in 1* (pp. 566–567). Philadelphia: Elsevier.

3-12. **(C)** COPD patients can demonstrate isolated elevations in PA pressures because of compensatory hypoxemic vasoconstriction, which increases pressures in the pulmonary circulation. To diagnose pulmonary hypertension, the mean PAP must be greater than 25 mm Hg at rest. The mean PAP can be calculated as follows: PA systolic + 2(PA diastolic) ÷ 3. Option A shows elevation across all hemodynamic variables, a finding often associated with pericardial tamponade. Option B shows uniformly low hemodynamic pressures, a pattern that may be observed in patients with hypovolemia. Option D shows an isolated elevation in the PAOP, a finding associated with left ventricular failure.

> **Reference:** Storzer, D. N. (2018). Pulmonary System. In T. M. Hartjes (Ed.), *AACN core curriculum for high acuity, progressive, and critical care nursing* (7th ed.). St. Louis: Elsevier.

3-13. **(C)** Early mobilization is critical to prevent delirium; however, there are exclusion criteria for early mobilization. Stable vital signs are required to safely mobilize a patient, but additional requirements are listed in an early mobility safety screening. Exclusion criteria for early mobilization include FiO_2 greater than 0.6, PEEP greater than 10 cm H_2O, SpO_2 less than 88% at rest, vasopressor dose change in the past 2 hours, acute CVA, abnormal ICP, and acute arrhythmia in past 12 hours. In addition, hospitals have institution-specific exclusion criteria for early mobilization.

> **References:** Chapa, D., & Akintade, B. (2018). Psychosocial aspects of critical care. In T. M. Hartjes (Ed.), *AACN core curriculum for high acuity, progressive, and critical care nursing* (7th ed.). St. Louis: Elsevier.
> Bounds, M. (2016). Effect of ABCDE bundle implementation on prevalence of delirium in intensive care unit patients. *American Journal of Critical Care, 25*(6), 535–544. http://dx.doi.org/10.4037/ajcc2016209.

3-14. **(C)** This patient has low levels of ability to participate in care related to her vision impairment. Data support that case management planning and coordination of care has the potential to reduce patient readmission rates. Option A is not correct at this time because all other options should be explored before removing the patient from her home. Option B is incorrect because it does not address the patient's visual problem, although it would have been part of the solution if the patient were lacking understanding of how to administer insulin. Option D is not correct because there is no indication that family members can be relocated to care for the patient at home.

> **References:** Dermenchyan, A. (2018). Professional caring and ethical practice. In T. M. Hartjes (Ed.), *AACN core curriculum for high acuity, progressive, and critical care nursing* (7th ed.). St. Louis: Elsevier.

3-15. **(D)** Identification and treatment of the underlying source of inflammation or infection is the most important element in reducing mortality associated with SIRS/MODS. Medical and surgical interventions to remove sources of infection or contamination may limit the inflammatory response and improve the patient's chances of recovery. Pain and associated anxiety can increase the patient's oxygen consumption, and narcotic pain medications must be used judiciously to prevent further hypotension. Maintenance of tissue oxygenation by focusing on interventions that decrease oxygen demand and increase oxygen delivery will preserve organ function until the underlying problem (infectious process or inflammatory condition) is corrected or resolved. Hypermetabolism in SIRS/MODS results in profound weight loss, cachexia, and loss of organ function. The goal of nutritional and metabolic support is to preserve organ structure and function. Nutrition will prevent generalized nutritional deficiencies and preserve gut integrity.

Reference: Johnson, A. (2018). Multisystem: multiple organ dysfunction syndrome. In T. M. Hartjes (Ed.), *AACN core curriculum for high acuity, progressive, and critical care nursing* (7th ed.). St. Louis: Elsevier.

3-16. **(B)** Surgery represents a major stress to the respiratory system. Although all the selections are potential serious complications of abdominal surgery, pneumonia and pulmonary complications are the most common cause of postoperative morbidity. Changes in pulmonary function occur in the immediate postoperative period, including a reduction in forced vital capacity, lung compliance, and functional residual capacity. Microatelectasis takes place and is the most common cause of postoperative hypoxemia. Pain, splinting, aspiration, obesity, decreased consciousness, somnolence-inducing pain medications, supine positioning, and the patient's comorbidities further complicate pulmonary recovery. Thoracic and abdominal surgery is especially hazardous to patients at risk. Hyperglycemia can be controlled with an insulin infusion. Strict handwashing and antibiotics can help prevent infection. Although perioperative myocardial infarction is a potentially serious complication, the patient is at greatest risk for pulmonary complications.

References: Storzer, D. N. (2018). Pulmonary system. In T. M. Hartjes (Ed.), *AACN core curriculum for high acuity, progressive, and critical care nursing* (7th ed.). St. Louis: Elsevier.

Yang, C., Teng, A., Lee, D., & Rose, K. (2015). Pulmonary complications after major abdominal surgery: National Surgical Quality Improvement Program analysis. *Journal of Surgical Research, 198*(2), 441–449. http://dx.doi.org/10.1016/j.jss.2015.03.028.

3-17. **(A)** When providing care for bariatric patients, the nurse should expect to find a high incidence of low self-esteem and negative body image because of the social stigma of obesity. This population will likely benefit from clear and feasible goals established frequently with considerable amounts of encouragement distributed generously during the postoperative period. Although some bariatric patients may have needs related to dependence versus independence, personal autonomy, and trusting others, these have not been identified in the literature as characteristic of the bariatric patient.

References: Benefield, A. (2018). Critical care patients with special needs: bariatric patients. In T. M. Hartjes (Ed.), *AACN core curriculum for high acuity, progressive, and critical care nursing* (7th ed.). St. Louis: Elsevier.

Yusufov, M., Dairymple, K., & Bernstein, M. (2017). Body mass index, depression, and suicidality: the role of self-esteem in bariatric surgery candidates. *Journal of Affective Disorders, 208,* 238–247.

3-18. **(C)** COPD is characterized by permanent impairment in airflow, so cessation of smoking will not restore "normal lungs" to this patient. Stopping smoking will, however, slow continuing COPD damage to the lungs, reduce the likelihood of exacerbations of COPD, and diminish the patient's risk of developing both lung cancer and coronary heart disease. Smoking cessation is a major component in preventing progression and exacerbation of COPD. Alpha-1–related emphysema is caused by an inherited lack of the protective protein alpha-1 antitrypsin. Cessation of smoking in patients with this disorder accrues comparable benefits as those with emphysema from other causes and, similarly, does not restore normal lungs.

References: Storzer, D. N. (2018). Pulmonary system. In T. M. Hartjes (Ed.), *AACN core curriculum for high acuity, progressive, and critical care nursing* (7th ed.). St. Louis: Elsevier.

Orisasami, I., & Ojo, O. (2016). Evaluating the effectiveness of smoking cessation in the management of COPD. *British Journal of Nursing, 25*(14), 786–791.

3-19. **(B)** Paralytic ileus is the most common cause of intestinal pseudoobstruction. It occurs after abdominal surgery or abdominal trauma. Patients should receive nothing by mouth. If the bowel is distended, initiation of nasogastric suction with low intermittent suctioning is appropriate because bowel distention can result in nausea, vomiting, and an increased risk of aspiration. Hypovolemia occurs secondary to nausea, vomiting, and the NPO status. Sepsis would be associated with a subnormal or elevated temperature. GI hemorrhage would likely present as hematemesis or melena. An SpO_2 of 94% does not indicate impending respiratory failure.

References: Radovich, P. (2018). Gastrointestinal system. In T. M. Hartjes (Ed.), *AACN core curriculum for high acuity, progressive, and critical care nursing* (7th ed.). St. Louis: Elsevier.

Menard-Katcher, P., & Lichtenstein, G. (2014). Ileus. In P. Lanken, S. Manaker, B. Kohl, & C. Hanson (Eds.), *Intensive care unit manual* (pp. 405–409). Philadelphia: Elsevier Saunders.

3-20. **(C)** When contrast dye will be administered, it is recommended that administration of metformin be temporarily halted because it has been associated with nephrotoxicity and lactic acidosis. In patients with renal failure (acute or chronic), the renal clearance of metformin is decreased, and there is an associated risk of lactic acidosis, which has a mortality rate of up to 50%. Some patients who receive intravenous contrast may experience a deterioration of renal function (contrast-induced nephropathy). Clopidogrel must be given to prevent stent restenosis. Enoxaparin and IV pantoprazole are not contraindicated at this time.

References: Boling, B. (2018). Renal system. In T. M. Hartjes (Ed.), *AACN core curriculum for high acuity, progressive, and critical care nursing* (7th ed.). St. Louis: Elsevier.

Baerlocher, M., Asch, M., & Myers, A. (2013). Metformin and intravenous contrast. *CMAJ: Canadian Medical Association Journal, 185*(1), E78. http://dx.doi.org/10.1503/cmaj.090550.

3-21. **(B)** The nurse is demonstrating caring practices with concern over adequacy of comfort measures. One of the main concerns of family members when a patient is at end of life is the comfort of their loved one. Assessing comfort can be challenging in an unresponsive patient. The BIS monitor can assist in the assessment and management of analgesic effectiveness. BIS monitoring provides information about the effects of pain medication and sedation. It involves placing an external sensor on a patient's forehead. No internal wires are required. Option A is incorrect because BIS monitoring does not alarm when the patient is brain dead. Option C is incorrect because BIS monitoring does not measure ICP. Option D is incorrect because BIS monitoring is not used on all comatose patients.

References: Wyckoff, M., Hartjes, T. M. (2018). Critical care patients with special needs: palliative and end-of life care in the ICU. In T. M. Hartjes (Ed.), *AACN core curriculum for high acuity, progressive, and critical care nursing* (7th ed.). St. Louis: Elsevier.

Masman, A., van Dijk, M., van Rosmalen, J., Blussé van Oud-Alblas, H., Ista, E., Baar, F., & Tibboel, D. (2016). Bispectral index monitoring in terminally ill patients: a validation study. *Journal of Pain & Symptom Management, 52*(2), 212–220.e3. http://dx.doi.org/10.1016/j.jpainsymman.2016.01.011.

3-22. **(C)** Reexpansion pulmonary edema is a complication associated with thoracentesis. Reexpansion pulmonary edema can occur when a large amount of effusion fluid (approximately 1000–1500 mL) is removed from the pleural space. Removal of the fluid increases the negative intrapleural pressure, which can lead to edema when the lung does not reexpand to fill the space. The patient experiences severe coughing and shortness of breath. This is an indication to discontinue the thoracentesis.

References: Stacy, K. (2018). Pulmonary diagnostic procedures. In L. Urden, K. Stacy, & M. Lough (Eds.), *Critical care nursing: diagnosis and management* (pp. 507–508). St. Louis, MO: Mosby/Elsevier.

Perricone, G., & Mazzarelli, C. (2014). Images in clinical medicine. Reexpansion pulmonary edema after thoracentesis. *New England Journal of Medicine, 370*(12), e19. http://dx.doi.org/10.1056/NEJMicm1309844.

3-23. **(B)** Several scoring systems and other methods have been developed to help guide clinicians to predict prognosis. The Ranson criteria, which are of historical interest only, have been replaced by APACHE (Acute Physiology and Chronic Health Evaluation) II and by more simplified systems using multiple-factor scoring. Practice guidelines suggest a cutoff of greater than eight APACHE II points as the definition of severe disease. An APACHE-II score of 24 or higher predicts a mortality of at least 80%. A markedly elevated-reactive protein (CRP) can also assist the clinician to predict the severity of the disease. Neither serum amylase nor arterial oxygen is used as a prognostic indicator for pancreatitis. CRP is a highly sensitive but not specific marker for the inflammatory processes associated with acute pancreatitis.

References: Radovich, P. (2018). Gastrointestinal system. In T. M. Hartjes (Ed.), *AACN core curriculum for high acuity, progressive, and critical care nursing* (7th ed.). St. Louis: Elsevier.

Kuo, D., Rider, A., Estrada, P., Kim, D., & Pillow, M. (2015). Acute pancreatitis: What's the score? *Journal of Emergency Medicine (0736-4679), 48*(6), 762–770. http://dx.doi.org/10.1016/j.jemermed.2015.02.018.

3-24. **(C)** Higher levels of PEEP can elevate pulmonary pressures and escalate the risk for additional pneumothorax or air leaks. Prompt ventilator weaning and aggressive pulmonary toilet are essential for reducing the risk of ventilator-associated pneumonia and barotrauma/volutrauma. Adequate pain management enhances the patient's ability to perform coughing, deep breathing, and incentive spirometry.

References: Storzer, D. N. (2018). Pulmonary system. In T. M. Hartjes (Ed.), *AACN core curriculum for high acuity, progressive, and critical care pursing* (7th ed.). St. Louis: Elsevier.

3-25. **(B)** Idiopathic pulmonary fibrosis (IPF) is a progressive disease with median survival from 2 to 7 years. Palliative care is an important part of patient care as lung transplantation is not an option for most patients. The majority of IPF patients die in a hospital with ongoing life-prolonging procedures until death. Studies demonstrate that the frequent use of opioids is an indicator of an intention to relieve symptoms, but end-of-life decisions were still made very late. Early integrated palliative care with advance care plan could improve the end-of-life care for dying IPF patients. Incentive spirometry has not been demonstrated to improve long-term outcomes for idiopathic pulmonary fibrosis. Anxiolytics may be required for patients to cope with the diagnosis but will not affect any long-term improvement for the condition. Prophylactic antibiotics are not required.

References: Wyckoff, M., & Hartjes, T. M. (2018). critical care patients with special needs: palliative and end-of life care in the ICU. In T. M. Hartjes (Ed.), *AACN core curriculum for high acuity, progressive, and critical care nursing* (7th ed.). St. Louis: Elsevier.

Rajala, K., Lehto, J., Saarinen, M., Sutinen, E., Saarto, T., & Myllärniemi, M. (2016). End-of-life care of patients with idiopathic pulmonary fibrosis. *BMC Palliative Care,* ***151–156. http://dx.doi.org/10.1186/s12904-016-0158-81.

3-26. **(A)** Disseminated intravascular coagulation (DIC) is a complex, consumptive coagulopathy that occurs in patients with a variety of disorders. It manifests as an overstimulation of the normal coagulation process and results in microvascular clotting and hemorrhage in organ systems that lead to thrombosis and fibrinolysis. Clotting factor derangements precipitate further inflammation, and thrombosis and microvascular damage leads to additional organ injury. Cell injury and damage to the endothelium activate the intrinsic and extrinsic coagulation pathways. Low platelet counts and elevated D-dimer concentrations and fibrin degradation products are clinical indicators of DIC. A prothrombin time (PT) longer than 12.5 seconds and an activated partial thromboplastin time (aPTT) longer than 40 seconds are also key laboratory findings with DIC.

References: Dressler, D. (2018). Hematological and immunological systems. In T. M. Hartjes (Ed.), *AACN core curriculum for high acuity, progressive, and critical care nursing* (7th ed.). St. Louis: Elsevier.

3-27. **(C)** Systems thinking is the body of knowledge and tools that allow the nurse to manage whatever environmental and system resources that exist for the patient, family, and staff, within or across health care systems and non–health care systems. The patient satisfaction improvement team is utilizing the hospital system to improve the patients' experiences. The unit clinical practice committee uses the information from these surveys and utilizes a variety of resources as necessary to optimize patient outcomes. Assisting patients to complete another survey (Option A) may help to identify unit specific problem areas. However, many patients are still very ill and unable to complete the survey when they are transferred from the unit. In addition, patients may feel pressured to provide positive survey responses in the presence of their caregivers. Patient satisfaction involves the all-inclusive experience with care. Nursing care (Option B) is only one aspect of that experience. Implementing practices identified by the clinical practice committee (Option D) recognizes the patient as isolated in the environment of the unit. Systems thinking recognizes interrelationships that exist within and across both health care and non–health care systems.

References: Dermenchyan, A. (2018). Professional caring and ethical practice. In T. M. Hartjes (Ed.), *AACN core curriculum for high acuity, progressive, and critical care nursing* (7th ed.). St. Louis: Elsevier.

Swickard, S., Swickard, W., Reimer, A., Lindell, D., & Winkelman, C. (2014). Adaptation of the AACN synergy model for patient care to critical care transport. *Critical Care Nurse, 34*(1), 16–29. http://dx.doi.org/10.4037/ccn2014573.

3-28. **(C)** A patient with respiratory failure will demonstrate hypoxia and respiratory acidosis. Hypoxemic respiratory failure is characterized by an arterial oxygen tension (PaO_2) lower than 60 mm Hg with a normal or low arterial carbon dioxide tension ($PaCO_2$). This is the most common form of respiratory failure. Hypercapnic respiratory failure is characterized by a $PaCO_2$ greater than 50 mm Hg. Option A indicates respiratory alkalosis. Option B indicates metabolic acidosis. Option D indicates compensated respiratory acidosis.

References: Storzer, D. N. (2018). Pulmonary system. In T. M. Hartjes (Ed.), *AACN core curriculum for high acuity, progressive, and critical care nursing* (7th ed.). St. Louis: Elsevier.

3-29. **(B)** A pneumonectomy may be followed by a rise in central venous pressure. With the loss of one lung, the right ventricle must empty its stroke volume into a vascular bed that has been reduced by 50%. The workload of the right ventricle increases because of the higher pressure system that has been created. This can precipitate right ventricular failure. Additional preload provided by IV normal saline can then worsen right ventricular failure. Positioning the patient on the operative side (Option A) promotes splinting of the incision and facilitates deep-breathing exercises. The surgeon will usually indicate when free side-to-side turning is safe. Pain can be a major problem after thoracic surgery (Option C). Aggressive pain management is required. Chest tube management (Option D) is important to remove air and fluid postoperatively.

References: Storzer, D. N. (2018). Pulmonary system. In T. M. Hartjes (Ed.), *AACN core curriculum for high acuity, progressive, and critical care nursing* (7th ed.). St. Louis: Elsevier.

Stacy, K. (2018). Pulmonary therapeutic management. In L. Urden, K. Stacy, & M. Lough (Eds.), *Critical care nursing: diagnosis and management*. St. Louis, MO: Mosby/Elsevier.

3-30. **(C)** ITP is a deficiency of platelets with measurable amounts of antiplatelet antibodies resulting in bleeding into the skin and other organs. Acute ITP is generally a disease that affects children, whereas chronic ITP is generally experienced by adolescents and adults. Because of blood loss, replacing circulating blood volume is the primary goal when managing patients with idiopathic thrombocytopenic purpura. Changes in the airway and respiratory function arise only when volume replacement is not adequate and shock occurs. Although coping with the bruises and purpura is a challenge for the patient, this is not a major focus of nursing interventions.

References: Dressler, D. (2018). Hematological and immunological systems. In T. M. Hartjes (Ed.), *AACN core curriculum for high acuity, progressive, and critical care nursing* (7th ed.). St. Louis: Elsevier.

Stacy, K. (2018). Hematologic disorders and oncologic emergencies. In L. Urden, K. Stacy, & M. Lough (Eds.), *Critical care nursing: diagnosis and management*. St. Louis, MO: Mosby/Elsevier.

3-31. **(B)** The hypothalamus is responsible for thermoregulation. Damage to the hypothalamus can lead to hyperthermia after head trauma. The neurologic effects of fever are significant as increased temperature in the postinjury period has been associated with increased local cytokine activity, increased infarct size, and poorer outcomes in the acute phase of injury. Hyperthermia, from fever or other sources, when high enough (higher than 43°C), has been reported to cause neuronal injury in normal brain, and lengthy periods of moderate (40°C) hyperthermia have been reported to alter brain structure and functioning.

References: Blissitt, P.A. (2018). Neurologic system. In T. M. Hartjes (Ed.), *AACN core curriculum for high acuity, progressive, and critical care nursing* (7th ed.). St. Louis: Elsevier.

3-32. **(B)** The patient has pulmonary hemorrhage, which requires a return to the operating room for exploration and definitive treatment. Insertion of a second chest tube would help evacuate the blood, but stopping the hemorrhage is a higher priority than removing the blood from the pleural space and could add more trauma to the area. Dopamine is not needed at this time because this patient requires fluid resuscitation. Using a positive inotropic agent can increase myocardial workload and cause myocardial ischemia in patients with reduced preload. A bronchoscopy will not likely be helpful in identifying the source of this rapid bleeding, as it may exist outside the tracheobronchial tree.

References: Holleran, R. (2018). Multisystem: multisystem trauma. In T. M. Hartjes (Ed.), *AACN core curriculum for high acuity, progressive, and critical care nursing* (7th ed.). St. Louis: Elsevier.

Bouzat, P., Raux, M., David, J. S., Tazarourte, K., Galinski, M., Desmettre, T., & Michelet, P. (2017). Chest trauma: first 48 hours management. *Anaesthesia Critical Care & Pain Medicine*. http://dx.doi.org/10.1016/j.accpm.2017.01.004.

3-33. **(C)** Cerebral arterial vasospasm is the most common cause of neurologic deterioration 4 to 7 days after SAH in both operated and nonoperated patients. It can be definitively diagnosed with either CT or traditional angiography as well as by clinical examination and transcranial Doppler ultrasonography. Nimodipine is the only medication shown to prevent vasospasm and improve patient outcome after aneurysmal SAH. Administration of this calcium channel blocking agent has become a standard practice for vasospasm prevention. Because of the vasodilator effect of nimodipine, BP should be carefully monitored. Triple-H therapy (hypertensive-hypervolemic-hemodilution [HHH]) increases cardiac output and BP with aggressive intravascular volume loading and vasopressor medications. Fluid loading usually leads to hemodilution. Vasoactive drugs are administered to increase BP if intravascular volume expansion alone is inadequate. Filling pressures (CVP or PCWP) are also monitored to guide volume dosing. Fluid restriction (Option B) is contraindicated in this patient population. Lumbar puncture (Option D) is not indicated at this time because cerebral vasospasm is the most likely cause of the patient's symptoms. If the patient had other signs or symptoms of meningitis, then LP would be indicated.

References: Blissitt, P. A. (2018). Neurologic system. In T. M. Hartjes (Ed.), *AACN core curriculum for high acuity, progressive, and critical care nursing* (7th ed.). St. Louis: Elsevier.

Danière, F., Gascou, G., Champfleur, N., Machi, P., Leboucq, N., Riquelme, C., & Costalat, V. (2015). Complications and follow up of subarachnoid hemorrhages. *Diagnostic and Interventional Imaging, 96*(7–8), 677–686. http://dx.doi.org/10.1016/j.diii.2015.05.006.

3-34. **(B)** The process of weaning from mechanical ventilation can be challenging and complex, especially for older patients with numerous chronic comorbidities. Data suggest that improved outcomes can result when collaborative decision-making processes are used (e.g., by ventilator teams who focus on patients such as this who need extra support). Discharge to a long-term care facility may not be appropriate, particularly for a patient with compromised pulmonary status. The patient is not sufficiently strong for discharge home, and no family members are mentioned to provide this care. Although optimizing the patient's nutritional status will surely benefit him, it does not afford a promising avenue for any near-term solution to the weaning problem.

References: Dermenchyan, A. (2018). Professional caring and ethical practice. In T. M. Hartjes (Ed.), *AACN core curriculum for high acuity, progressive, and critical care nursing* (7th ed.). St. Louis: Elsevier.

3-35. **(D)** Clinical inquiry is the ongoing process of questioning and evaluating practice and providing informed practice. Clinical inquiry creates changes through evidence-based practice, research utilization, and experiential knowledge. Options A, B, and C are all appropriate, but change in practice will require evidence-based protocols to be presented to the physicians, respiratory therapists, and nursing management.

References: Dermenchyan, A. (2018). Professional caring and ethical practice. In T. M. Hartjes (Ed.), *AACN core curriculum for high acuity, progressive, and critical care nursing* (7th ed.). St. Louis: Elsevier.

Danckers, M., Grosu, H., Jean, R., Cruz, R., Fidellaga, A., Han, Q., & Khouli, H. (2013). Nurse-driven, protocol-directed weaning from mechanical ventilation improves clinical outcomes and is well accepted by intensive care unit physicians. *Journal of Critical Care, 28*(4), 433–441. http://dx.doi.org/10.1016/j.jcrc.2012.10.012

3-36. **(D)** The patient with DKA is dehydrated and may have lost 5% to 10% of body weight in fluids. Aggressive IV fluid replacement is required to prevent circulatory collapse. Even though the patient's admitting glucose is only 200 mg/dL, the patient is experiencing dehydration and an anion gap leading to a DKA; therefore, administration of NPH insulin will not provide a timely reduction of serum glucose. Absorption of insulin through the subcutaneous route would be impaired because of diminished circulation associated with hypovolemia. Oral fluids should also be discouraged because they are unlikely to be absorbed and may result in nausea and emesis. Delaying treatment for a period of hours as a specimen is obtained and sent to the laboratory and the results reported could have potentially lethal consequences for this patient.

References: MacDermott, J. (2018). Endocrine system. In T. M. Hartjes (Ed.), *AACN core curriculum for high acuity, progressive, and critical care nursing* (7th ed.). St. Louis: Elsevier.

Atkinson, M. (2016). Type 1 diabetes mellitus. In S. Melmed, K. Polonsky, P. Larsen & H. Kronenberg (Eds.), *Williams textbook of endocrinology* (13th ed.). (pp. 1451–1483). Philadelphia: Elsevier Saunders.

3-37. **(C)** After a patient has died, Orthodox Jewish tradition directs that burial happen within 24 hours and that there be no autopsy (unless it is mandated by the medical examiner). The family may request that a family member or representative constantly accompany (watch over and guard) the body until he or she is buried. This is the ritual of "Shemira."

References: Dermenchyan, A. (2018). Professional caring and ethical practice. In T. M. Hartjes (Ed.), *AACN core curriculum for high acuity, progressive, and critical care nursing* (7th ed.). St. Louis: Elsevier.

Gabbay, E., McCarthy, M., & Fins, J. (2017). The care of the ultra-orthodox Jewish patient. *Journal of Religion & Health, 56*(2), 545–560. http://dx.doi.org/10.1007/s10943-017-0356-6.

3-38. **(D)** Terminal sedation is an option to treat otherwise intractable symptoms in patients imminently dying. Terminal sedation is an option for easing suffering in a terminally ill patient whose suffering is overwhelming. Although consulting palliative care is an option (Option C), the patient will continue to suffer until palliative care can see the patient and intervene. Option A and B are incorrect as laws state that the physician has not committed assisted suicide or homicide if the pain medications were ordered to relieve pain and suffering during palliative care.

References: Wyckoff, M., & Hartjes, T. M. (2018). Critical care patients with special needs: palliative and end-of life care in the ICU. In T. M. Hartjes (Ed.), *AACN core curriculum for high acuity, progressive, and critical care nursing* (7th ed.). St. Louis: Elsevier.

Ho, A., & Tsai, D. (2016). Making good death more accessible: end-of-life care in the intensive care unit. *Intensive Care Medicine, 42*(8), 1258–1260. http://dx.doi.org/10.1007/s00134-016-4396-2.

3-39. **(D)** Patients with the best outcome after a traumatic arrest are those who are promptly transported to a trauma care facility where appropriate interventions can be initiated. The focus of prehospital and hospital resuscitation should be to safely extricate and stabilize the patient and to minimize interventions that will delay transport to definitive care at a trauma center. The primary and secondary surveys, including exposure of the patient to determine the extent of injury, are performed within minutes of the patient arriving at the tertiary care facility. Aggressive fluid resuscitation is now recommended only for patients with isolated head or extremity trauma, either blunt or penetrating. It is not recommended for penetrating trauma, especially in the urban setting, because it is likely to increase blood pressure and accelerate the rate of blood loss.

References: Holleran, S. (2018). Critical care patients with special needs: patient transport. In T. M. Hartjes (Ed.), *AACN core curriculum for high acuity, progressive, and critical care nursing* (7th ed.). St. Louis: Elsevier.

Holleran, R. (2018). Multisystem: multisystem trauma. In T. M. Hartjes (Ed.), *AACN core curriculum for high acuity, progressive, and critical care nursing* (7th ed.). St. Louis: Elsevier.

3-40. **(A)** In the setting of noncardiac surgery, the diagnosis of myocardial infarction (MI) is confirmed with an elevated cardiac biomarker (usually troponin). Troponins are specific to cardiac tissue and are not affected by skeletal muscle injury. Creatinine kinase is found in skeletal muscle and is therefore a nonspecific indicator of MI in the surgical patient. C-reactive protein is synthesized in the liver in response to inflammation and is used to determine risk of cardiovascular disease. C-reactive protein levels less than 1.0 mg/L indicate a patient has a low risk of developing cardiovascular disease, whereas a level higher than 3.0 mg/L identifies a patient at high risk of cardiovascular disease. Myoglobin levels increase in skeletal muscle injury and are therefore unreliable indicators of myocardial infarction in the surgical patient.

References: Efre, A., & Boling, B. (2018). Cardiovascular system. In T. M. Hartjes (Ed.), *AACN core curriculum for high acuity, progressive, and critical care nursing* (7th ed.). St. Louis: Elsevier.

Devereaux, P. (2016). Perioperative myocardial infarction after noncardiac surgery. Available from http://www.uptodate.com/home.

3-41. **(B)** Critical care nurses who provide care for persons with HIV/AIDS face many complexities related to the administration of antiretrovirals. Potential interactions between antiretroviral drugs and commonly administered ICU medications—including antiarrhythmics, benzodiazepines, H2 antagonists, proton pump inhibitors, and anticoagulants—must be considered in planning nursing care. Many antiretroviral therapies are not available in intravenous form (Option C). Some medications, when given enterally, may be inadequately absorbed, especially when administered with H2 receptor antagonists (Option A). This may lead to drug resistance. ICU nurses must also observe for serious toxic reactions to the agents prescribed, such as hypersensitivity or pancreatitis. Option D does not exhibit sensitivity to the patient's concerns. Antiretroviral therapy has resulted in rare but potentially life-threatening toxic effects, such as hypersensitivity reactions, pancreatitis, and lactic acidosis, but these conditions are not related to the onset of critical illness but rather to the medications themselves.

References: Dressler, D. (2018). Hematological and immunological systems. In T. M. Hartjes (Ed.), *AACN core curriculum for high acuity, progressive, and critical care nursing* (7th ed.). St. Louis: Elsevier.

DeFreitas, A., D'Souza, T. Lazaro, G., Windes, E., Johnson, M., & Relf, M. (2013). Pharmacological considerations in human immunodeficiency virus-infected adults in the intensive care unit. *Critical Care Nurse, 33*(2), 46–57. http://dx.doi.org/10.4037/ccn2013854.

3-42. **(C)** Evidence-based practice provides nurses with a method to use critically appraised and scientifically proven evidence for delivering quality health care to a specific population. If clinical studies support best patient outcomes with early mobility, discussing the concerns with the surgeon (Option A) will not be helpful for best patient outcomes. Documentation of patient's pain experience upon increased mobility (Option B) does not improve patient outcomes because pain is an expected experience after cardiac surgery. Evidence-based practice protocols provide guidance for patient care so the clinician does not have to "judge" what would be best for the patient (Option D).

References: Dermenchyan, A. (2018). Professional caring and ethical practice. In T. M. Hartjes (Ed.), *AACN core curriculum for high acuity, progressive, and critical care nursing* (7th ed.). St. Louis: Elsevier.

3-43. **(C)** There are many approaches to problem solving, depending on the nature of the problem and the people involved, but most approaches involve clarifying the nature and extent of the problem, analyzing causes, identifying alternatives, assessing each alternative, choosing one, implementing it, and evaluating whether the problem was solved. The most effective approach to defuse this situation is to begin problem identification by asking the surgeon to explain what happened and describe the reason(s) underlying his comments. This fact finding will help to isolate the problem(s) and lend clarity to determining its possible causes and appropriate solutions. Option A delays dealing with the physician's concerns and defers problem solving to the nurse manager. Option B is inappropriate because there is no basis currently established to question the efficacy of existing unit standards. Option D applies an instructional solution to a problem yet to be identified.

References: Dermenchyan, A. (2018). Professional caring and ethical practice. In T. M. Hartjes (Ed.), *AACN core curriculum for high acuity, progressive, and critical care nursing* (7th ed.). St. Louis: Elsevier.

3-44. **(B)** Maintaining activity levels is a key component of pulmonary rehabilitation because it prevents many of the physical and psychological complications common to patients with COPD. Bronchitis exacerbations may be associated with many environmental factors, only one of which is increased physical activity. Supplemental oxygen and bronchodilators are interventions that may make resumption of physical activity easier for the patient and should be considered, but only if indicated.

References: Storzer, D. N. (2018). Pulmonary system. In T. M. Hartjes (Ed.), *AACN core curriculum for high acuity, progressive, and critical care nursing* (7th ed.). St. Louis: Elsevier.

Spruit, M., Pitta, F., McAuley, E., ZuWallack, R., & Nici, L. (2015). Pulmonary rehabilitation and physical activity in patients with chronic obstructive pulmonary disease. *American Journal of Respiratory & Critical Care Medicine, 192*(8), 924–933. http://dx.doi.org/10.1164/rccm.201505-0929CI.

3-45. **(D)** Ventricular dyssynchrony can impair ventricular pump function. Cardiac resynchronization therapy (CRT) involves simultaneous pacing of both ventricles (biventricular or BiV pacing) or of one ventricle in patients with bundle branch block to reduce dyssynchrony. Resynchronization

may improve pump performance, reduce functional mitral regurgitation, and reverse the deleterious process of ventricular remodeling in patients with heart failure and systolic dysfunction. CRT is not beneficial and can cause harm in patients with heart failure (HF) and a QRS duration less than 120 ms.

References: Efre, A., Boling, B. (2018). Cardiovascular system. In T. M. Hartjes (Ed.), *AACN core curriculum for high acuity, progressive, and critical care nursing* (7th ed.). St. Louis: Elsevier.

Chinitz, J., d'Avila, A., Goldman, M., Reddy, V., & Dukkipati, S. (2014). Cardiac resynchronization therapy: who benefits? *Annals of Global Health, 80*(1), 61–68. http://dx.doi.org/10.1016/j.aogh.2013.12.003.

3-46. **(A)** Studies have demonstrated that massage, music therapy, and therapeutic touch promotes relaxation and comfort in critically ill patients. Environmental interventions are safe and logical interventions to use to help patients sleep. Options B and C are not recommended for sleep promotion in critically ill patients because the safety data related to aromatherapy and alternative sedatives (e.g., valerian, melatonin) are unclear. Progressive muscle relaxation has been extensively studied and shown to be effective in enhancing sleep in persons with insomnia, but it requires that patients consciously relax specific muscle groups and practice these techniques. This may be challenging for many critically ill patients and impossible for others.

References: Chapa, D., Akintade, B. (2018). Psychosocial aspects of critical care. In T. M. Hartjes (Ed.), *AACN core curriculum for high acuity, progressive, and critical care nursing* (7th ed.). St. Louis: Elsevier.

Hu, R., Jiang, X., Chen, J., Zeng, Z., Chen, X. Y., & Li, Y. (2015). Nonpharmacological interventions for sleep promotion in the intensive care unit. *Protocols Cochrane Database of Systematic Reviews.* http://dx.doi.org/10.1002/14651858.cd008808.

3-47. **(A)** The critical care nurse should provide activities that can support a sense of normalcy to the individual and their loved ones within a setting that they are often unfamiliar. The patient will benefit from being involved in performing his or her

ADLs. Research has shown that music can be beneficial for patients with dementia and can trigger memories of the past (Option B). Puzzles, games, and cards can make the patient feel more involved through offering mind-stimulating activities (Option C). Sleep deprivation in the ICU can cause delirium and worsened dementia (Option D).

References: Chapa, D., Akintade, B. (2018). Psychosocial aspects of critical care. In T. M. Hartjes (Ed.), *AACN core curriculum for high acuity, progressive, and critical care nursing* (7th ed.). St. Louis: Elsevier.

Volland, J., Fisher, A., & Drexler, D. (2015). Delirium and dementia in the intensive care unit. *Dimensions of Critical Care Nursing, 34*(5), 259–264. http://dx.doi.org/10.1097/DCC.00000 00000000133.

3-48. **(D)** Selective serotonin reuptake inhibitors (SSRIs) are frequently prescribed to elderly patients for depression. Gastrointestinal bleeding has been described in patients taking these medications and may result in hospitalization. This risk is significantly elevated when SSRI medications are used in combination with NSAIDS. The patient's hemoglobin and hematocrit values will afford a good initial estimate of possible bleeding. Because the patient is taking digoxin, the heart rate may not increase as a compensatory response to the bleeding. Signs of increased intracranial pressure include a widening pulse pressure and bradycardia. The patient's pulse pressure is not widened, and the bradycardia is more likely attributable to taking digoxin. Because the bradycardia is medication induced, it does not require intervention. Although the patient's diet and nutritional support may need attention at some point, this is not currently a pressing need.

References: Radovich, P. (2018). Gastrointestinal system. In T. M. Hartjes (Ed.), *AACN core curriculum for high acuity, progressive, and critical care nursing* (7th ed.). St. Louis: Elsevier.

Anglin, R., Yuan, Y., Moayyedi, P., Tse, F., Armstrong, D., & Leontiadis, G. (2014). Risk of upper gastrointestinal bleeding with selective serotonin reuptake inhibitors with or without concurrent nonsteroidal antiinflammatory use: a systematic review and meta-analysis. *Am J Gastroenterol, 109*(6), 811–819. http://dx.doi.org/10.1038/ajg.2014.82.

3-49. **(C)** Both the tricuspid and pulmonary valves are right heart structures. Septic emboli released from diseased valves would lodge in the pulmonary tree and cause ventilation/perfusion mismatch and potentially prevent adequate oxygenation. Endocarditis associated with right heart valves is frequently associated with intravenous drug abuse, but this patient is at low risk for seizures because of administration of lorazepam. Antibiotic therapy reduces the risk of septicemia. Stroke would be a potential complication of endocarditis affecting left heart valves.

References: Lough, M. (2018). Cardiovascular disorders. In L. Urden, K. Stacy, & M. Lough (Eds.), *Critical care nursing: diagnosis and management* St. Louis, MO: Mosby/Elsevier.

Swaminath, D., Yaqub, Y., Narayanan, R., Paone, R., Nugent, K., & Arvandi, A. (2013). Isolated pulmonary valve endocarditis complicated with septic emboli to the lung causing pneumothorax, pneumonia, and sepsis in an intravenous drug abuser. *Journal of Investigative Medicine High Impact Case Reports, 1*(4). http://dx.doi.org/10.1177/2324709613514566.

3-50. **(C)** There are many barriers to compliance with a medical regimen. These barriers are personal and specific to each patient. The critical care nurse is responsible for working on another's behalf and representing the concerns of the patient and family. The nurse should not assume that financial concerns or age are barriers specific to this patient (Option B and D). Compliance suggests unintentional act of subjection to authority. Engaging in an open discussion about barriers to adherence will facilitate learning and demonstrate a nonjudgmental approach to changing the patient's behavior. Education about the possible effects of nonadherence can be part of the discussion. However, it should be presented in a less threatening manner (Option A).

References: Dermenchyan, A. (2018). Professional caring and ethical practice. In T. M. Hartjes (Ed.), *AACN core curriculum for high acuity, progressive, and critical care nursing* (7th ed.). St. Louis: Elsevier.

Brown, M., Bussell, J., Dutta, S., Davis, K., Strong, S., & Mathew, S. (2016). Medication adherence: Truth and consequences. *The American Journal of the Medical Sciences, 351*(4), 387–399. http://dx.doi.org/10.1016/j.amjms.2016.01.010.

3-51. **(C)** The patient is exhibiting signs of meningitis, which include headache, chills, fever, nausea, vomiting, photophobia, back pain, and generalized seizures. Signs of meningeal irritation may include stiff neck (nuchal rigidity), Brudzinski sign (adduction/flexion of legs as examiner flexes neck), and Kernig sign (after examiner adducts thigh against abdomen, examiner's attempts to extend the leg are met with resistance). Common CSF findings in meningitis include high protein, low glucose, and an elevated white blood cell count. Bacterial meningitis is most commonly caused by *Staphylococcus* and is most appropriately treated with antibiotics. Meningitis is diagnosed with lumbar puncture for CSF evaluation after head CT scan is obtained. CT is the preferred scan in this population, and MRI (Option A) to rule out any intracranial pathology such as a mass lesion (e.g., brain tumor) is not indicated. Plasmapheresis (Option B) is indicated for patients with Guillain-Barré syndrome when IV immune globulin (IVIG) is not used. It is generally used every other day for 10 to 15 days and works by removing detrimental immune factors. There is no basis for serial LPs (Option D) in this scenario. Typically, CSF findings for patients with meningitis include elevated protein and low glucose. Another population with clinical findings of meningeal irritation is patients who have had a subarachnoid hemorrhage (SAH). LP is typically done only if SAH is suspected but head CT is negative. LP in SAH commonly includes elevated cell count (particularly RBCs) and xanthochromia but neither elevated protein nor low glucose.

References: Blissitt, P. A. (2018). Neurologic system. In T. M. Hartjes (Ed.), *AACN core curriculum for high acuity, progressive, and critical care nursing* (7th ed.). St. Louis: Elsevier.

3-52. **(D)** Normal cardiac output is 4 to 8 L/min but is dependent on multiple factors such as stroke volume and heart rate. The normal mixed venous oxygen saturation (SVO$_2$) is 60% to 80%. Decreased SVO$_2$ indicates hypovolemia, decreased hemoglobin, or increased oxygen consumption by the tissues. Normal systemic vascular resistance (SVR) is 800 to 1200 dynes/sec/cm^{-5}. Increased SVR indicates that peripheral vasoconstriction is occurring to support cardiac output, an indication that fluid resuscitation is not adequate. Increased SVR indicates the patient needs more volume to maintain cardiac output.

References: Efre, A., Boling, B. (2018). Cardiovascular system. In T. M. Hartjes (Ed.), *AACN core curriculum for high acuity, progressive, and critical care nursing* (7th ed.). St. Louis: Elsevier.

Stacy, K. (2018). Shock, sepsis, and multiple organ dysfunction syndrome. In L. Urden, K. Stacy, & M. Lough (Eds.), *Critical care nursing: diagnosis and management*. St. Louis, MO: Mosby/Elsevier.

3-53. **(B)** Tachyphylaxis is a rapidly diminishing response to successive doses of a drug. It is a common issue that arises with vasopressor use. The responsiveness to these drugs can decrease over time, and doses must be constantly titrated to adjust for this phenomenon and for changes in the patient's clinical condition.

References: Use of vasopressors and inotropes. (2016). Available from http://www.uptodate.com/contents/use-of-vasopressors-and-inotropes.

Bangash, M., Kong, M., & Pearse, R. (2012). Use of inotropes and vasopressor agents in critically ill patients. *British Journal of Pharmacology, 165*(7), 2015–2033. http://dx.doi.org/10.1111/j.1476-5381.2011.01588.x.

3-54. **(C)** In acute respiratory failure, the oxygen content in the blood (available for tissue use) is reduced to a level at which the possibility of end-organ dysfunction increases markedly. Acute respiratory failure is defined by a PaO$_2$ lower than 55 mm Hg or a PaCO$_2$ higher than 50 mm Hg. The additional finding of respiratory acidosis indicates an acute respiratory condition. Patients with chronic respiratory conditions may compensate for their chronically low PaO$_2$ or elevated PaCO$_2$ with a pH greater than 7.45. These patients may benefit from low-flow oxygen or noninvasive modes of ventilation. Metabolic acidosis is indicated by a low pH and low PaCO$_2$.

References: Storzer, D. N. (2018). Pulmonary system. In T. M. Hartjes (Ed.), *AACN core curriculum for high acuity, progressive, and critical care nursing* (7th ed.). St. Louis: Elsevier.

Larkin, B., & Zimmanck, R. (2015). Interpreting arterial blood gases successfully. *AORN Journal, 102*(4), 343–357. http://dx.doi.org/10.1016/j.aorn. 2015.08.002.

3-55. **(C)** When administered within 2 weeks of exposure, immunoglobulin will help provide antibodies to prevent active hepatitis B infection. Acetaminophen administration will stress the liver and, in large enough quantities, can produce chemical hepatitis or liver failure. IV penicillin is used to treat syphilis exposure. Transfusions would not be useful, as the infected person would not acquire immunity, and transfusion would subject the recipient to unnecessary risks, including contracting viruses, circulatory overload, or even hemolytic reactions related to clerical and patient identity errors.

References: Radovich, P. (2018). Gastrointestinal system. In T. M. Hartjes (Ed.), *AACN core curriculum for high acuity, progressive, and critical care nursing* (7th ed.). St. Louis: Elsevier.

3-56. **(B)** CT scan of the head is useful for looking at bone and blood and is the best imaging study to view most intracranial processes, including trauma, intracerebral hemorrhage, and hydrocephalus. MRI (Option A) is useful for evaluating tumors, spinal pathology, spinal cord injury, and other processes. It is most helpful for looking at tissue, structures, and perfusion. MRI is not the first imaging tool in suspected abusive head trauma because it has lower sensitivity for acute hemorrhage than CT and is more difficult to perform because of the length of the procedure, sensitivity to patient motion, and need for sedation and compatible monitoring equipment. However, MRI may be used after the acute period after TBI has passed, when it can help identify injuries such as diffuse axonal injury and shearing injuries. An LP (Option C) is contraindicated until intracranial pathology has been ruled out and is not useful in the initial evaluation of TBI. An LP assists in detection of infection or increased ICP. Cerebral angiography (Option D) is valuable for evaluating and managing cerebral aneurysms, arteriovenous malformations, and cerebral vasospasm. Angiography may also be used to identify carotid artery dissection in some traumatic cases.

References: Blissitt, P.A. (2018). Neurologic system. In T. M. Hartjes (Ed.), *AACN core curriculum for high acuity, progressive, and critical care nursing* (7th ed.). St. Louis: Elsevier.

3-57. **(D)** Reviewing relevant research findings related to the nature and scope of support that family members of ICU patients need can afford a sound and evidence-based approach to identifying family-friendly and visitor-friendly features that should be incorporated into waiting areas. The nurse member of the design team can provide valuable input by gathering, compiling, and summarizing the findings of this research. Facilitating visitor comfort can then operate in conjunction with open visitation policies to provide additional elements in the patient support system. Summarizing these findings is well within the capability of a single nurse, so involvement of the nurse manager or another group of nurses is not necessary. Waiting until the next meeting to mention these concerns unnecessarily delays addressing the problem.

References: Dermenchyan, A. (2018). Professional caring and ethical practice. In T. M. Hartjes (Ed.), *AACN core curriculum for high acuity, progressive, and critical care nursing* (7th ed.). St. Louis: Elsevier.

Bjuresäter, K., & Athlin, E. (2016). Improvement of nursing care by means of the evidence based practice process: the facilitator role. *JNEP Journal of Nursing Education and Practice, 6*(11),61–72. http://dx.doi.org/10.5430/jnep.v6n11p61.

3-58. **(B)** The critical care nurse must facilitate learning using clinical inquiry and evidence-based research. Research shows that beta blockers are not associated with a substantial increase in the incidence of sexual dysfunction. Many patients are noncompliant with their blood pressure medications because of the fear of sexual dysfunction. Patients who experience sexual dysfunction with chronic disease may be able to use Viagra, but that must be determined on a case-by-case basis by the patient's physician. The patient should be encouraged never to stop taking his medications unless advised by the physician.

References: Efre, A., Boling, B. (2018). Cardiovascular system. In T. M. Hartjes (Ed.), *AACN core curriculum for high acuity, progressive, and critical care nursing* (7th ed.). St. Louis: Elsevier.

Aggarwal, V., Shore, S., Galindo, R., & Zolty, R. (2012). Incidence of depression, chronic fatigue and sexual dysfunction with beta-blocker use: a meta-analysis of randomized control trials. *Journal of the American College of Cardiology,* *59*(13)***. http://dx.doi.org/10.1016/s0735-109 7(1261462-4).

3-59. **(C)** The patient is currently on hemodialysis, and it would be continued. Hemodialysis is the most effective of all of the renal replacement therapies and is considered the "gold standard" for the treatment of acute and chronic renal failure. Hemodialysis is contraindicated in patients with hemodynamic instability, hypovolemia, coagulation disorders, or vascular access problems. Slow continuous ultrafiltration is used for patients with fluid volume excess and some degree of renal function. It has minimal effect on urea and creatinine levels. Continuous venovenous hemodialysis is used for patients who are hemodynamically unstable and unable to tolerate the rapid fluid and electrolyte shifts that occur with hemodialysis. Peritoneal dialysis is slower and less effective than hemodialysis.

References: Boling, B. (2018). Renal system. In T. M. Hartjes (Ed.), *AACN core curriculum for high acuity, progressive, and critical care nursing* (7th ed.). St. Louis: Elsevier.

3-60. **(D)** Malnutrition affects wound healing, especially protein malnutrition. Patients who follow a low-carbohydrate diet have adequate protein for healing. Diabetes affects wound healing; however, many people follow low-carbohydrate diets for health reasons and not diabetes. Smoking affects oxygen delivery to the wound and causes vasoconstriction. Chronic venous insufficiency affects blood circulation to the wound area. Sickle cell disease represents another form of local tissue ischemia at the specific location of the wound. It is also obstructive in nature, similar to chronic peripheral artery disease, but is caused by dysmorphic red blood cells physically occluding small vessels, usually of the lower extremities.

References: Urden, L. (2018). The older adult patient. In L. Urden, K. Stacy, & M. Lough (Eds.), *Critical care nursing: diagnosis and management.* St. Louis, MO: Mosby/Elsevier.

Wound healing and risk factors for non-healing. (2016). Available from http://www.uptodate.co m/contents/wound-healing-and-risk-factors-for-non-healing.

3-61. **(A)** ST and T-wave changes indicate myocardial ischemia. ST and T-wave changes occur in dilated, restrictive, and hypertrophic cardiomyopathies that affect the left ventricle and are associated with inadequate coronary filling during diastole, resulting in ischemia. Arrhythmogenic right ventricular cardiomyopathy causes right ventricular dilation and signs of right ventricular failure and is associated with right bundle branch block and ventricular tachycardia. Bundle branch blocks are associated with QRS, ST, and T-wave abnormalities that reflect altered conduction rather than ischemia. ST segment elevation in the precordial leads occurs in pericarditis but does not reflect the severity of this disorder.

References: Efre, A., & Boling, B. (2018). Cardiovascular system. In T. M. Hartjes (Ed.), *AACN core curriculum for high acuity, progressive, and critical care nursing* (7th ed.). St. Louis: Elsevier.

Lough, M. (2018). Cardiovascular disorders. In L. Urden, K. Stacy, & M. Lough (Eds.), *Critical care nursing: diagnosis and management.* St. Louis, MO: Mosby/Elsevier.

3-62. **(A)** The focus should be on restoring circulating volume and preventing the complications of hypovolemia. Signs and symptoms of early hypovolemic shock include diminished level of consciousness, which can manifest as agitation or restlessness; cool, clammy skin; tachycardia; and vasoconstriction. The patient is having an acute deterioration in his cardiovascular status. After fluid resuscitation is instituted, the nurse can complete the abdominal assessment. Although the patient's fever may be contributing to his tachycardia and vasodilation, it is not the cause of this acute change and so is of lesser importance now. Initiation of fluid resuscitation should be the first intervention with cultures and cooling measures following. It is important to identify the patient's current medications; however, this can be delegated to another member of the nursing staff until cardiovascular stabilization is achieved.

References: Efre, A., & Boling, B. (2018). Cardiovascular system. In T. M. Hartjes (Ed.), *AACN core curriculum for high acuity, progressive, and critical care nursing* (7th ed.). St. Louis: Elsevier.

3-63. **(C)** The clinical scenario describes pneumococcal pneumonia. Pleuritic chest pain is a common occurrence with pneumococcal pneumonia and needs to be treated to improve the patient's ventilation. Pleural effusions, pneumothoraces, and pulmonary edema are not consistent with the patient's clinical presentation (Options A, B, and D).

References: Storzer, D. N. (2018). Pulmonary system. In T. M. Hartjes (Ed.), *AACN core curriculum for high acuity, progressive, and critical care nursing* (7th ed.). St. Louis: Elsevier.

3-64. **(A)** Rebound pulmonary hypertension may occur when nitric oxide is discontinued. Patients on nitric oxide may develop methemoglobinemia, which prevents release of oxygen to tissues, falsely elevating SpO_2 and thus making SpO_2 an unreliable indicator of oxygenation status. Although hypotension is common with the administration of nitric oxide (because it causes vasodilation), it can be readily treated with vasopressors or by titration of nitric oxide delivery rates and so is not a major concern. Nitric oxide may cause coagulation defects, including thrombocytopenia and bleeding disorders.

References: Storzer, D. N. (2018). Pulmonary system. In T. M. Hartjes (Ed.), *AACN core curriculum for high acuity, progressive, and critical care nursing* (7th ed.). St. Louis: Elsevier.

Hill, N., Preston, I., & Roberts, K. (2015). Inhaled therapies for pulmonary hypertension…includes discussion by Willson, Hill, MacIntyre, Berlinski, DiBlasi, Restrepo, Hess. *Respiratory Care, 60*(6), 794–805. http://dx.doi.org/10.4187/respcare.03927.

3-65. **(A)** Four conditions of negligence must be present for nurses to be judged guilty of malpractice: (1) the nurse owes the patient a duty, (2) the nurse has breached that duty or standard of care, (3) harm or damage has resulted and can be linked to the duty owed, and (4) the breached duty is the proximate cause of the harm or damage. This scenario contains all the elements of malpractice. In this scenario, the nurse owed the patient a duty to verify the placement of the feeding tube based on the AACN standard of care for verification of feeding tube placement in adults. The nurse breached the duty when the tube was not verified before use. The harm was the aspiration caused by misplacement of the tube. The cause of the harm (aspiration and eventual death) was

caused by the breach of duty. Malpractice includes Options B, C, and D, which are included in the scenario.

References: Dermenchyan, A. (2018). Professional caring and ethical practice. In T. M. Hartjes (Ed.), *AACN core curriculum for high acuity, progressive, and critical care nursing* (7th ed.). St. Louis: Elsevier.

Watson, E. (2014). Nursing malpractice: costs, trends, and issues. *Journal of Legal Nurse Consulting, 25*(1), 26–31.

3-66. **(A)** The approach that will best serve this patient's needs is for the ICU team to collaborate with the perinatal team, with the perinatal CNS serving as the initial bridge between those patient care areas by providing immediate support in establishing priorities of care, particularly for aspects of maternal and fetal monitoring unfamiliar to the ICU nurse. After the basic plan of care is developed and procedures are reviewed, the perinatal team may continue their consulting involvement less directly on a more as-needed basis. Collaboration between perinatal and ICU teams in caring for critically ill pregnant women works best to promote the best possible outcomes for mothers and babies. Option B is not optimal because the ICU nurse likely does not have competency to initiate and manage fetal heart monitoring without more direct assistance and needs to know much more about this patient's care than just fetal monitoring. Although both ED nurses and neurosurgical CNSs could lend some support to the ICU nurse, neither has the unique expertise and skills required for optimal care of this patient that the prenatal CNS has.

References: Dermenchyan, A. (2018). Professional caring and ethical practice. In T. M. Hartjes (Ed.), *AACN core curriculum for high acuity, progressive, and critical care nursing* (7th ed.). St. Louis: Elsevier.

Houston, J. F. (2018). Critical care patients with special needs: high-risk obstetric patients. In T. M. Hartjes (Ed.), *AACN core curriculum for high acuity, progressive, and critical care nursing* (7th ed.). St. Louis: Elsevier.

3-67. **(D)** Losing a loved one in the ICU is a stressful experience for the family and friends of the patient. Nursing care has a profound effect on families' memories of the end-of-life care provided to their loved one who is dying. Communication is shown to be the factor that most influences the families' perceptions of the end-of-life care provided for their loved one. Options A, B, and C are all important aspects of end-of-life care. However, many institutions have barriers to executing these options. Follow-up meetings after the patient dies are not available in many institutions. Most ICU designs make it difficult to foster privacy and proximity for the family. Also, family presence during all procedures and care can be difficult to achieve if the policy and culture of the unit do not support unlimited family presence. When good communication across the ICU staff is a reality and when family members are involved in end-of-life conversations and communication, decisions to limit medical care can be made in a timely manner. Thus, the dying patient's suffering is not prolonged.

References: Wyckoff, M., & Hartjes, T. M. (2018). Critical care patients with special needs: palliative and end-of life care in the ICU. In T. M. Hartjes (Ed.), *AACN core curriculum for high acuity, progressive, and critical care nursing* (7th ed.). St. Louis: Elsevier.

Fridh, I. (2014). Caring for the dying patient in the ICU—the past, the present and the future. *Intensive & Critical Care Nursing, 30*(6), 306–311. http://dx.doi.org/10.1016/j.iccn.2014.07.004.

3-68. **(C)** Nurses are accountable and responsible for the assignment or delegation of nursing activities. Nurses may not delegate responsibilities such as assessment and evaluation. Nurses must not knowingly assign or delegate to any member of the nursing team a task for which they are not qualified. A patient assessment should not be delegated to an unlicensed technician. In addition, the patient requires specialty assessment skills because of the support technology (ventricular support devices).

References: Dermenchyan, A. (2018). Professional caring and ethical practice. In T. M. Hartjes (Ed.), *AACN core curriculum for high acuity, progressive, and critical care nursing* (7th ed.). St. Louis: Elsevier.

3-69. **(C)** The behavior described in the visitors' complaints is a comfort gesture between two people. Although some visitors may not personally like the gesture, there is nothing inherent in the behavior that warrants convening a team conference or moving the patient to a different cubicle. Option B puts visitors' needs and preferences before those of a patient and does not support caring practices (i.e., creating a compassionate and therapeutic environment) toward that patient.

References: Dermenchyan, A. (2018). Professional caring and ethical practice. In T. M. Hartjes (Ed.), *AACN core curriculum for high acuity, progressive, and critical care nursing* (7th ed.). St. Louis: Elsevier.

3-70. **(B)** In order to determine whether this patient is experiencing acute rejection, preparation for liver biopsy is essential, as this provides definitive diagnosis of rejection. Later during treatment, should rejection be ruled out, magnetic resonance imaging or a CT scan may be employed in an effort to detect lesions. Cardiovascular instability unresponsive to less invasive treatment is not mentioned, so neither a central nor a PA line requires insertion at this point. Abdominal girth measurement should have been performed with the admission assessment. There is no indication that this patient has ascites or other basis for intraabdominal pressure monitoring.

References: Lough, M. (2018). Organ donation and transplantation. In L. Urden, K. Stacy, & M. Lough (Eds.), *Critical care nursing: diagnosis and management.* St. Louis, MO: Mosby/Elsevier.

3-71. **(C)** Short-term noninvasive positive-pressure ventilation (NIPPV) can help to relieve the patient's suffering as his palliative medications are adjusted. The nurse acts as the patient advocate by suggesting short-term use of NIPPV to palliate severe refractory dyspnea in an actively dying patient who was not responding well to usual palliative treatments with opioids and benzodiazepines. In this case, the patient was physiologically tolerant to the usual symptomatic treatments and was having a crescendo of symptoms that were not responding to a rapid escalation in dosage. The nurse is responsible for promoting comfort and preventing unnecessary suffering. Short-term intubation will prolong the suffering by providing life support to a patient with a terminal illness. High-dose IV propofol will cause respiratory suppression and could be considered a form of euthanasia. Encouraging the patient to withdraw the DNR will prolong the suffering of both the patient and the family because of the terminal nature of his illness.

References: Dermenchyan, A. (2018). Professional caring and ethical practice. In T. M. Hartjes (Ed.), *AACN core curriculum for high acuity, progressive, and critical care nursing* (7th ed.). St. Louis: Elsevier.

Quill, C., & Quill, T. (2014). Palliative use of non-invasive ventilation: Navigating murky waters. *Journal of Palliative Medicine, 17*(6), 657–661. http://dx.doi.org/10.1089/jpm.2014.0010.

3-72. **(A)** One of the predictors for successful weaning from the ventilator is a maximum inspiratory pressure of −20 to −25 cmH$_2$O or lower. A spontaneous VT greater than 5 mL/kg is a recommended parameter for ventilator liberation. Low PEEP and FiO$_2$ requirements also indicate potential for a successful extubation. Other criteria include, but are not limited to, stable cardiovascular status, adequate hemoglobin, stable vital signs, ABG within normal limits preextubation, and absence of muscle weakness.

References: Storzer, D. N. (2018). Pulmonary system. In T. M. Hartjes (Ed.), *AACN core curriculum for high acuity, progressive, and critical care nursing* (7th ed.). St. Louis: Elsevier.

Zein, H., Baratloo, A., Negida, A., & Safari, S. (2016). Ventilator weaning and spontaneous breathing trials: an educational review. *Emergency, 4*(2), 65–71.

3-73. **(D)** Acute blood loss results in the development of hypovolemic shock, which occurs as a result of inadequate fluid volume in the intravascular space. When this occurs, the kidneys will increase retention of sodium, thereby conserving both sodium and body water and increasing circulating volume. The pulse pressure narrows when systolic pressure is low, and the diastolic blood pressure is rising because of compensatory vasoconstriction. Arterial vasodilation would worsen the shock state and diminish oxygen delivery to tissues, as vasoconstriction increases systemic vascular resistance and systolic blood pressure, thereby improving tissue perfusion. The heart rate increases in response to increased sympathetic nervous system stimulation.

References: Efre, A., & Boling, B. (2018). Cardiovascular system. In T. M. Hartjes (Ed.), *AACN core curriculum for high acuity, progressive, and critical care nursing* (7th ed.). St. Louis: Elsevier.

Rivers, E. (2016). Approach to the patient with shock. In L. Goldman (Ed.), *Goldman-Cecil medicine* (25th ed.) (pp. 672–681). Philadelphia: Elsevier Saunders.

3-74. **(B)** Although pulmonary complications are a significant risk after esophageal surgery, pain control is essential in ensuring good pulmonary toilet. Pain control is a key in the patient who has undergone an esophageal surgical procedure. Without optimal pain control, many of the other interventions to prevent complications (e.g., pulmonary toilet) cannot be performed effectively. Patients who undergo esophageal surgical procedures are susceptible to noncardiogenic pulmonary edema. Major fluid shifts occur in the first few days after surgery, however; because of the reduced clearance of lymph, patients are predisposed to interstitial pulmonary edema, so large volumes of IV fluid would not be appropriate. Although a feeding tube is placed during surgery, these patients may not receive tube feedings for 2 to 3 days after surgery to allow sufficient time for peristalsis to return.

References: Alderden, J. (2018). Critical care patients with special needs: geriatric patients. In T. M. Hartjes (Ed.), *AACN core curriculum for high acuity, progressive, and critical care nursing* (7th ed.). St. Louis: Elsevier.

Ramly, E., Kaafarani, H., & Velmahos, G. (2015). The effect of aging on pulmonary function: Implications for monitoring and support of the surgical and trauma patient. *Surgical Clinics of North America, 95*(1), 53–69. http://dx.doi.org/10.1016/j.suc.2014.09.009.

3-75. **(A)** Isolated, mild deficits (NIH Stroke Scale score of 1 or less) represent a contraindication to rt-PA therapy. Although a seizure at the onset of stroke is a contraindication, a history of epilepsy or seizure disorder (Option B), in itself, would not constitute a contraindication. Another stroke, intracranial surgery, or serious head trauma within the past 3 months would exclude a patient from rt-PA use, but a mild TBI 6 months prior would not (Option C). Current use of anticoagulants or an INR greater than 1.7 would qualify as a contraindication, but an INR of 1.3 (Option D) would be acceptable.

References: Blissitt, P.A. (2018). Neurologic system. In T. M. Hartjes (Ed.), *AACN core curriculum for high acuity, progressive, and critical care nursing* (7th ed.). St. Louis: Elsevier.

Fugate, J., & Rabinstein, A. (2015). Absolute and relative contraindications to IV rt-PA for acute ischemic stroke. *The Neurohospitalist, 5*(3), 110–121. http://dx.doi.org/10.1177/1941874415578532.

3-76. **(A)** Subglottic suctioning can prevent ventilator-associated pneumonia (VAP) or a ventilator-associated event (VAE). The prevention is enhanced by the addition of the VAP or VAE bundle along with the subglottic suction endotracheal tube. Endotracheal tubes are available with integrated suction lines running along their edges, with fenestrations lower than the level of the vocal cords and just higher than the endotracheal tube cuff. Attaching the line to wall suction or a syringe can remove contaminated oral secretions pooling above the tube cuff, before they are aspirated by the patient. The initiation of nutrition (Option B) is important; however, at this point, the intubated patient is at highest risk for VAEs and not malnutrition. Early mobilization (Option C) is critical, but the patient would be best served to be given the opportunity to rest for a period after an acute exacerbation of her illness. DVT prophylaxis (Option D) does not require IV heparin.

References: Stacy, K. (2018). Pulmonary therapeutic management. In L. Urden, K. Stacy, & M. Lough (Eds.), *Critical care nursing: diagnosis and management.* St. Louis, MO: Mosby/Elsevier.

Damas, P., Frippiat, F., Ancion, A., Canivet, J., Lambermont, B., Layios, N., & Ledoux, D. (2015). Prevention of ventilator-associated pneumonia and ventilator-associated conditions: a randomized controlled trial with subglottic secretion suctioning. *Critical Care Medicine, 43*(1), 22–30. http://dx.doi.org/10.1097/CCM.0000000000000674.

3-77. **(B)** The code of ethics for nurses states that nurses must be alert to and must take appropriate action in all instances of incompetent, unethical, illegal, or impaired practice or actions that place the rights or best interests of the patient in jeopardy. When a nurse becomes aware of inappropriate or questionable practice, the concern must be expressed to the person involved, focusing on the patient's best interests as well as on the integrity of nursing practice. The arterial line is intermittently positional and at times may be accurate during which an alarm would indicate a critical situation for the patient. The code of ethics states that if the practice threatens the welfare of the patient, nurses should express their concern to the responsible manager. In this situation, the ICU nurse addressed the colleague, who continued to ignore the alarm. The nursing code of ethics would then have the ICU nurse report to a manager. Asking the intensivist to change the line would expose the patient to significant discomfort and potential complications. Troubleshooting the line may fix the positional readings. Ignoring an alarm is never an option.

References: Dermenchyan, A. (2018). Professional caring and ethical practice. In T. M. Hartjes (Ed.), *AACN core curriculum for high acuity, progressive, and critical care nursing* (7th ed.). St. Louis: Elsevier.

Ross, J. (2015). Alarm fatigue: are you tuning out? *Journal of Perianesthesia Nursing, 30*(4), 351–353. http://dx.doi.org/10.1016/j.jopan.2015.05.007.

3-78. **(C)** The nurse should delegate tasks to ensure that priority patient care needs are met in a timely fashion and that staff needs for instruction are accommodated in accordance with patient care priorities. A nurse who must devote full attention to patient care needs to seek a colleague who may be in a better position to lend support to the new nurse. In deciding the best course of action, the nurse should consider that both patients would benefit from assessments performed by the same provider to ensure continuity of care. Hourly glucose checks on a young patient with DKA reflect a patient whose care requires close and frequent nursing supervision that should not be disrupted unnecessarily. Hourly neurologic checks should be performed only by a skilled RN. A new nurse should not be asked to review a staffing schedule, as this requires considerable experience and knowledge of other staff members' competency.

References: Dermenchyan, A. (2018). Professional caring and ethical practice. In T. M. Hartjes (Ed.), *AACN core curriculum for high acuity, progressive, and critical care nursing* (7th ed.). St. Louis: Elsevier.

National guidelines for nursing delegation. (2016). *Journal of Nursing Regulation, 7*(1), 5–14.

3-79. **(B)** Fat embolism syndrome can occur as a complication of orthopedic trauma. The clinical onset of fat embolism syndrome ranges from 12 to 72 hours after injury. The presence of fat in the pulmonary circulation injures the endothelial lining of the capillary, increasing capillary permeability and resulting in alveolar flooding. The skin rash, diminished level of consciousness, and reduction in platelet count are indications of fat emboli most likely associated with the femur fracture. A thrombus resulting from venous stasis or deep vein thrombosis is more likely to cause a pulmonary embolus. The bronchociliary clearance mechanisms are protective mechanisms usually affected in cases of aspiration or pneumonia. Although they could be affected in this patient, there is no evidence of this in the scenario described. The shunting of blood through poorly ventilated areas of pulmonary consolidation can produce hypoxia, but this scenario does not describe a patient who has aspirated or developed pneumonia.

References: Lough, M. (2018). Trauma. In L. Urden, K. Stacy, & M. Lough (Eds.), *Critical care nursing: diagnosis and management*. St. Louis, MO: Mosby/Elsevier.

Weinhouse, G. (2016). Fat embolism syndrome. Available from http://www.uptodate.com/contents/fat-embolism-syndrome.

3-80. **(C)** This patient is at high risk for reintubation because of his history of multiple intubations with extubation failure. Studies show that high-flow nasal cannula immediately after scheduled extubation was not inferior to noninvasive mechanical ventilation for risk of reintubation and postextubation respiratory failure in patients at high risk of reintubation. High-flow nasal cannula improves oxygenation and ventilation and decreases the work of breathing. High-flow nasal cannula is tolerated better by patients and can be sustained longer with more comfort than noninvasive positive pressure ventilation. Patients can perform activities of daily living, including eating while sustaining high-flow nasal cannula. A partial rebreather mask will not provide the level of respiratory support that is provided by NPPV and high-flow nasal cannula.

References: Stacy, K. (2018). Pulmonary therapeutic management. In L. Urden, K. Stacy, & M. Lough (Eds.), *Critical care nursing: diagnosis and management*. St. Louis, MO: Mosby/Elsevier.

Hernández, G., Vaquero, C., Colinas, L., Cuena, R., González, P., Canabal, A., & Fernández, R. (2016). Effect of postextubation high-flow nasal cannula vs noninvasive ventilation on reintubation and postextubation respiratory failure in high-risk patients: a randomized clinical trial. *JAMA, 316*(15), 1565–1574. http://dx.doi.org/10.1001/jama.2016.14194.

3-81. **(A)** Intravenous infusions of norepinephrine and dobutamine are indicated for this patient based on the provided hemodynamic parameters. Norepinephrine will increase the patient's mean arterial pressure. Dobutamine is an inotropic agent that will increase myocardial contractility, cardiac output, and cardiac index. Both agents will increase tissue perfusion and subsequent oxygen delivery. Fluid administration with intravenous dopamine is not warranted for this patient because both the pulmonary artery pressure and the central venous pressure indicate adequate intravascular volume. Sodium bicarbonate is generally not indicated unless the patient is experiencing severe acidosis with a pH less than 6.9.

References: Johnson, A. (2018). Multisystem: systemic inflammatory response syndrome and septic shock. In T. M. Hartjes (Ed.), *AACN core curriculum for high acuity, progressive, and critical care nursing* (7th ed.). St. Louis: Elsevier.

Gelinas, J., & Russell, J. (2016). Vasopressors during sepsis. *Clinics in Chest Medicine, 37*(2), 251–262. http://dx.doi.org/10.1016/j.ccm.2016.01.008.

3-82. **(B)** Leveling the transducer air–fluid interface to the left atrium corrects for changes in hydrostatic pressure in vessels above and below the heart. Data suggest that in the supine position, the external landmark for the left atrium is the phlebostatic axis (fourth ICS/half AP diameter of the chest). Option A is incorrect because a square wave test is only performed on the initial system setup and then at least once each shift, after opening the catheter system (e.g., for rezeroing, drawing blood, or changing tubing) and whenever the PAP waveform appears to be damped or distorted. Option C is not a requirement because data support that the head of the bed elevation can be at any angle from 0 degrees (flat) to 60 degrees for measurement. Accurate measurements require reading pressure waveforms during end expiration, so Option D is incorrect.

References: Efre, A., & Boling, B. (2018). Cardiovascular system. In T. M. Hartjes (Ed.), *AACN core curriculum for high acuity, progressive, and critical care nursing* (7th ed.). St. Louis: Elsevier.

Bridges, E., Barros, L., Cockerham, M., Greco, S., Herrera, F., & Solvang, N. (2016). Pulmonary artery/central venous pressure monitoring in adults. *Critical Care Nurse, 36*(4). http://dx.doi.org/10.4037/ccn2016268.

3-83. **(B)** Aneurysms located at the anterior communicating artery are the most common site of aneurysmal SAH. The anterior communicating artery is located near the optic nerve. Aneurysm arising in this area can produce visual symptoms such as visual dimness, unilateral visual field defect, or unilateral visual loss.

References: Blissitt, P. A. (2018). Neurologic system. In T. M. Hartjes (Ed.), *AACN core curriculum for high acuity, progressive, and critical care nursing* (7th ed.). St. Louis: Elsevier.

3-84. **(C)** Diagnostic studies are needed to evaluate for pulmonary embolism or bleeding from the aorta. Although the patient's clinical picture has deteriorated, neither intubation (Option A) nor emergency surgery (Option D) is indicated without diagnostic evaluation. The patient may require sedation and analgesia (Option B), but further workup needs to precede administration of these agents so the cause of her acute decompensation can be determined.

Reference: Storzer, D. N. (2018). Pulmonary system. In T. M. Hartjes (Ed.), *AACN core curriculum for high acuity, progressive, and critical care nursing* (7th ed.). St. Louis: Elsevier.

3-85. **(B)** This patient is experiencing severe leukopenia. Identification of the underlying cause and treatment of the cause is a priority for this patient. Certain medications, especially schizophrenia and psychosis medications, can cause leukopenia. Medication-induced leukopenia is a first suspicion for this patient. Eliminating these medications is a priority. HIV testing and blood cultures are important to rule out other possible causes of leukopenia because of the patient's high risk for infection from IV drug abuse. Bone marrow biopsy to rule out leukemia is invasive and should only be completed once less invasive testing rules out other causes.

References: Dressler, D. (2018). Hematological and immunological systems. In T. M. Hartjes (Ed.), *AACN core curriculum for high acuity, progressive, and critical care nursing* (7th ed.). St. Louis: Elsevier.

Abanmy, N., Al-Jaloud, A., Al-Jabr, A., Al-Ruwaisan, R., Al-Saeed, W., & Fatani, S. (2014). Clozapine-induced blood dyscrasias in Saudi Arab patients. *International Journal of Clinical Pharmacy, 36*(4), 815–820. http://dx.doi.org/10.1007/s11096-014-9967-0.

3-86. **(B)** Encephalopathy is not a disease itself but always occurs as the end result of another disease process. Evaluation for these disease processes—often infectious or metabolic— should be considered first. For example, diabetic ketoacidosis may precipitate encephalopathy and be evidenced by headache and lethargy, which suggest cerebral edema. A second disorder, water intoxication, may be ruled out by checking serum osmolality, and a third, hepatic encephalopathy, can be determined by checking serum ammonia. Level of consciousness is most important in monitoring these patients. The nurse should look for signs of increased ICP (e.g., hypertension, increased muscle tone in extremities, hyperventilation, dilated pupils). ICP monitoring (Option A) would be indicated in stage III hepatic encephalopathy but would not be a first-line action in this patient. Lumbar puncture (LP) (Option C) is not indicated in this patient. If ICP were elevated, LP could be harmful. Immunoassay is not indicated for this patient, and a CT of the head would be a more appropriate diagnostic study than cerebral angiography (Option D).

References: Radovich, P. (2018). Gastrointestinal system. In T. M. Hartjes (Ed.), *AACN core curriculum for high acuity, progressive, and critical care nursing* (7th ed.). St. Louis: Elsevier.

Chalkely, J. (2017). Encephalopathy. In F. Ferri, *2017 Ferri's clinical advisor: 5 books in 1* (pp. 421–422). Philadelphia: Elsevier Saunders.

3-87. **(B)** Maintenance of renal perfusion pressure and renal blood flow remain the mainstay of perioperative management during cardiac surgery. Increasing the cardiac index to greater than 2.2 L/min/m^2 will increase renal blood flow and enhance renal tissue perfusion. If MAP, PAOP, PAD, and CVP are within normal limits, then the patient has achieved outcome criteria. Other outcome criteria include electrolytes within normal limits, normalization of acid-base balance, lungs clear on auscultation, normal level of consciousness, BUN and creatinine within normal limits, urine output within normal limits or patient stable on dialysis, stable hemoglobin and hematocrit values. In Options A, C, and D, the patient's CVP, MAP, and PAOP are low, indicating decreased renal blood flow and tissue perfusion.

References: Boling, B. (2018). Renal system. In T. M. Hartjes (Ed.), *AACN core curriculum for high acuity, progressive, and critical care nursing* (7th ed.). St. Louis: Elsevier.

3-88. **(D)** The nurse's primary commitment is to the patient and family. Federal and state laws require that certain individuals, particularly those who work in health care, with older adults, children, and other vulnerable populations, have an affirmative duty to report to a specified state agency when violence occurs against those populations. Nurses are designated as mandatory reporters of child abuse. When a mandatory duty to report violence against an individual or individuals exists, there is no exception to the directive: one must report without fail. This translates into no excuse for not doing so. Thus nurse–patient confidentiality, another staff member or administrator telling you not to report your concerns, or a family member pleading with you not to report your observations do not affect your duty to report. If a nurse fails to report an instance of violence when required to do so, the nurse could face professional disciplinary action by the state board of nursing, a loss of any certifications, and criminal prosecution (usually a misdemeanor).

References: Dermenchyan, A. (2018). Professional caring and ethical practice. In T. M. Hartjes (Ed.), *AACN core curriculum for high acuity, progressive, and critical care nursing* (7th ed.). St. Louis: Elsevier.

3-89. **(B)** Overwedging is usually caused by migration of the PA catheter forward into the pulmonary capillaries. For a catheter that has migrated to a more distal position, it is possible for overwedging to occur without balloon inflation. The overwedge pressure is devoid of pulsatility, is higher than expected, and increases continuously because of the continuous flush pressure. This should be corrected by catheter

withdrawal. The overwedge result is completely inaccurate and should not be treated. The PA catheter can be repositioned if it has a sterile sleeve so it does not need to be discontinued.

References: Efre, A., & Boling, B. (2018). Cardiovascular system. In T. M. Hartjes (Ed.), *AACN core curriculum for high acuity, progressive, and critical care nursing* (7th ed.). St. Louis: Elsevier.

Schroeder, B., Barbeito, A., Bar-Yosef, S., & Mark, J. (2015). In R. Miller & N. Cohen (Eds.), *Miller's anesthesia* (8th ed.). (pp. 1345–395). Philadelphia, PA: Elsevier Saunders.

3-90. **(C)** By providing correct and appropriate information, the nurse is helping to promote a caring environment for the family during a potentially stressful time. Several physiologic changes will likely be manifested by the patient after withdrawal of mechanical ventilation, some of which may be distressing to the family unless they know about them beforehand. The anticipated time frame to death is variable and cannot be predicted with any confidence. The name of the person performing the procedure will not likely be relevant to the family or contribute to promoting a caring environment to the family. Secretions associated with a "death rattle" do not cause discomfort to the patient. This fluid should not be suctioned, as suctioning can cause discomfort to the patient.

References: Dermenchyan, A. (2018). Professional caring and ethical practice. In T. M. Hartjes (Ed.), *AACN core curriculum for high acuity, progressive, and critical care nursing* (7th ed.). St. Louis: Elsevier.

3-91. **(C)** The nurse observed a Cheyne-Stokes respiratory pattern. This respiratory pattern is a frequent finding in patients with heart failure. It is a form of nonhypercapnic central sleep apnea. This pattern can exist during sleep and wakefulness in heart failure patients. Cheyne-Stokes breathing is a normal finding for a patient with heart failure, and the pulse oximetry result is normal; no further testing would be required.

References: Storzer, D. N. (2018). Pulmonary system. In T. M. Hartjes (Ed.), *AACN core curriculum for high acuity, progressive, and critical care nursing* (7th ed.). St. Louis: Elsevier.

3-92. **(C)** The critical care nurse knows that heart failure patients are prone to depression. An

Indian patient may not be able to communicate depression. In many areas throughout the world, people avoid seeking treatment for psychological disorders because of the stigma associated with mental illness. This is true in India, where informing people that someone has a psychological disorder can negatively affect that person's way of life. Some of the concerns Indian people may have are unique to their culture, and other concerns are shared by many cultures. Social standing is highly valued in Indian communities, so some concerns deal with the loss of status and respect in society. Indian people be afraid to reveal emotional or psychological problems because they are afraid to cause pain or worry for the persons they disclose their problems to. They tend to be especially concerned about the effect of their problem on their spouses and other family members. People in India who have depression most often present with somatic symptoms initially. These individuals identify the most troubling aspects of their disorder to be aches and pains. A trip outside to see a favorite pet may help to lift the patient's spirits. Distraction is also a nonpharmacologic treatment for pain, anxiety, and depression. Antidepressants (Option A) may help Mr. Patel, but their peak effect can take up to 6 weeks. Informing the patient's family (Option C) of suspected depression could violate Mr. Patel's privacy and cause concern about the effect on the family. Providing a favorite meal (Option D) is not helpful if the patient has lost his appetite secondary to depression.

References: Dermenchyan, A. (2018). Professional caring and ethical practice. In T. M. Hartjes (Ed.), *AACN core curriculum for high acuity, progressive, and critical care nursing* (7th ed.). St. Louis: Elsevier.

Roberts, L., Mann, S., & Montgomery, S. (2016). Mental health and sociocultural determinants in an Asian Indian community. *Family & Community Health, 39*(1), 31–39. http://dx.doi.org/10.1097/FCH.0000000000000087.

3-93. **(D)** Tumor necrosis factor (TNF)-α is released from macrophages and lymphocytes in response to endotoxin, tissue injury, viral agents, and interleukins. Cellular responses to TNF include increased formation of oxygen radicals; recruitment and activation of neutrophils, macrophages, and lymphocytes; increased cytokine production; initial hyperglycemia followed by hypoglycemia, hypotension, metabolic acidosis, and coagulopathy; fever and increased oxygen consumption; increased capillary permeability, vasodilation, microvascular vasoconstriction, and noncardiac pulmonary edema; activation of the coagulation cascade; and production of nitric oxide.

References: Johnson, A. (2018). Multisystem: systemic inflammatory response syndrome and septic shock. In T. M. Hartjes (Ed.), *AACN core curriculum for high acuity, progressive, and critical care nursing* (7th ed.). St. Louis: Elsevier.

3-94. **(C)** Definitive treatment for a persistent air leak can include bronchoscopy to introduce endobronchial glue, obliteration of the pleural space with chemical irritants such as antibiotics, or surgical decortication with removal of the pleural lining. Progressive advancement of the chest tube would not be included among the treatments for air leak; that intervention is used to treat empyemas.

References: Stacy, K. (2018). Pulmonary disorders. In L. Urden, K. Stacy, & M. Lough (Eds.), *Critical care nursing: diagnosis and management*. St. Louis, MO: Mosby/Elsevier.

3-95. **(B)** This patient is experiencing one of the clinical findings of uremic syndrome. Intensive dialysis is indicated for true uremic pericarditis. Four hours of hemodialysis needs to be done daily because the patient is manifesting symptomatic uremic pericarditis. Management of this disorder includes increasing the duration and frequency of hemodialysis. The goals of care would be to decrease the BUN below 60 mg/dL or lower than the level at which patient no longer demonstrates uremic symptoms. Peritoneal dialysis would not be considered for management in this case, as the patient is already on hemodialysis.

References: Boling, B. (2018). Renal system. In T. M. Hartjes (Ed.), *AACN core curriculum for high acuity, progressive, and critical care nursing* (7th ed.). St. Louis: Elsevier.

Black, R. (2015). Pericarditis in renal failure. Available from http://www.uptodate.com/contents/pericarditis-in-renal-failure.

3-96. **(B)** The need for clergy support is a specific psychosocial need of family members, and is not a psychosocial need for **all** families of the critically ill. Specific needs vary depending on patient characteristics, family characteristics, and the patient's status on the health-to-illness continuum. Families need to be with their family members when they are in the hospital. They require support and reassurance from the medical team to feel confident in the care of their loved one. Also, they need frequent information about the progress, plan of care, and interventions for their loved one.

> **References:** Chapa, D., & Akintade, B. (2018). Psychosocial aspects of critical care. In T. M. Hartjes (Ed.), *AACN core curriculum for high acuity, progressive, and critical care nursing* (7th ed.). St. Louis: Elsevier.

3-97. **(D)** This patient may have posttraumatic stress disorder (PTSD). Many veterans have PTSD and are four times more likely to have suicidal tendencies. Some of these suicidal tendencies manifest in risk-taking behavior such as reckless driving, drug use, unsafe sex, gambling, and drinking. The patient admits to reckless driving and excessive drinking. He demonstrates signs of PTSD such as nightmares and insomnia. A psychiatry consult could immediately help identify his psychological state and if he is suicidal or needs referral to an alcohol abuse program or veterans support program. Benzodiazepines can worsen symptoms of PTSD and are not recommended to be given in combination with narcotic pain control.

> **References:** Chapa, D., & Akintade, B. (2018). Psychosocial aspects of critical care. In T. M. Hartjes (Ed.), *AACN core curriculum for high acuity, progressive, and critical care nursing* (7th ed.). St. Louis: Elsevier.
>
> Strom, T., Leskela, J., James, L., Thuras, P., Voller, E., Weigel, R., & Holz, K. (2012). An exploratory examination of risk-taking behavior and PTSD symptom severity in a veteran sample. *Military Medicine, 177*(4), 390–396.

3-98. **(B)** Furosemide has also been found to cause temporary and sometimes permanent cases of hearing loss. Permanent hearing loss has been reported in certain adults treated with furosemide. Plasma levels of furosemide greater than 50 mg/L have been associated with hearing loss, and sensorineural hearing loss may be accompanied by tinnitus and vertigo.

The incidence of ototoxicity with furosemide was reported to be approximately 6% in a small series of patients. Clinical studies suggest that the ototoxicity of furosemide may be reduced by infusing the drug at rates of less than 15 mg/min. Hypotension can occur after furosemide administration but it is not related to how quickly it was administered. AKI associated with IV furosemide occurs commonly in patients hospitalized with pulmonary edema because of acute heart failure but is associated with multiple independent risk factors. Diuretic-induced hypokalemia can be monitored and treated and is not related to the speed of furosemide administration but rather to the response to the diuretic.

> **References:** Efre, A., Boling, B. (2018). Cardiovascular system. In T. M. Hartjes (Ed.), *AACN core curriculum for high acuity, progressive, and critical care nursing* (7th ed.). St. Louis: Elsevier.
>
> Rybak, L., & Brenner, M. (2015). Vestibular and auditory ototoxicity. In P. Flint, B. Haughey, V. Lund, J. Niparko, M. Richardson, K. Robbins & J. Thomas (Eds.), *Cummings otolaryngology* (pp. 2369–2382). Philadelphia: Elsevier Saunders.

3-99. **(A)** The symptoms described by the patient are indicative of hemorrhage in the cerebellum. Hemorrhagic pontine stroke is distinguished by contralateral hemiparesis and, with more extensive hemorrhage, quadriparesis and "locked-in" syndrome, impaired lateral eye movement, poorly reactive pupils, and abnormal respiratory patterns. Thalamus hemorrhage causes contralateral hemiparesis and sensory loss equal in the face, arm, and leg or hemisensory loss alone. Hemorrhagic damage to the putamen causes contralateral hemiparesis, sensory loss, and dysarthria.

> **References:** Blissitt, P.A. (2018). Neurologic system. In T. M. Hartjes (Ed.), *AACN core curriculum for high acuity, progressive, and critical care nursing* (7th ed.). St. Louis: Elsevier.
>
> Rocco, T., & Goldstein, J. (2014). Stroke. In J. Marx, P. Rosen, & H. Bessen (Eds.), *Rosen's emergency medicine* (8th ed.). (pp. 1363–1374). Philadelphia: Elsevier Saunders.

3-100. **(C)** Waterhouse-Frideichsen syndrome involves adrenal hemorrhage. It may be seen in fulminating meningococcal meningitis. It results in adrenal insufficiency, subsequent hypotension, respiratory distress, DIC, and circulatory collapse. Korsakoff syndrome is a chronic memory disorder caused by severe deficiency of thiamine (vitamin B_1). Korsakoff syndrome is most commonly caused by alcohol misuse, but certain other conditions also can cause the syndrome. Brudzinski sign is one of the physically demonstrable symptoms of meningitis. Severe neck stiffness causes a patient's hips and knees to flex when the neck is flexed. Patients with Brown-Séquard syndrome have ipsilateral upper motor neuron paralysis and loss of proprioception, as well as contralateral loss of pain and temperature sensation. A zone of partial preservation or segmental ipsilateral lower motor neuron weakness and analgesia may be noted.

References: Blissitt, P. A. (2018). Neurologic system. In T. M. Hartjes (Ed.), *AACN core curriculum for high acuity, progressive, and critical care nursing* (7th ed.). St. Louis: Elsevier.

3-101. **(A)** Rudolf Virchow described the triad of venous stasis, vein (endothelial) injury, and a hypercoagulable state as risk factors for the development of pulmonary emboli. Pelvic fractures require immobility; lower extremity trauma that results in swelling reduces blood flow, and the need for blood replacement products heightens this patient's risk for thrombi. Recognition of these risks provides the greatest opportunity for prevention of the complication of pulmonary embolism. Intravascular cannulation can lead to vein injury, and dehydration can result in venous stasis, but this patient's age is not a factor in the triad. Hypoxia and interstitial edema result from rather than cause development of pulmonary embolus. Right ventricular dysfunction, pulmonary artery hypertension, and atelectasis are complications seen in the critically ill patient but do not increase a patient's risk for pulmonary embolism

References: Storzer, D. N. (2018). Pulmonary system. In T. M. Hartjes (Ed.), *AACN core curriculum for high acuity, progressive, and critical care nursing* (7th ed.). St. Louis: Elsevier.

Benrashid, E., Youngwirth, L. M., Turley, R. S., & Mureebe, L. (2017). Venous thromboembolism: prevention, diagnosis, and treatment. In A. M. Cameron & J. L. Cameron (Eds.), *Current*

surgical therapy (pp. 1091–1098). Philadelphia: Elsevier Saunders.

3-102. **(D)** Bed rest is common practice in ICUs worldwide, especially for mechanically ventilated patients. ICU-acquired weakness is an increasingly recognized problem, with sequelae that may last for months and years after ICU discharge. Bed rest can lead to rapid deconditioning, catabolism, insulin resistance, and muscle atrophy. The combination of critical illness and bed rest results in substantial muscle wasting during an ICU stay. When initiated shortly after the start of mechanical ventilation, mobilization and rehabilitation can play an important role in decreasing the duration of mechanical ventilation and hospital stay and improving patients' return to functional independence. Such weakness of the extremities as occurs with ICU-acquired weakness is also associated with respiratory muscle weakness and prolonged weaning from mechanical ventilation. Despite the potential concerns about mobilizing mechanically ventilated patients, many studies have repeatedly demonstrated its safety and feasibility, with very low rates of potential safety events.

References: Hashem, M., Nelliot, A., & Needham, D. (2016). Early mobilization and rehabilitation in the ICU: moving back to the future. *Respiratory Care, 61*(7), 971–979. http://dx.doi.org/10.4187/respcare.04741.

Dos Santos, C., Herridge, M., & Batt, J. (2016). Early goal directed mobility in the ICU: 'Something in the way you move'. *Journal of Thoracic Disease, 8*(8), E784–E787. http://dx.doi.org/10.21037/jtd.2016.05.96.

3-103. **(A)** The patient already demonstrates hypotension and tachycardia related to hypovolemia, so attaining the primary goal of replacing renal function via ultrafiltration while obtaining solute removal via convection that will not further compromise hypotension represents the rationale for selecting this mode of renal replacement therapy. Patients treated with CVVH are not less vulnerable to developing complications such as clotting and infection. This patient would be expected to benefit from CVVH because she is experiencing acute (rather than chronic) renal failure because of perioperative hypotension associated with hypovolemia related to operative blood loss. In acute renal failure, the BUN level does not elevate to the same level as it does in chronic renal failure, when BUN is over 100 mg/dL.

References: Boling, B. (2018). Renal system. In T. M. Hartjes (Ed.), *AACN core curriculum for high acuity, progressive, and critical care nursing* (7th ed.). St. Louis: Elsevier.

Kobrin, S. (2014). Renal replacement therapy. In P. Lanken, S. Manaker, B. Kohl & C. Hanson (Eds.), *Intensive care unit manual* (2nd ed.). (pp. 205–214). Philadelphia: Elsevier Saunders.

3-104. **(D)** The nurse will advocate for the family by facilitating the wife's request with the physician and then identifying the best location for the wife. The advantage to the wife's staying is consistent with a holistic family-centered approach to care that sees the patient and family as the unit of care. Family presence during ICU procedures, when the patient and family member both desire it, fulfills the mandates of patient-centered care. Family inclusion increases family engagement, improves patient and family satisfaction, and may decrease psychological distress in patients and family members based on studies of open visitation and family presence during cardiopulmonary resuscitation. Denying the request because of unit policy (Option A) does not advocate for the family. Option B seems to approach refusal by attempting to intimidate the wife. Option C fails to advocate for the family and attempts to harness the notion of sterility as the reason the family should not stay.

References: Dermenchyan, A. (2018). Professional caring and ethical practice. In T. M. Hartjes (Ed.), *AACN core curriculum for high acuity, progressive, and critical care nursing* (7th ed.). St. Louis: Elsevier.

Guzzetta, C. (2016). Family presence during resuscitation and invasive procedures. *Critical Care Nurse, 36*(1), e11–e14. http://dx.doi.org/10.4037/ccn2016980.

3-105. **(A)** Damaged endothelial cells secrete a protein that converts the inactive form of plasmin (plasminogen) to its active form (plasmin) so that degradation of a fibrin clot can begin. The degradation of fibrin is called fibrinolysis. As the clot is degraded, fibrin split products can be detected in the blood. Thrombin (Option B) is produced by the enzymatic cleavage of two

sites on prothrombin by activated factor X. Thrombin is an important part of the coagulation cascade causing the formation of blood clots. Antithrombin III (Option C) is a circulating plasma protein that inactivates thrombin. It can prevent the progression of clot formation but does not enhance clot degradation. Phospholipid (Option D) is a component of the platelet cell membrane that initiates the coagulation cascade.

References: Dressler, D. (2018). Hematological and immunological systems. In T. M. Hartjes (Ed.), *AACN core curriculum for high acuity, progressive, and critical care nursing* (7th ed.). St. Louis: Elsevier.

Draxler, D. F., & Medcalf, R. L. (2015). The fibrinolytic system—More than fibrinolysis? *Transfusion Medicine Reviews, 29*(2), 102–109. http://dx.doi.org/10.1016/j.tmrv.2014.09.006.

3-106. **(B)** Administration of fluid bolus is indicated to treat hypotension. Hypotension in the mechanically ventilated patient may be related to increased intrathoracic pressure from high PEEP levels that decrease venous return. High PEEP levels are indicated in ARDS to improve oxygenation, and lowering PEEP would likely cause a further decrease in PaO_2. Norepinephrine may be administered if volume replacement is insufficient to increase blood pressure to acceptable levels but would not be given before the volume replenishment. Tidal volumes for patients with ARDS should be maintained at 5 to 7 mL/kg.

References: Storzer, D. N. (2018). Pulmonary system. In T. M. Hartjes (Ed.), *AACN core curriculum for high acuity, progressive, and critical care nursing* (7th ed.). St. Louis: Elsevier.

Vieillard-Baron, A., Matthay, M., Teboul, J., Bein, T., Schultz, M., Magder, S., & Marini, J. (2016). Experts' opinion on management of hemodynamics in ARDS patients: focus on the effects of mechanical ventilation. *Intensive Care Medicine, 42*(5), 739–749. http://dx.doi.org/10.1007/s00134-016-4326-3.

3-107. **(C)** Hyperthermia causes a shift to the right of the oxyhemoglobin disassociation curve. More oxygen is unloaded for a given PaO_2, which thus increases the oxygen delivery to the tissues. These shifts are also caused by acidosis, $PaCO_2$ increase, and increased levels of 2,3-diphosphoglycerate. A shift to the left of the curve occurs during which oxygen is not dissociated from hemoglobin until tissue and capillary oxygen levels are very low. This is caused by alkalosis, decreased $PaCO_2$ levels, hypothermia, carbon monoxide poisoning, and decreased levels of 2,3-diphosphoglycerate.

References: Storzer, D. N. (2018). Pulmonary system. In T. M. Hartjes (Ed.), *AACN core curriculum for high acuity, progressive, and critical care nursing* (7th ed.). St. Louis: Elsevier.

Hooley, J. (2015). Decoding the oxyhemoglobin dissociation curve. *American Nurse Today, 10*(1), 18–23.

3-108. **(B)** Autonomy and self-determination are ethical principles that refer to the potential to be self-determining. Patients must be clinically supported through the informed consent process that will facilitate decision making that is individualized based on the patient's own values. A competent adult patient has the right to make his or her own health care decisions. There are different types of consent. Implied consent is implied by the patient's behavior (such as presenting an arm to a practitioner to have blood drawn). This patient cannot verbalize or write her consent or refusal because of her medical condition. She has refused the second set of blood cultures by refusing to extend her arm. The patient should not be forced into complying (Option A) nor should another practitioner persuade the patient to comply (Option C). The intensivist may choose to speak to the patient to further the informed consent process and provide more explanation to reinforce that the patient is making an informed decision. Blood cultures obtained from a central line (Option D) have a higher contamination rate and may lead to false-positive results.

References: Dermenchyan, A. (2018). Professional caring and ethical practice. In T. M. Hartjes (Ed.), *AACN core curriculum for high acuity, progressive, and critical care nursing* (7th ed.). St. Louis: Elsevier.

Bull, E., & Sørlie, V. (2016). Ethical challenges when intensive care unit patients refuse nursing care. *Nursing Ethics, 23*(2), 214–222. http://dx.doi.org/10.1177/0969733014560931.

3-109. **(A)** For patients with COPD, goals of care related to ABGs are based on the patient's baseline values, not on textbook definitions of normal values. Some environmental or situational triggers that lead to exacerbations may be identifiable but not avoidable, and others may be unknown. Antibiotics may be used for these patients but would not be arbitrarily based on WBC counts because these are less reliable indicators in older patients. Bronchodilators are commonly used early in the care of these patients to relax the airways and reduce the work of breathing.

References: Storzer, D. N. (2018). Pulmonary system. In T. M. Hartjes (Ed.), *AACN core curriculum for high acuity, progressive, and critical care nursing* (7th ed.). St. Louis: Elsevier.

3-110. **(C)** Adenosine triphosphate (ATP) is a nucleoside triphosphate, a small molecule used in cells as a coenzyme. It is often referred to as the "molecular unit of currency" of intracellular energy transfer. ATP transports chemical energy within cells for metabolism. Cerebrospinal fluid provides all the listed functions for the brain. In addition, it provides support and buoyancy for the brain, decreasing the weight on the skull; cerebrospinal fluid also compensates for increases in intracranial volume and pressure.

References: Blissitt, P. A. (2018). Neurologic system. In T. M. Hartjes (Ed.), *AACN core curriculum for high acuity, progressive, and critical care nursing* (7th ed.). St. Louis: Elsevier.

3-111. **(D)** Basophils are nonphagocytic cells that attract immunoglobulin E (IgE) antibodies to their cell membranes. When the IgE binds antigen, the basophils release histamine, bradykinin, serotonin, heparin, and slowly reacting substances of anaphylaxis, triggering a massive inflammatory response.

Reference: Dressler, D. (2018). Hematological and immunological systems. In T. M. Hartjes (Ed.), *AACN core curriculum for high acuity, progressive, and critical care nursing* (7th ed.). St. Louis: Elsevier.

3-112. **(C)** The ethical principle of beneficence demands that the medical team "always act in the best interest of the patient." When members of the medical team feel conflict about further life-prolonging aggressive medical interventions and if they are in the best interest of the patient, it is important to note that life-prolonging medical treatments such as CPR, defibrillation, intubation with mechanical ventilation, and prolonged artificial nutrition are "ethically neutral." That means, independently, they are neither good nor bad. It is only in the context of a patient scenario that these treatments can be defined as either "beneficial" or "harmful." The family clearly and consistently expressed the perceived value of full interventions even after receiving detailed and complete information from the medical team. It is at this time that the medical professional may need to ask themselves, "Whose life, and subsequent death, is this?" A hospital ethics consult might not be helpful as the family is clearly acting according to the expressed wishes of the patient. The patient cannot be placed in hospice without his or his family's consent. Also, treatments cannot be withdrawn against the patient's wishes to receive complete life support as that would not support the ethical oath of "do no harm."

References: Dermenchyan, A. (2018). Professional caring and ethical practice. In T. M. Hartjes (Ed.), *AACN core curriculum for high acuity, progressive, and critical care nursing* (7th ed.). St. Louis: Elsevier.

Koesel, N., & Link, M. (2014). Conflicts in goals of care at the end of life. *Journal of Hospice & Palliative Nursing, 16*(6), 330–337. http://dx.doi.org/10.1097/NJH.0000000000000068.

3-113. **(B)** Pericardial tamponade may occur in radiofrequency ablation from coronary artery perforation or dissection. Pericardial tamponade restricts myocardial pumping and may result in cardiogenic shock or pulseless electrical activity. Second-degree AV block is not life threatening unless the rate is so slow it is considered to be symptomatic bradycardia. Second-degree block may become life threatening if it progresses to third-degree AV block. Cardiac valve damage is generally not severe enough from the ablation catheter to cause immediate threat to life. Microemboli may cause TIA or CVA.

References: Efre, A., & Boling, B. (2018). Cardiovascular system. In T. M. Hartjes (Ed.), *AACN core curriculum for high acuity, progressive, and critical care nursing* (7th ed.). St. Louis: Elsevier.

Mujović, N., Marinković, M., Marković, N., Kocijančić, A., Kovačević, V., Simić, D., & Stanković, G. (2016). Management and outcome of periprocedural cardiac perforation and tamponade with radiofrequency catheter ablation of cardiac arrhythmias: a single medium-volume center experience. *Advances in Therapy, 33*(10), 1782–1796. http://dx.doi.org/10.1007/s12325-016-0402-x.

3-114. **(B)** This question illustrates the nurse's competency for response to diversity. Asian culture has been defined as possessing a high power distance index (PDI). The PDI refers to the distance or level of respect that an individual must afford to a superior, and this ideal is reflected in Asian conformance to a strict social hierarchy. Thus, physicians are viewed as authority figures, and it is proper to nod or smile to indicate polite deference. However, showing respect and "buying in" to treatment recommendations are entirely different matters. Cultural factors make it difficult for patients to openly disagree with physician recommendations without feeling as though they have been disrespectful. The patient may have nodded and smiled, but that does not mean he consents to the surgery. A hospital-provided language service member can provide translation to assure that the patient consents to the procedure. Refusing to sign the consent does not advocate for this patient who needs surgical intervention. Health care providers and family members are not permitted by law to act as translators for medical translation and legal documentation.

References: Dermenchyan, A. (2018). Professional caring and ethical practice. In T. M. Hartjes (Ed.), *AACN core curriculum for high acuity, progressive, and critical care nursing* (7th ed.). St. Louis: Elsevier.

Juckett, G., Nguyen, C., & Shahbodaghi, S. (2014). Caring for Asian immigrants: tips on culture that can enhance patient care. *Journal of Family Practice, 63*(1), E1–9.

3-115. **(C)** The herniation description is that of central transtentorial herniation. Option A is a unilateral cerebral lesion that shifts brain tissue laterally across the midline, which causes distortion of the cingulate gyrus under the falx cerebri. In Option B, the expanding lesion forces the uncus of the medial temporal lobe over the edge of the tentorium. Option D is described by posterior fossa contents—particularly the cerebellar tonsils are displaced through the foramen magnum, which causes brainstem distortion.

References: Blissitt, P. A. (2018). Neurologic system. In T. M. Hartjes (Ed.), *AACN core curriculum for high acuity, progressive, and critical care nursing* (7th ed.). St. Louis: Elsevier.

3-116. **(C)** Intracuff pressure should not exceed the capillary filling pressure of the trachea (≤25 cm H_2O or ≤20mmHg) to avoid tracheal mucosa injury. Regardless of cuff design or pressure characteristics, all cuff pressures should be routinely measured at least every 8 to 12 hours and whenever the cuff is reinflated or the tube position is changed.

References: Storzer, D. N. (2018). Pulmonary system. In T. M. Hartjes (Ed.), *AACN core curriculum for high acuity, progressive, and critical care nursing* (7th ed.). St. Louis: Elsevier.

Khan, M., Khokar, R., Qureshi, S., Zahrani, T., Aqil, M., & Shiraz, M. (2016). Measurement of endotracheal tube cuff pressure: instrumental versus conventional method. *Saudi Journal of Anesthesia*, 10(4), 428. http://dx.doi.org/10.4103/1658-354x.179113.

3-117. **(A)** Patients older than 65 years who have an advanced stage of chronic kidney disease (stage 3 or higher), diabetes, or chronic heart failure are at higher risk for hyperkalemia. The patient needs an immediate IV administration of insulin and glucose because he is demonstrating clinical signs of acute hyperkalemia. Clinical manifestations of hyperkalemia include irritability, restlessness, anxiety, nausea, vomiting, abdominal cramps, weakness, numbness, tingling, and cardiac irregularities. The presence of insulin forces potassium out of the serum and into the cells on a temporary basis, thereby protecting the heart from the effects of elevated serum potassium. In a patient with ESRD, potassium levels rise quickly because of the complete loss of kidney function. Sodium polystyrene sulfonate (Kayexalate) is an ion resin that exchanges sodium for potassium in the bowel so that excessive amounts of potassium can be excreted via the feces. Although this is an effective means of eliminating excess potassium, its effects take longer to produce, making it a later option for management of hyperkalemia. Lidocaine and amiodarone are used to treat ventricular dysrhythmias and play no role in treating hyperkalemia.

References: Boling, B. (2018). Renal system. In T. M. Hartjes (Ed.), *AACN core curriculum for high acuity, progressive, and critical care nursing* (7th ed.). St. Louis: Elsevier.

Dunn, J., Benton, W., Orozco-Torrentera, E., & Adamson, R. (2015). The burden of hyperkalemia in patients with cardiovascular and renal disease. *American Journal of Managed Care*, S307–S315.

3-118. **(D)** Normal ICP range is 0 to 15 mm Hg. Thresholds for treating sustained ICP elevations vary, but 20 mm Hg is the upper limit beyond which intervention is recommended in patients with traumatic brain injury. ICP will rise in response to stimuli (coughing, turning, suctioning) but should return to baseline after the stimuli is removed. A failure to return to baseline after stimuli would require immediate physician notification.

References: Blissitt, P. A. (2018). Neurologic system. In T. M. Hartjes (Ed.), *AACN core curriculum for high acuity, progressive, and critical care nursing* (7th ed.). St. Louis: Elsevier.

3-119. **(B)** Patients should receive nonbenzodiazepine sedatives whenever possible. The use of dexmedetomidine could be associated with a shorter duration of mechanical ventilation, less delirium during ICU stay, and better cognitive performance after the recovery of critical illness. Dexmedetomidine is an anxiolytic, sedative, and analgesic medication. It is a selective agonist of α_2-adrenergic receptor notable for its ability to provide sedation without risk of respiratory depression. Compared with benzodiazepines and propofol, the pharmacologic profile of dexmedetomidine allows effective light to moderate sedation with earlier emergence from sedation, minimal respiratory depression, and absence of active metabolites and systemic accumulation after prolonged infusions. Maintenance of lighter levels of sedation is associated with improved clinical outcomes in critically ill patients, such as shorter durations of mechanical ventilation and ICU lengths of stay. One of the characteristics of the sedation with dexmedetomidine is that it mirrors natural sleep and, as such, provides less amnesia than benzodiazepines (Options A and D). Among ICU patients receiving prolonged mechanical ventilation, dexmedetomidine reduced duration of mechanical ventilation compared with midazolam and improved patients' ability to communicate pain compared with midazolam and propofol. Vecuronium (Option C) is a paralytic and not a sedative; it not indicated at this time.

References: Makic, M. (2018). Critical care patients with special needs: sedation in critically ill patients. In T. M. Hartjes (Ed.), *AACN core curriculum for high acuity, progressive, and critical care nursing* (7th ed.). St. Louis: Elsevier.

Zaal, I., Devlin, J., Hazelbag, M., Klein Klouwenberg, P., Kooi, A., Ong, D., & Slooter, A. (2015). Benzodiazepine-associated delirium in critically ill adults. *Intensive Care Medicine, 41*(12), 2130–2137. http://dx.doi.org/10.1007/s00134-015-4063-z.

3-120. **(B)** The nurse is demonstrating a clinical inquiry, collaboration, and systems thinking approach to solving a critical patient care issue that interferes in the caring practices necessary to meet the needs of the bariatric patient population. The nurse understands how patient care relates to the health care system and how to use that system to improve the quality and safety of patient care. In Option A, an ethics committee consult is not appropriate, and the purchase of bariatric equipment may not be cost-effective for this hospital. The physician should be aware of issues that affect patient care, but physician notification does not provide a solution to the ongoing issue. Incident reports can document an unsafe patient care issue; however, they only document a problem but do not provide a solution.

References: Benefield, A. (2018). Critical care patients with special needs: bariatric patients. In T. M. Hartjes (Ed.), *AACN core curriculum for high acuity, progressive, and critical care nursing* (7th ed.). St. Louis: Elsevier.

Broome, C., Ayala, E., Georgeson, K., Heidrich, S., Karnes, K., & Wells, J. (2015). Nursing care of the super bariatric patient: Challenges and lessons learned. *Rehabilitation Nursing, 40*(2), 92–99. http://dx.doi.org/10.1002/rnj.165.

3-121. **(C)** Hypoglossal neurapraxia caused by damage to the hypoglossal nerve during intubation is a rare but serious finding. The hypoglossal nerve innervates the muscles of the tongue. This nerve is involved in controlling tongue movements required for speech and swallowing. The abducens nerve, trochlear nerve, and oculomotor nerves all have sensory or motor functions that involve the eyes.

References: Blissitt, P. A. (2018). Neurologic system. In T. M. Hartjes (Ed.), *AACN core curriculum for high acuity, progressive, and critical care nursing* (7th ed.). St. Louis: Elsevier.

Haslam, B., & Collins, S. (2013). Bilateral hypoglossal neurapraxia following endotracheal intubation for total shoulder arthroplasty. *AANA Journal, 81*(3), 233–236.

3-122. **(C)** Persons receiving enteral nutrition are at increased risk for developing hyperglycemic hyperosmolar nonketotic coma because these solutions provide high carbohydrate nourishment. Assessment findings indicate polyuria resulting in dehydration. Without a history of diabetes, it is unlikely the patient has developed ketoacidosis. No bruising or other signs of trauma have been found, so there is little possibility the patient has developed diabetes insipidus. Syndrome of inappropriate antidiuretic hormone is caused by malignant disease processes, central nervous system disease processes, neurogenic stimuli, certain pulmonary diseases, endocrine disturbances and certain medications.

References: MacDermott, J. (2018). Endocrine system. In T. M. Hartjes (Ed.), *AACN core curriculum for high acuity, progressive, and critical care nursing* (7th ed.). St. Louis: Elsevier.

3-123. **(D)** Erikson proposed a lifespan model of development, taking in five stages up to the age of 18 years and three further stages beyond, well into adulthood. Erikson suggests that there is still plenty of room for continued growth and development throughout one's life. The last stage, acquisition of wisdom (integrity versus despair) applies to people aged 65 and older. The developmental tasks involve the acceptance of one's own life as significant and others' as important. The patient feels responsible for his or her own life, and life has dignity and love. Emotional integration provides the strength to deal with life as it is right now. Option D is an approach important in the stage that applies to 13- to 20-year-old patients.

Reference: Chapa, D., & Akintade, B. (2018). Psychosocial aspects of critical care. In T. M. Hartjes (Ed.), *AACN core curriculum for high acuity, progressive, and critical care nursing* (7th ed.). St. Louis: Elsevier.

3-124. **(A)** The balloon is set to inflate after the aortic valve closure (which corresponds to the dicrotic notch on the arterial waveform) and deflate immediately before the opening of the aortic valve (which corresponds to the point just before the upstroke on the arterial pressure waveform).

References: Efre, A., & Boling, B. (2018). Cardiovascular system. In T. M. Hartjes (Ed.), *AACN core curriculum for high acuity, progressive, and critical care nursing* (7th ed.). St. Louis: Elsevier.

Parissis, H., Graham, V., Lampridis, S., Lau, M., Hooks, G., & Mhandu, P. (2016). IABP: history-evolution-pathophysiology-indications: what we need to know. *Journal of Cardiothoracic Surgery*, 111–113. http://dx.doi.org/10.11 86/s13019-016-0513-0.

3-125. **(B)** Chemotherapy regimens for leukemia such as methotrexate can have the side effect of gastrointestinal bleeding. Gastrointestinal perforation can occur. Dark-colored stools, fatigue, and the development of hypotension are symptomatic of a gastrointestinal bleed. Although malnutrition is a possibility in patients receiving chemotherapy, this patient does not exhibit evidence of that condition. The patient experiencing bleeding may well experience anemia, but stopping this patient's bleeding is a higher priority need than treating the anemia. Patients on chemotherapy will incur immunosuppression, but that is not a pressing concern at this time.

References: Radovich, P. (2018). Gastrointestinal system. In T. M. Hartjes (Ed.), *AACN core curriculum for high acuity, progressive, and critical care nursing* (7th ed.). St. Louis: Elsevier.

Tsukada, T., Nakano, T., Miyata, T., & Sasaki, S. (2013). Life-threatening gastrointestinal mucosal necrosis during methotrexate treatment for rheumatoid arthritis. *Case Reports in Gastroenterology*, 7(3), 470–475. http://dx.doi.org/10.1159 /000356817.

3-126. **(B)** A patient with shallow respirations does not move air effectively in and out of the lungs. Diminished ventilation increases the volume of dead space or air that does not contribute to gas exchange. The patient with increased dead space effectively rebreathes carbon dioxide, causing a rise in $PaCO_2$. The amount of dead space affects the $PaCO_2$ value. Administration of oxygen to a hypercapnic patient may actually increase $PaCO_2$ because the higher amount of oxygen diminishes respiratory drive, thereby slowing the respiratory rate, which increases the

$PaCO_2$. Oxygen administration does not increase the work of breathing, but administration of 100% oxygen in a patient relying on hypoxia for respiratory drive should be avoided. In addition, excess oxygen administration causes a loss of hypoxic pulmonary vasoconstriction (HPV) (i.e., redirection of blood flow from relatively well-ventilated units to poorly ventilated units). HPV normally serves to improve the matching between blood flow and ventilation. This compensatory response improves V/Q matching and decreases physiologic dead space. The effect of loss of HPV is most pronounced in patients with a low initial $PaCO_2$. Not all hypercapnic patients require hypoxia to stimulate ventilation; that response pattern is usually seen in patients with chronic rather than acute pulmonary disease. Decreased hemoglobin levels in anemia do not change the ratio of oxygen to carbon dioxide and therefore will not affect $PaCO_2$. The A-a gradient is the difference in partial pressure of oxygen between arterial and alveolar blood. The normal value is 5 to 25 mm Hg or

$$\left[\frac{(Age + 10)}{4}\right].$$

High A-a gradients result from impaired diffusion or the presence of shunting. A higher A-a gradient worsens the diffusion defect. The A-a gradient reflects oxygenation and is independent of CO_2 levels.

References: Storzer, D. N. (2018). Pulmonary system. In T. M. Hartjes (Ed.), *AACN core curriculum for high acuity, progressive, and critical care nursing* (7th ed.). St. Louis: Elsevier.

Preventing acute hypercapnic respiratory failure in COPD patients. (2013). *Nursing Standard*, 27(47), 35–41. http://dx.doi.org/10.7748/ns2013 .07.27.47.35.e7339.

3-127. **(B)** The SPICES tool can help identify syndromes particular to the geriatric population in an ICU. In Option B, incontinence is represented by the letter "I." The letter "P" represents problems with eating or feeding, and the last letter, "S," identifies skin breakdown as a common geriatric syndrome. Geriatric patients are more likely to experience problems with sleeping, eating, feeding, elimination, incontinence, confusion, falls, and skin breakdown. The presence of these conditions alone or in combination can lead to increased death rates, higher costs, and longer hospitalizations. Research suggests that as a screening tool used within 24 hours of admission, SPICES is both valid and predictive of adverse events.

References: Alderden, J. (2018). Critical care patients with special needs: geriatric patients. In T. M. Hartjes (Ed.), *AACN core curriculum for high acuity, progressive, and critical care nursing* (7th ed.). St. Louis: Elsevier.

Aronow, H., Borenstein, J., Haus, F., Braunstein, G., & Bolton, L. (2014). Validating SPICES as a screening tool for frailty risks among hospitalized older adults. *Nursing Research and Practice, 2014*, 1–5. http://dx.doi.org/10.1155/2014/846759.

3-128. **(C)** Patients with sudden-onset neurologic deficiencies and persistent focal neurologic deficits should be considered for rt-PA therapy. Patients with persistent symptoms after 1 hour have an 85% risk of stroke with only a 15% chance of full recovery. Patients whose symptoms resolve rapidly are most likely having a TIA and should not receive rt-PA. It is essential to identify the time of the onset of symptoms or at least the last time the patient was seen without deficits. For therapy to be effective, it must begin within 3 hours of symptom onset but can be extended up to 4.5 hours based on new data. Therapy should not be based on arrival to the hospital (Option A). Patient allergies are important to identify (Option B) but are not the most important factor. The time window of treatment options is the primary limiting factor in treatment of these patients. Bleeding at a noncompressible site such as a central vein (Option D) should be avoided, so a peripheral IV line is preferred to a central line.

References: Blissitt, P. A. (2018). Neurologic system. In T. M. Hartjes (Ed.), *AACN core curriculum for high acuity, progressive, and critical care nursing* (7th ed.). St. Louis: Elsevier.

Lew, W., & Weaver, F. (2014). Thrombolytic agents. In R. Rutherford, J. Cronenwett & K. Wayne (Eds.), *Rutherford's vascular surgery* (8th ed.). (pp. 567–581). Philadelphia: Elsevier Saunders.

3-129. **(B)** Aortic stenosis can best be heard at the second intercostal space, right sternal border radiating to the neck and apex. Option A describes tricuspid stenosis. Option C is pulmonary insufficiency or regurgitation. Option D describes mitral insufficiency or regurgitation.

References: Efre, A., & Boling, B. (2018). Cardiovascular system. In T. M. Hartjes (Ed.), *AACN core curriculum for high acuity, progressive, and critical care nursing* (7th ed.). St. Louis: Elsevier.

Mc Gee, S. (2017). *Evidence-based physical diagnosis.* Philadelphia: Elsevier Saunders.

3-130. **(D)** If a patient is scheduled for a procedure that may cause pain or discomfort, premedication is appropriate. Recent studies demonstrate that cold application before chest tube removal can also provide some relief of the pain and discomfort associated with chest tube removal. A chest tube should not be clamped (Option A) unless ordered by a physician. Consent for chest tube removal (Option B) is not required. The original informed consent for chest tube placement also covers chest tube removal. Chest tube removal after pneumothorax (Option C) is not an indication for blood transfusion.

References: Storzer, D. N. (2018). Pulmonary system. In T. M. Hartjes (Ed.), *AACN core curriculum for high acuity, progressive, and critical care nursing* (7th ed.). St. Louis: Elsevier.

Claeys, K., Hammel, S., & Wolf, S. (2015). EB77 chest tube removal by nurses. *Critical Care Nurse, 35*(2), e37–38.

3-131. **(C)** Critically ill older patients exhibit delayed resolution of swallowing impairment post extubation. A fiberoptic endoscopic evaluation of swallowing should be considered in older patients after prolonged endotracheal intubation. Although other consults (Options A and B) may be required, they can be delayed until the patient's respiratory status is assured. Option D is incorrect because the presence of laryngeal edema will be assessed before extubating the patient. Evaluation of the patient's ability to swallow is essential to help prevent postextubation aspiration.

References: Storzer, D. N. (2018). Pulmonary system. In T. M. Hartjes (Ed.), *AACN core curriculum for high acuity, progressive, and critical care nursing* (7th ed.). St. Louis: Elsevier.

Tsai, M., Ku, S., Wang, T., Hsiao, T., Lee, J., Chan, D., & Chen, C. (2016). Swallowing dysfunction following endotracheal intubation: age matters. *Medicine, 95*(23), e3871. http://dx.doi.org/10.1097/MD.0000000000003871.

3-132. **(C)** Aortic regurgitation results in dilation and noncompliance of the left ventricle.

Vasopressor support with alpha-adrenergic agents such as norepinephrine (Levophed) increases the force of contraction and compliance of the left ventricle and constricts peripheral vessels to improve blood pressure. Volume boluses are often insufficient to improve BP and CO in a dilated, non-compliant left ventricle. In addition, PCWP and urine output indicate intravascular volume is adequate. Although dobutamine's beta-adrenergic effects on the myocardium would increase LV contractility and heart rate, its beta$_2$ effects may dilate the peripheral vasculature, thereby lowering BP. Increasing the pacing rate without enhancing circulating volume would add further myocardial workload.

References: Efre, A., & Boling, B. (2018). Cardiovascular system. In T. M. Hartjes (Ed.), *AACN core curriculum for high acuity, progressive, and critical care nursing* (7th ed.). St. Louis: Elsevier.

Williams, J. B., Milano, C. A., & Smith, P. K. (2016). Critical care for the adult cardiac patient. In F. Sellke (Ed.), *Sabiston and spencer's surgery of the chest* (pp. 1026–1050). Elsevier.

3-133. **(D)** Most signs and symptoms of alcohol withdrawal are caused by rapid removal of the depressant effects of alcohol in the central nervous system. Alcohol withdrawal syndrome (AWS) usually occurs within 24 hours of the last drink and results in autonomic hyperreactivity (tremors, nausea, vomiting, sweating) and neuropsychiatric alterations (agitation, anxiety, auditory disturbances, clouding of sensorium, disturbances in visual or tactile senses). The worst form of AWS is called alcohol withdrawal delirium, or delirium tremens, a life-threatening medical emergency that typically occurs 48 to 72 hours after the last drink. The autonomic hypersensitivity symptoms of delirium include hypertension, tachycardia, tachypnea, seizures, and tremors. Neuropsychiatric indications of delirium include hallucination, disorientation, and impaired attention. The cornerstone of pharmacologic management to halt progression of AWS and prevent DTs is administration of benzodiazepines, which provide CNS depression. Haldol is not indicated for the management of neuropsychiatric alterations associated with AWS. Restraints should not be applied, as they may intensify the neuropsychiatric alterations, and they do not prevent DTs. The visual and auditory images associated with television may contribute to a patient's confusion and hallucinations.

References: Chapa, D., & Akintade, B. (2018). Psychosocial aspects of critical care. In T. M. Hartjes, (Ed.), *AACN core curriculum for high acuity, progressive, and critical care nursing* (7th ed.). St. Louis: Elsevier.

Schmidt, K., Doshi, M., Holzhausen, J., Natavio, A., Cadiz, M., & Winegardner, J. (2016). Treatment of severe alcohol withdrawal. *Annals of Pharmacotherapy, 50*(5), 389–401. http://dx.doi.org/10.1177/1060028016629161.

3-134. **(C)**, The presence of heart disease, cerebrovascular disease, lung disease, liver failure, anemia, shock, and morbid obesity may indicate dangerous risk factors for conscious sedation. Patients at increased risk for developing complications during procedural sedation need a preprocedural consult with an appropriate specialist. The disadvantages of conscious sedation mainly are the lack of airway control and the risk of airway obstruction or aspiration. Several potential problems can arise from airway management in morbidly obese patients, including difficult mask ventilation and difficult intubation. Severely compromised patients should have an anesthesia provider administer sedation with equipment (video laryngoscope) to assist with emergency intubation if complications arise. The nurse's role as a patient advocate involves providing a safe experience during this procedure and preventing possible complications.

References: Benefield, A. (2018). Critical care patients with special needs: bariatric patients. In T. M. Hartjes, (Ed.), *AACN core curriculum for high acuity, progressive, and critical care nursing* (7th ed.). St. Louis: Elsevier.

Hodgson, E. (2016). Airway management of the morbidly obese patient. *Journal of Perioperative Practice, 26*(9), 196–200.

Berrios, L. (2016). The ABCDs of managing morbidly obese patients in intensive care units. *Critical Care Nurse, 36*(5), 17–26. http://dx.doi.org/10.4037/ccn201667.

3-135. **(C)** By seeking clarification and not readily implementing the order, the nurse is acting as an advocate for the patient. This is indicated as the patient's family has not agreed to a do-not-resuscitate order and the ordered ventilator change is not clinically indicated. Option B could place the family in the middle between the patient and the physician and does not reflect caring practices. The nurse should recognize that to change a patient from receiving maximal ventilator support to a room-air level of oxygen support (Option A) when the patient's oxygen saturation is low is not physiologically sound and could cause discomfort to the patient. The nurse will need to perform an ongoing patient assessment for presence of pain and discomfort and administer the medications based on that assessment. Administration of medications, as suggested in Option D, is not indicated until an assessment is completed.

References: Dermenchyan, A. (2018). Professional Caring and Ethical Practice. In Hartjes, T.M. (ed.), *AACN Core Curriculum for High Acuity, Progressive, and Critical Care Nursing* (7th ed.). St. Louis: Elsevier.

Lucatorto, M., Thomas, T., & Siek, T. (2016). Registered nurses as caregivers: influencing the system as patient advocates. *Online Journal of Issues in Nursing, 21*(3), 5. http://dx.doi.org/10.3912/OJIN.Vol21No03Man02.

3-136. **(A)** The nurse in this case has an ethical obligation to call the organ procurement organization, despite the objection of the intensivist. The referral to organ procurement can be made by any member of the care team. Referral is a legal obligation in cases of imminent death. In this case referral has already been made but the organ procurement organization must be notified of the new clinical decline. Notifying the agency early enables potential discussions to be planned and not rushed. The organ procurement organization can then have a follow-up discussion with the family that will be sensitive to the distress they are experiencing. The opportunity to donate their son's organs may provide the family with a sense of purpose and closure instead of causing further upset. Delaying the call to the organ procurement organization is detrimental to future donor recipients and deprives the family of their one final autonomous decision on behalf of their son.

References: Dermenchyan, A. (2018). Professional caring and ethical practice. In T. M. Hartjes (Ed.), *AACN core curriculum for high acuity, progressive, and critical care nursing* (7th ed.). St. Louis: Elsevier.

Milliken, A., & Wall, A. (2014). Duty, distress, and organ donation. *Hastings Center Report, 44*(6), 9–10. http://dx.doi.org/10.1002/hast.381.

3-137. **(A)** Elevation of a pulseless extremity will decrease perfusion and is therefore contraindicated. Reverse Trendelenburg poisitioning places the foot in a dependent position that would increase blood flow. Heparin could aid in resolving a clot that could be causing occlusion. Vasodilator medications would assist in promoting circulation to the foot and toe.

References: Efre, A., Boling, B. (2018). Cardiovascular system. In T. M. Hartjes (Ed.), *AACN core curriculum for high acuity, progressive, and critical care nursing* (7th ed.). St. Louis: Elsevier.

Creager, M., & Libby, P. (2015). Peripheral artery diseases. In D. Mann & L. Mauri (Eds.), *Braunwald's heart disease: A textbook of cardiovascular medicine* (10th ed.). (pp. 1312–1335). Philadelphia: Elsevier Saunders.

3-138. **(D)** The nurse supervising the task must ensure that the task is appropriately documented. The evaluation of the intervention provided and the documentation of that evaluation may not be within the scope of practice for the assistive personnel. For example, a patient experiencing fear, anxiety, and pain may benefit greatly from a back rub administered by unlicensed assistive personnel. However, unlicensed assistive personnel are not permitted to document an assessment of the patient's symptoms, the effectiveness of the intervention, or an evaluation of the task.

References: Dermenchyan, A. (2018). Professional caring and ethical practice. In T. M. Hartjes (Ed.), *AACN core curriculum for high acuity, progressive, and critical care nursing* (7th ed.). St. Louis: Elsevier.

3-139. **(C)** The most likely cause of these findings is a pneumothorax, and the physician will assess the situation and probably insert a chest tube. If the opening in the chest wall is smaller than the diameter of the trachea, the patient may have minimal subjective symptoms. To do nothing and continue with the bath will delay management of a recognizable condition that requires treatment and could pose some risk to the patient. Application of an occlusive dressing could convert this pneumothorax into a potential tension pneumothorax, a serious and possibly lethal problem that could result in cardiac arrest. At this time, the patient does not appear to be in any pulmonary distress, so intubation is not warranted.

References: Storzer, D. N. (2018). Pulmonary system. In T. M. Hartjes (Ed.), *AACN core curriculum for high acuity, progressive, and critical care nursing* (7th ed.). St. Louis: Elsevier.

Kong, V., Liu, M., Sartorius, B., & Clarke, D. (2015). Open pneumothorax: the spectrum and outcome of management based on advanced trauma life support recommendations. *European Journal of Trauma & Emergency Surgery, 41*(4), 401–404. http://dx.doi.org/10.1007/s00068-014-0469-5.

3-140. **(C)** The identified structures are the right and left bundle branches. The conduction system begins with the SA (sinoatrial) node, and the AV (atrioventricular) node is lower than the SA node. The His bundle is next followed by the right and left bundle branches and terminates in the Purkinje fibers.

References: Efre, A., & Boling, B. (2018). Cardiovascular system. In T. M. Hartjes (Ed.), *AACN core curriculum for high acuity, progressive, and critical care nursing* (7th ed.). St. Louis: Elsevier.

3-141. **(D)** Transport needs of the critically ill must be determined by the specific needs of the patient. The Synergy Model for Patient Care helps guide those specific needs based on patient resiliency, vulnerability, stability, complexity, resource availability, participation in care, participation in decision making, and predictability. Matching the patient's needs with the appropriate provider and resources can reduce the risk of adverse outcomes during transport. Outcomes are further improved by utilizing evidence-based practice. Evidence-based quality improvement and health care transformation underscores the need for redesigning care that is effective, safe, and efficient. Options A, B, and C are all appropriate, and they demonstrate patient advocacy. However, the tool should be created using evidence-based practice first.

References: Holleran, S. (2018). Critical care patients with special needs: patient transport. In T. M. Hartjes (Ed.), *AACN core curriculum for high acuity, progressive, and critical care nursing* (7th ed.). St. Louis: Elsevier.

Swickard, S., Swickard, W., Reimer, A., Lindell, D., & Winkelman, C. (2014). Adaptation of the AACN synergy model for patient care to critical care transport. *Critical Care Nurse, 34*(1), 16–28. http://dx.doi.org/10.4037/ccn2014573.

3-142. **(C)** This patient is experiencing atrial fibrillation that spontaneously terminates and is followed by a pause before sinus rhythm resumes. This is indicative of sick sinus syndrome and indicates the need for a permanent pacemaker. A transvenous pacemaker will provide an effective temporary intervention until a permanent pacemaker can be placed. A transcutaneous pacemaker could be used when the heart rate slows but would not be effective when tachycardia appears. Atropine is not an appropriate treatment for a dysrhythmia that alternates between bradycardia and tachycardia. Continuous monitoring is indicated for this patient but is not sufficient for management and places the patient at risk for syncopal episodes that may result in patient injury.

References: Efre, A., & Boling, B. (2018). Cardiovascular system. In T. M. Hartjes (Ed.), *AACN core curriculum for high acuity, progressive, and critical care nursing* (7th ed.). St. Louis: Elsevier.

Doran, A., & Frisch, D. (2017). Sick sinus syndrome. In F. Ferri, *2017 Ferri's clinical advisor: 5 books in 1* (pp. 1173–1174). Philadelphia: Elsevier.

3-143. **(C)** In this case, ECMO is viewed by the medical team to be an intervention with no reasonable likelihood of returning a patient to normal functioning or consciousness. The ICU team determines that ECMO would be a futile therapy that should not be initiated, although the patient's family may judge the fact that the intervention keeps the patient alive (even if only in a biological sense) as confirmation that the therapy is not futile. A clinician is not ethically required to provide a treatment that he or she reasonably perceives as not medically or ethically appropriate. Thus, withholding a treatment, even contrary to the wishes of a patient or surrogate, is widely perceived as ethically justified. The hospital ethics committee can intervene to assist with the ethically appropriate goals of care for this patient. The family can request transfer to a different physician or facility if so desired. Option C is inappropriate because the ethics of withdrawal of existing treatment can seem different as it involves an action (removing already functioning technology), as opposed to a refusal to act. The ethical implications of discontinuing ECMO in 24 hours if the patient does not respond may cause the family more distress and intensify the patient's suffering.

References: Dermenchyan, A. (2018). Professional caring and ethical practice. In T. M. Hartjes (Ed.), *AACN core curriculum for high acuity, progressive, and critical care nursing* (7th ed.). St. Louis: Elsevier.

Chung, G., Yoon, J., Rasinski, K., & Curlin, F. (2016). U.S. physicians' opinions about distinctions between withdrawing and withholding life-sustaining treatment. *Journal of Religion & Health, 55*(5), 1596–1606. http://dx.doi.org/10.1007/s10943-015-0171-x.

3-144. **(D)** Initial treatment for mild to moderate *C. difficile* infection (CDI) is metronidazole 500 mg orally three or four times daily for 10 to 14 days. Metronidazole is not contraindicated for patients with a vancomycin allergy. Perpetual dysbiosis seems to be the key driver in multiple recurrent CDI, restoring a healthy colonic microbiota after treatment of CDI can break the dysbiotic cycle. With multiple courses of antimicrobials, the colonic microbiome loses its diversity and its function. Subsequent alterations in bile acids, sugar alcohols, and fatty acids can promote growth of *C. difficile*. The bulk of evidence for FMT exists for multiple recurrent CDI. In this setting, FMT is highly effective for treating multiple recurrent CDIs with a nearly 90% cure rate in many observational studies.

References: AACN. (2017). Liubakka, A., & Vaughn, B. (2016). Clostridium difficile infection and fecal microbiota transplant. *AACN Advanced Critical Care, 27*(3), 324–337. http://dx.doi.org/10.4037/aacnacc2016703.

Han, S., Shannahan, S., & Pellish, R. (2016). Fecal microbiota transplant. *Journal of Intensive Care Medicine (Sage Publications Inc.), 31*(9), 577–586. http://dx.doi.org/10.1177/0885066615594344.

3-145. **(A)** A narrowed pulse pressure, tachycardia, location of the stab wound, and chest x-ray demonstrating an enlarged cardiac silhouette strongly suggest pericardial tamponade is present. A 10% pneumothorax is not sufficient to cause hypotension, and the condition is treated appropriately with chest tube placement. At least 250 mL of blood is needed in most cases to be visible as a hemothorax on chest x-ray; however, even a 250-mL loss would have been treated appropriately by the 500-mL bolus in the ED. There is no apparent source of excessive bleeding causing hypovolemia on chest x-ray, wound dressing, or in the chest tube collection chamber. Hypovolemia would cause hypotension and tachycardia but not an enlarged cardiac silhouette.

References: Efre, A., & Boling, B. (2018). Cardiovascular system. In T. M. Hartjes (Ed.), *AACN core curriculum for high acuity, progressive, and critical care nursing* (7th ed.). St. Louis: Elsevier.

3-146. **(C)** Post–intensive care syndrome (PICS), which includes physical, psychological, and cognitive impairments, develops in many ICU survivors. Listening to music is highlighted as a nonpharmacologic, adjunctive intervention to reduce anxiety associated with mechanical ventilation. Music therapy is effective in reducing ventilator-associated anxiety and reduces the need for higher doses of sedation and deliriogenic medications. Option A is incorrect because PICS usually affects patients after discharge from the hospital and can persist for years after a patient leaves the ICU, adversely affecting patients and their families. Many individuals do not return to work because of functional or cognitive impairments because they have substantial ongoing medical problems that require expensive treatment, and they often have substantial reductions in quality of life. Medication management strategies (Option B) in the ICU, upon transition to the medical-surgical unit and after hospitalization, are critical to preventing and treating PICS. Delirium prevention and treatment and avoidance or proper dosage adjustment of deliriogenic or neuromuscular weakness-inducing medications are all strategies to prevent PICS. The choice and duration of sedatives in the ICU can lead to the development of PICS. Nursing care has a direct effect (Option D) on the development of PICS. Early mobilization, daily sedation cessation, delirium prevention, comfort measures, ventilator weaning, infection prevention, sleep promotion, and early discharge planning can prevent or improve some of the symptoms.

References: Alexander, E., Susla, G., Stollings, J., Bloom, S., Huggins, E., Grayson, S., & Sevin, C. (2016). Medication management to ameliorate post-intensive care syndrome. *AACN Advanced Critical Care, 27*(2), 133–140. http://dx.doi.org/10.4037/aacnacc2016931.

Chlan, L. (2016). Engaging critically ill patients in symptom management: thinking outside the box! *American Journal of Critical Care, 25*(3), 202–202. http://dx.doi.org/10.4037/ajcc2016671.

3-147. **(B)** Administration of insulin will help to correct the hyperglycemia associated with steroid administration and stress. This intervention should be followed by administration of IV fluids and electrolytes, as the patient has likely been experiencing polyuria. A low-dose insulin drip will require a greater period of time to correct the metabolic alterations but may be desirable at a later time. Although the bicarbonate level is slightly decreased, administration of bicarbonate is not appropriate at this time, as this value will return to normal as fluids and electrolytes are replaced. This level of carbon dioxide may be a normal value for this patient, whose underlying respiratory disease may result in carbon dioxide retention.

References: MacDermott, J. (2018). Endocrine system. In T. M. Hartjes (Ed.), *AACN core curriculum for high acuity, progressive, and critical care nursing* (7th ed.). St. Louis: Elsevier.

Baldwin, D., & Apel, J. (2013). Management of hyperglycemia in hospitalized patients with renal insufficiency or steroid-induced diabetes. *Current Diabetes Reports, 13*(1), 114–120. http://dx.doi.org/10.1007/s11892-012-0339-7t7.

3-148. **(C)** Although it is common to maintain CSF pressure at 10 mm Hg after thoracic aortic aneurysm repair, there is only about 150 mL of CSF in the system at one time. If CSF is drained too rapidly or in too large a volume, the patient is at risk of subdural hemorrhage. Fluid administration may be used to maintain blood pressure after TAA repair and is used in conjunction with nitroglycerin administration to decrease systolic BP because many of these patients have preexisting hypertension. FFP and platelets are commonly administered to these patients to replace coagulation factors and prevent coagulopathy.

References: Blissitt, P. A. (2018). Neurologic system. In T. M. Hartjes (Ed.), *AACN core curriculum for high acuity, progressive, and critical care nursing* (7th ed.). St. Louis: Elsevier.

3-149. **(C)** NPPV works by increasing inspiratory pressure to expand tidal volume and minute ventilation. Increased tidal volume, in turn, enhances alveolar recruitment and diminishes the atelectasis caused by hypoventilation. Care must be exercised in use of NPPV, however, to avoid inadvertently increasing expiratory pressures as well. This is a particular concern for patients with COPD, who already have excessively high expiratory pressures because of airway collapse on expiration with air-trapping in distal alveoli. Further increases in expiratory pressure from NPPV would then magnify one of the fundamental pathophysiologic effects of COPD. NPPV has minimal effects on V/Q matching and has no effect on mucous production in distal airways.

References: Storzer, D. N. (2018). Pulmonary system. In T. M. Hartjes (Ed.), *AACN core curriculum for high acuity, progressive, and critical care nursing* (7th ed.). St. Louis: Elsevier.

Mahmoodpoor, A., & Golzari, S. (2015). Noninvasive positive-pressure ventilation. *New England Journal of Medicine, 373*(13), 1279. http://dx.doi.org/10.1056/NEJMc1508384#SA1.

3-150. **(B)** *Paternalism* is the term used when health care providers make the decisions for the patient based on the rationale that it is in the patient's best interest. This practice denies the patient the autonomy to make his or her own decisions. In this scenario, the patient has refused surgery. However, the physician consults the surgeons against the patient's wishes. Beneficence is the principle that the competent patient is the best judge of the patient's best interests. Nonmaleficence is the principle to "do no harm." The patient is competent to decide his own outcomes, and determining a different outcome for the patient may do harm. Patient autonomy is a principle that a competent adult patient has the right to make his or her own health care decision.

References: Dermenchyan, A. (2018). Professional caring and ethical practice. In T. M. Hartjes (Ed.), *AACN core curriculum for high acuity, progressive, and critical care nursing* (7th ed.). St. Louis: Elsevier.

Credits

CORE REVIEW TEST 1

Figure, pg. 3

From Slutzman, J., Curley, D., Macias-Konstan-topoulos, W., & Brown, D. F. (2015). Altered mental status and tachycardia. *Journal of Emergency Medicine, 48*(5), 597-602. doi: 10.1016/j.jemermed.2014.12.021.

Figure, pg. 7

From Habis, M., & Paul, J. (2010). Multidetector computed tomography of right ventricular acute myocardial infarction. *Archives of Cardiovascular Diseases, 103*(2), 131-132. doi:10.1016/j.acvd.2009.09.012.

Figure, pg. 14

Surawicz, B., Knilans, T. K., & Chou, T. (2008). *Chou's electrocardiography in clinical practice: Adult and pediatric* (6th ed.). Philadelphia: Saunders/Elsevier.

Figure, pg. 19

From Ufberg, J. W., & Clark, J. S. (2006). Bradydysrhythmias and atrioventricular conduction blocks. *Emergency Medicine Clinics of North America, 24*(1), 1-9. doi:10.1016/j.emc.2005.08.006.

Figure, pg. 19

Ibrahim, A. W., Riddell, T. C., & Devireddy, C. M. (2014). Acute myocardial infarction. *Critical Care Clinics, 30*(3), 341-364. doi: http://dx.doi.org/10.1016/j.ccc.2014.03.010.

CORE REVIEW TEST 2

Figure, pg. 69

From Saksena, S., & Camm, A. J. (2011). *Electrophysiological disorders of the heart* (2nd ed.). Philadelphia: Saunders.

Figure, pg. 75

From Schwartz, P. J., & Woosley, R. L. (2016). Predicting the unpredictable: Drug-induced QT prolongation and torsades de pointes. *Journal of the American College of Cardiology, 67*(13), 1639-1650. doi:10.1016/j.jacc.2015.12.063.

Figure, pg. 75

From Samadov, F., Akaslan, D., Cincin, A., Tigen, K., & Sarı, I. (2014). Acute proximal left anterior descending artery occlusion with de Winter sign. *The American Journal of Emergency Medicine, 32*(1). doi:10.1016/j.ajem.2013.08.024.

Figure, pg. 76

From Vincent, J. L., Abraham, E., Kochanek, P. M., Moore, F. A., & Fink, M. P. (2011). *Textbook of critical care* (6th ed.). Philadelphia: Saunders.

CORE REVIEW TEST 3

Figure, pg. 135

From Weinberger, S. B., Cockrill, B. A., & Mandel, J. (2014). *Principles of pulmonary medicine* (6th ed.). Philadelphia: Saunders.

Figure, pg. 140

From Liang, X., Evans, S. M., & Sun, Y. (2015). Insights into cardiac conduction system formation provided by HCN4 expression. *Trends in Cardiovascular Medicine, 25*(1), 1-9. doi:10.1016/j.tcm.2014.08.009.

Figure, pg. 141

From Issa, Z., & Miller, J. M. (2012). *Clinical arrhythmology and electrophysiology: A companion to Braunwald's heart disease* (2nd ed.). Philadelphia: Saunders.